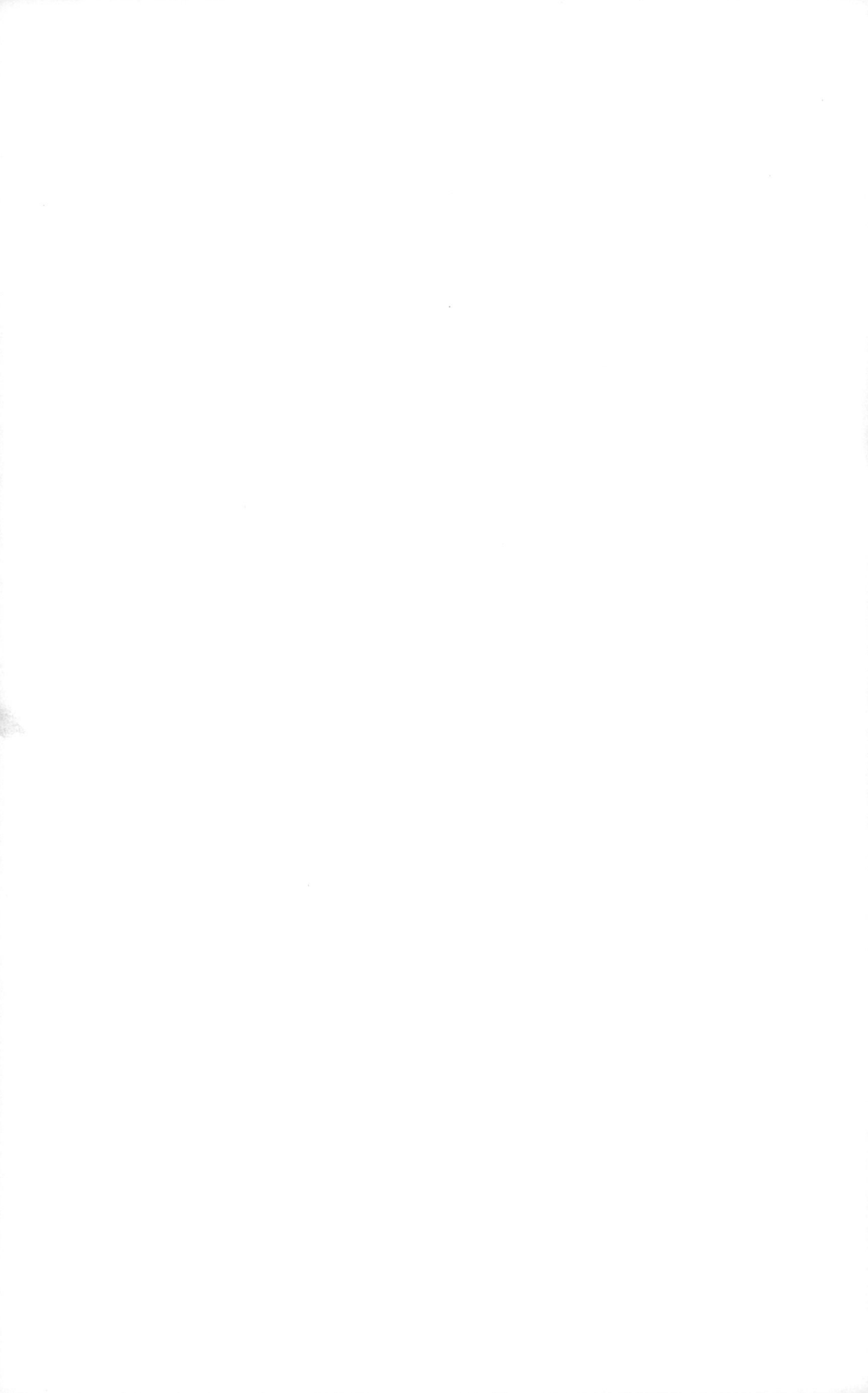

Social Indicators Research Series

Volume 72

This series aims to provide a public forum for single treatises and collections of papers on social indicators research that are too long to be published in our journal *Social Indicators Research*. Like the journal, the book series deals with statistical assessments of the quality of life from a broad perspective. It welcomes the research on a wide variety of substantive areas, including health, crime, housing, education, family life, leisure activities, transportation, mobility, economics, work, religion and environmental issues. These areas of research will focus on the impact of key issues such as health on the overall quality of life and vice versa. An international review board, consisting of Ruut Veenhoven, Joachim Vogel, Ed Diener, Torbjorn Moum, Mirjam A.G. Sprangers and Wolfgang Glatzer, will ensure the high quality of the series as a whole.

More information about this series at http://www.springer.com/series/6548

Andreas M. Krafft
Pasqualina Perrig-Chiello
Andreas M. Walker

Editors

Hope for a Good Life

Results of the Hope-Barometer International
Research Program

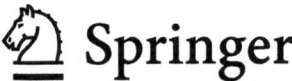 Springer

Editors
Andreas M. Krafft
Institute of Systemic Management
and Public Governance
University of St. Gallen
St. Gallen, Switzerland

Pasqualina Perrig-Chiello
Institute of Psychology
University of Bern
Bern, Switzerland

Andreas M. Walker
Swissfuture
Basel, Switzerland

ISSN 1387-6570   ISSN 2215-0099 (electronic)
Social Indicators Research Series
ISBN 978-3-319-78469-4   ISBN 978-3-319-78470-0 (eBook)
https://doi.org/10.1007/978-3-319-78470-0

Library of Congress Control Number: 2018942196

Printed on acid-free paper

This Springer imprint is published by the registered company Springer International Publishing AG part of Springer Nature.
The registered company address is: Gewerbestrasse 11, 6330 Cham, Switzerland

Contents

Introduction

In 2009, when the idea of launching the Hope-Barometer as a broad public survey on hope and other positive attributes and experiences was born, the research project was started as a "private" initiative among friends and colleagues around swissfuture, the Swiss Society for Futures Studies, a member of the Swiss Academy of Humanities and Social Sciences (SAGW). The basic motivation for initiating such a venture was the impression, that in Europe, especially in Germany and Switzerland, the attention of people and particularly of mass media has been much more focused on problems, risks, catastrophes, worries, and fears regarding the future than on opportunities and potentials. In order to empirically investigate the fundamental aspects, conditions, and interrelations of a positive attitude toward the future, and to be able to discuss the results in the public media, a multidisciplinary group was established. Members included representatives from different scientific fields such as future studies, sociology of religion, theology, psychotherapy, history, economy, management, and media. Based on the results of a broad literature review we came to the conclusion, that in contrast to the USA, hope was under-researched in German-speaking Europe.

Based on the first experiences and insights of the Hope-Barometer in 2009 and 2010, a summarizing report in the swissfuture magazine (2010/Issue 1) was published. During the following years, research collaboration with the University of St. Gallen and several other universities was established. Furthermore, contact with print and e-media in Switzerland, Germany, and successively also in other countries was extended. Since 2011, the annual results of the Hope-Barometer were regularly presented in the form of talks, symposia, and roundtables at the international congresses of the International Positive Psychology Association (IPPA) and the European Conference of Positive Psychology (ECPP). The interest in the Hope-Barometer among researchers from different countries has led to the establishment of an international research network. Consequently, the Hope-Barometer survey now takes place every year not only in Switzerland and Germany but also in France, the Czech Republic, Poland, Spain, India, Malta, Israel, and South Africa.

Particularly gratifying is the positive echo the Hope-Barometer has achieved in the mass media. Various newspapers offer their internet pages every year to promote the survey and to publish the link to the questionnaire in order to reach a large number of interested public. Consequently, thousands of people have been able to participate in the survey every year and by doing so, to reflect upon their own hopes for the future. Moreover, these and other newspapers and magazines have dedicated a prominent space to the results of the survey, both in their online and print issues. Thanks to the support of the Swiss Positive Psychology Association (SWIPPA) and the tight collaboration between swissfuture and the Institute of Psychology of the University of Bern (Switzerland), the first Swiss Conference on Hope was organized in 2015, with representatives of the international network of the Hope-Barometer, and the participation of other researchers, students, the media, and the general public.

This book presents selected results of the Hope-Barometer, focusing on the relationship of hope and the quest for a good life in several countries with different cultural backgrounds. The book is structured in three parts. In Part I, Krafft and Walker first provide an overview of the many psychological theories and conceptualizations of hope and introduce the reader to the methodological foundations of the Hope-Barometer (Chap. 1). Then, in Chap. 2, the authors present a review of research findings of the Hope-Barometer, based on research conducted in the last seven years in Germany and German-speaking Switzerland. The basic conclusion is that eudaimonic domains of well-being lead to cultivating a virtuous circle of hope, in which the principal sources of hope are at the same time the most-valued targets of hope, mutually reinforcing each other.

In the second part of the book, selected empirical contributions related to the levels and variations of hope across different population groups, and the relationship of hope with several measures of well-being, are presented.

In Chap. 3, Guse and Shaw study the relationship between dispositional and perceived hope, meaning in life and well-being in a sample of South African young adults. Their results indicate that meaning in life mediates the relationship between both dispositional and perceived hope and well-being, concluding that the quality of the relationship may be different in each case.

In Chap. 4, Perrig-Chiello et al. adopt a lifespan and gender perspective, analyzing to which extent dispositional hope, well-being, and age/gender are related among the Swiss-German population. They conclude that all well-being and dispositional hope (agency and pathways) parameters increase with age and highlight the particular role of agency, defined as will-power, for predicting life satisfaction and meaning in life over all age groups, especially for women. Furthermore, they discuss the special effect of optimism (stronger than dispositional hope) with regard to higher levels of happiness.

The impact of marital status on well-being and dispositional hope is the focus of Chap. 5. Spahni and Perrig-Chiello compare married, separated/divorced, and widowed individuals in German-speaking Switzerland and examine how subjective well-being and health are affected by the marital status and to what extent dispositional hope, optimism, and social resources can explain these outcomes. They come to the conclusion that, in different ways, dispositional hope and optimism are crucial personal characteristics associated with better well-being after facing separation, divorce, or death.

Although religiosity and spirituality are often considered to be important dimensions of hope in existing literature, research findings in Europe have shown rather low correlations between these constructs and hope. The objective of Chap. 6 is to explore the importance of religiosity and spirituality among different demographic groups (age, gender, etc.) of the Swiss population and their association with subjective well-being. Margelisch comes to the conclusion that religiosity and spirituality, both in general and particularly in terms of activities to promote hope, can play an important role in the context of critical life events and the adaptation to profound life transitions.

Part III includes three contributions on the comparison of elements and levels of hope across cultures.

In Chap. 7, Krafft and Choubisa outline the main ontological and epistemological propositions of Indian Psychology, its conceptualizations of the self and of a good and fulfilling life. They furthermore explore the notion of hope within the Eastern philosophical and spiritual tradition in contrast to the cognitive Western approach. The chapter concludes with empirical findings comparing a group of young adults in India to a similar sample in German-speaking Europe.

Slezáčková et al. compare two Czech and Maltese samples in Chap. 8. They explore the correlates and predictors of perceived hope among the two groups in terms of optimism, life satisfaction, positive relations, loneliness, generativity, and spirituality. Besides finding cultural differences with regard to demographic factors such as gender, age, family status, education level, religious beliefs, and engagement in voluntary activities, and the strong role of dispositional optimism in relation to hope, the researchers identified two different variables, which measure a facet of transcendence, as major predictors of perceived hope. Specifically, generativity predicted perceived hope in the Czech sample and spirituality in the Maltese group.

In Chap. 9, Flores-Lucas et al. introduce the concept of psychological capital, as well as its role and usefulness in relation to academic success. They furthermore analyze the relationship between hope, psychological capital, and other relevant variables that impact educational and future life success, comparing three samples of Spanish, German, and Indian students. The chapter attempts to highlight the effect of positive resources not only to improve the academic success in students but also to prepare them for successful integration in their future career.

The success of the Hope-Barometer and the publication of this book was only possible thanks to the commitment and the support of many people. The first working group led by Andreas M. Walker was composed by (in alphabetical order) Markus Baumgartner, Markus Merz, Francis Müller, Stephan Nüesch, Stefan Schwarz, and Stefan Siegrist. The international network led by Andreas M. Krafft includes (in alphabetical order) Carmel Cefai, Rajneesh Choubisa, Fabien Fenouillet, Liora Findler, María del Valle Flores-Lucas, Tharina Guse, Pawel Izdebski, Elzbieta Kasprzak, Charles Martin-Krumm, and Alena Slezáčková, some of them being authors of chapters in this book. We want to direct special acknowledgement and personal recognition and appreciation, to Shane Lopez, a pioneer in the field of hope research. The many talks with him were always very inspiring and finally triggered the formation of this international research network on hope. For their valuable collaboration, we also want to acknowledge the team led by Pasqualina Perrig-Chiello, namely Stefanie Spahni and Katja Margelisch, who also contributed to this book. Furthermore, we are especially grateful to Leo Bormans for his motivating and inspiring work to promote happiness and hope. For their long-standing support and their trust and encouragement, we want to express our gratefulness to Thomas Winkler, Fritz Peyer-Müller, and the Foundation for Education and Research. Likewise, we thank the support of swissfuture as well as of the Swiss Academy of Humanities and Social Sciences.

With the Hope-Barometer, we want to make a scientific contribution with a positive value for society, so that more and more people could be encouraged to adopt a positive view on the future, to believe in their own strengths and the goodness of the world, and by doing so, to attain their own dreams of a happy and fulfilling life.

The Authors

Carmel Cefai (PhD) is the director of the Centre for Resilience and Socio-Emotional Health, and Associate Professor at the Department of Psychology, at the University of Malta. His research interests include resilience, social and emotional well-being of children and young people, and mental health promotion in school. He is joint founding honorary chair of the European Network for Social and Emotional Competence (ENSEC) and founding co-editor of the International Journal of Emotional Education.

Rajneesh Choubisa (PhD) is Assistant Professor at the Department of Humanities and Social Sciences at BITS Pilani, Pilani Campus (Rajasthan), India. He is associated with international associations such as APA, IPPA, and IAAP and a founder member of National Positive Psychology Association of India.

Valle Flores-Lucas (PhD) is Lecturer in Developmental and Educational Psychology at the University of Valladolid. Her main research areas include language and developmental disorders and applications of positive psychology to education and to disability. She is a member of SEPP (Spanish Society on Positive Psychology) and ACIPE (Scientific Society of Psychology and Education).

Tharina Guse (PhD) is a counseling psychologist and Associate Professor in the Department of Psychology at the University of Johannesburg, South Africa. She is appointed as member of Professional Board for Psychology of the Health Professions Council of South Africa (HPCSA) and is a member of the Psychological Society of South Africa (PSYSSA). Her research focus on psychosocial well-being, positive psychology interventions, hypnosis for mental health promotion, and psychological strengths such as hope and gratitude.

Andreas M. Krafft (PhD) is Associate Researcher and Lecturer in the Institute for Systemic Management and Public Governance at the University of St. Gallen

(Switzerland) and Lecturer at the University of Zürich in the field of Work and Health. He is a member of the Executive Board of swissfuture, the Swiss Society of Futures Studies, and since 2011 responsible for the Hope-Barometer research program. He has a specialization in Social Psychology of Organizations as well as in Work and Health Psychology.

Katja Margelisch (PhD) studied Psychology at the University of Bern after her fifteen-year obligation as a primary school teacher and choir conductor. She graduated in 2015 (key aspects: Neuropsychology and Developmental Psychology). Along with her scientific obligation, Katja Margelisch works as a lecturer at the University of Teacher Education in Bern and at the Swiss Distance Learning University.

Raquel Martínez-Sinovas holds a PhD in Psychology. She is Associate Professor and Researcher in the Department of Developmental and Educational Psychology, University of Valladolid. Besides her focus on the psychology of physical activity and sport, she also interested in positive psychology and sense of humor.

Pasqualina Perrig-Chiello (PhD) is honorary professor at the University of Bern. Her research has been focused on topics of lifespan developmental psychology, especially individual differences in well-being and health and familial intergenerational relations. She is a member of the executive board of the Swiss Positive Psychology Association.

Tomáš Prošek participates at the Program of Psychology at the Faculty of Arts, Masaryk University in Brno, Czech Republic. His main area of interest is statistics and psychometrics.

Monique Chalize Shaw graduated with a Master of Arts in Counseling Psychology from the University of Johannesburg (UJ), South Africa. She is a registered counselling psychologist and completed her professional training at the Centre for Psychological Services and Career Assessment of UJ.

Alena Slezáčková (PhD) is Associate Professor of Psychology at the Department of Psychology of Masaryk University in Brno, Czech Republic. She is a founder and director of the Czech Positive Psychology Centre and the Academic Centre for Positive Psychology affiliated to Masaryk University. Her main research interests include hope, mental health, and well-being. She is a member of the Advisory Council of the International Positive Psychology Association (IPPA) and the Country Representative for the Czech Republic in the European Network for Positive Psychology (ENPP).

Stefanie Spahni (PhD) is a senior teaching and research associate at the University of Bern, Switzerland, in the area of health psychology and behavioral medicine in the Department of Psychology. Her teaching and research focus on partnership and sexuality across the lifespan, well-being, and adaptation to stressful life events.

Andreas M. Walker (PhD) is Co-president of Swissfuture, the Swiss Society for Futures Studies, and one of the leading futurists of Switzerland. In 2009, he was the founder of the Hope Barometer.

Part I
Theoretical Foundations and General Empirical Findings

Chapter 1
Exploring the Concept and Experience of Hope – Theoretical and Methodological Foundations

Andreas M. Krafft and Andreas M. Walker

Introduction and Purpose

Hope is a basic human phenomenon that has been the focus of inquiry of many different disciplines throughout history such as philosophy, theology, ethics, sociology and psychology (Krafft & Walker, 2018; Scioli & Biller, 2009). Although almost all related disciplines and scientific communities understand hope as a positive expectation towards a better future, many fundamental differences became evident in the meaning, roots and overall understanding of what hope is, where it comes from and which elements it contains. Reverting to distinct traditions and philosophies of hope, researchers in psychology and nursing research have conceptualized this term in different ways (see Eliott, 2005). Current concepts of hope differ fundamentally with regard to core aspects and elements contained in its definition (Slezáčková, 2017). Differences in the conceptualization of hope are not only rooted in the diverse disciplinary traditions, but also in the diversity of cultural, political, religious, economic and social backgrounds and beliefs not only of ordinary people but also of scientists and researchers (Averill & Sundararajan, 2005).

In the psychological context there are various perspectives regarding the conceptualization of hope and what it delimits this phenomenon from other constructs such as optimism and self-efficacy. Basically, hope has been the object of research within a cognitive-behavioral framework of goal-related theories (Snyder, 1994, 2002; Stotland, 1969) as well as embedded in broader theories of basic human emotions (Averill, Catlin, & Chon, 1990; Fredrickson, 1998, 2004; Scioli et al., 1997). Furthermore, hope has been seen as something merely individual or something that

A. M. Krafft (✉)
Institute of Systemic Management and Public Governance, University of St. Gallen, St. Gallen, Switzerland
e-mail: andreas.krafft@unisg.ch

A. M. Walker
Swissfuture, Lucerne, Switzerland

© Springer International Publishing AG, part of Springer Nature 2018
A. M. Krafft et al. (eds.), *Hope for a Good Life*, Social Indicators Research
Series 72, https://doi.org/10.1007/978-3-319-78470-0_1

is fundamentally related to others, be it other people or even a universal and transcendent higher power (Erikson, 1963; Godfrey, 1987; Marcel, 1951). Some theories highlight personal control and mastery over the outcomes hoped-for, while others emphasize exactly the opposite, namely the perception of helplessness when hoping for something out of our direct control (Pruyser, 1986). Main differences can also be found regarding the objects hoped-for, the sources of hope and the actions performed for its realization (Averill et al., 1990; Averill & Sundararajan, 2005). In recent years, discussions regarding the nature of hope have increased as well as the attempts to integrate more complex and multidimensional theories and measures into the many different facets the experience of hoping seems to entail.

Despite the increasing amount of international research and publications on hope, mass media and institutions in Europe, at least in the German speaking countries, have been more interested in the negative side of life, i.e. in the worries, fears and anxieties of the population. For example, for the past 30 years, two leading Swiss financial institutions have been conducting an annual Worry- and Fear-Barometer survey, asking the Swiss population about their greatest concerns (e.g. unemployment, retirement provision, healthcare, personal security, etc.) and how much (or how little) trust they have in those responsible for making political, business and social decisions. Against this background, swissfuture, the Swiss Association for Future Studies,[1] in cooperation with the University of St. Gallen started an annual survey on hope and several other positive attributes in 2009. The aim was to develop a new Hope-Barometer with the objective to explore the meaning, the sources, the targets and levels of hope among the population, not only for academic purposes but also for spreading hope throughout society (Walker & Müller, 2010).

Using data collected in the context of the Hope-Barometer in different countries, the purpose of this book is to present international results, especially the assessment of the concrete levels and cultural aspects of hope in relation to different dimensions of well-being. Accordingly, the book has three central aims that build successively on each other: (1) A discussion and evaluation of different conceptualizations of hope; (2) The presentation of new instruments to measure different aspects and elements of hope and (3) The presentation of results from different countries and the evaluation of specific cultural peculiarities.

Different Conceptualizations of Hope

Hope philosophers and nowadays the discipline of positive psychology have seen hope as an inner driving force towards a better life and world. Many authors refer to the work of Aristotle (1962) who defined a good life as a life lived in congruence with the human virtues and personal strengths, which he called Eudaimonia, i.e. happiness in accordance with one's good spirit. However, Aristotle did not consider

---

[1] A member of the Swiss Academy of Humanities and Social Sciences.

hope a human virtue. In Christian theology, hope is considered a divine virtue, with God as the first source and the final target of hope. According to Christian theologians and philosophers, Christian hope can be considered to be an absolute or fundamental hope, because it is based on the certainty the believer has regarding God's love and omnipotence (Godfrey, 1987; Marcel, 1951). For Kant the highest good is defined as the degree of happiness in accordance with our worthiness for it, based on our moral behavior, independently from any religious value system. His hopes are directed to this highest good not only for the individual but also in terms of an ethical commonwealth, which, however, only can be achieved thanks to the assistance and support of a benevolent God (Michalson, 1999). Moltmann (1968) is the German theologian for whom hope is the theological virtue that brings men closer to the kingdom of God already here on earth, and Bloch (1959) the secular philosopher who saw hope as the human capacity to anticipate a better life and world for oneself and for all human beings. For the existentialist philosopher Marcel (1951) hope is a creative and transcendent mysterious spiritual force that emerges in the intersubjective encounter between two human beings connected in love.

After centuries of philosophical and theological conceptualizations of hope, new psychological theories started to understand hope as a cognitive-behavioral phenomenon, defining it as "an expectation greater than zero of achieving a goal" (Stotland, 1969, p. 2) or the belief that a favorable outcome is likely to occur (Gottschalk, 1974). The main variables to asses if a person is hopeful or not became the level of perceived probability in the attainment of specific personal goals and the importance the person attributes to these goals, linked to the basic belief that the fulfilment of hopes is basically an effect of the person's own capabilities, actions and efforts. Currently, the most diffused cognitive theory of hope is that of Snyder (1994, 2000, 2002) and his colleagues (Lopez, Snyder, & Pedrotti, 2003), who characterize hope as individual mental will- and way-power towards the fulfilment of personal goals. Dispositional hope, as Snyder (2002) defined it, is a trait-like cognitive mindset involving two basic components: (1) Agency as the basic perception of one's determination and motivation to initiate and sustain actions (will-power) to reach defined personal goals and (2) Pathways, the belief in one's own capabilities to generate alternative routes in case of facing obstacles and setbacks (way-power).

Snyder's theory of hope has a self-centered character in that it refers to the person's perception in relation to his or her own efficacy to attain personal goals (Snyder et al., 1991). Key attributes of hopeful people are their tenacity and their active thinking and behaving towards ambitious personal goals. As he formulated it: "Hope is the essential process of linking oneself to potential success" (Snyder, 1994, p. 18). Very hopeful people perceive themselves in control of their lives and having a sense of self-direction. Hope is related to perceptions of personal mastery, the ability to solve problems and a higher level of self-esteem. Hopeful people are ambitious because they tend to have a greater number and more difficult goals than average people. The emphasis in Snyder's hope theory is on success, performance, achievement, resilience and coping (Snyder et al., 1991). The process of hoping is seen as a universal phenomenon largely neutral about the value of the goals and the probability of their attainment (Snyder, 2002). Thoughts and actions have predominance over feelings, and emotions are seen as an effect of successful or frustrated goal attainment. Relationships to other people are important, however primarily in the sense of supporting hopeful thinking and in taking into consideration the goals and perspectives of others to pursue one's own goals (Snyder, 2000).

A common criticism of Snyder's theory of hope is that it is conceptually similar to other psychological constructs (Bruininks & Malle, 2005; Rand & Cheavens, 2009; Tennen, Affleck, & Tennen, 2002; Tong, Fredrickson, Chang, & Lim, 2010). Snyder himself has noted the conceptual overlap between his theory of hope and other goal-oriented constructs such as optimism and self-efficacy (Snyder 2000, 2002). However, in his eyes, optimism (as defined by Scheier & Carver, 1987) and self-efficacy (Bandura 1977) are different from his definition of hope, since these constructs consider only one of the two relevant dimensions: Agency in the case of optimism (Snyder, Sympson, Michael, & Cheavens, 2001) and Pathways in the case of self-efficacy. There is a huge difference, he argues, between the "can" (capacity) in the case of self-efficacy and the "will" (intention) in the concept of agentic hope.

Alternative theories of hope want to overcome the limitations of the cognitive concept and intend to represent the complexity of the phenomenon by integrating different research findings and traditional philosophical reflections. The main differences in alternative theories of hope vis-à-vis the cognitive-behavioral paradigm can be found in the fundamental nature of hope as an emotion, in the degree of control the hopeful person has over the hoped-for outcome, in the interpersonal character of hope as well as in the intrinsic moral value of hope compared to other constructs such as optimism and wishing. Many authors relate to the work of Erikson (1963) who, within the framework of his developmental theory, recognized hope as the first and fundamental human virtue necessary for man's psychosocial development. The emergence and reinforcement of hope is grounded in the basic trust an individual has in people in his immediate social environment. For Erikson, hope, as a virtue, is not only the basis for effective action but also for ethical human behavior. Instead of being cognitive and rational, hope does not always depend on evidence or reason but is fundamentally based on trust (Eliott, 2005; Godfrey, 1987; Tennen et al., 2002).

This focus on trust and interpersonal relations is especially crucial when the individual does not seem to have enough possibilities to influence the event or situation he or she is hoping for. Inspired by the work of Marcel (1951) hope is categorically distinguished from optimism and expectation by its fundamental existential character (Pruyser, 1986). Hope comes into play when the person is confronted with a threatening or dreadful situation and does not feel capable of coping with it by means of his or her own resources alone. For these authors, hope deals with critical experiences in life and has a transformative character for the person involved. The central question related to hope is, how people make sense of and respond to these critical situations (Eliott, 2005). As in the work of Frankl (1959), hope presupposes the transcendence of one's own ego, a feeling of communion with other people and the belief in a benevolent higher power (Pruyser, 1986). For this reason, Peterson and Seligman (2004) included hope in their catalogue of character strengths common across cultures as belonging to the virtue of transcendence. For them, hope belongs to the virtue of transcendence because it goes beyond one's own knowledge and coping capabilities and allows us to build connections to something bigger than ourselves that provides us with meaning, purpose and basic beliefs. In their categorization, hope is linked to other character strengths such as gratitude, appreciation of beauty and excellence, humor and especially spirituality and religious faith. As a transcendent character strength, hope is linked to values which provide a moral framework that keeps the person committed to the expectation and pursuit of goodness.

Fredrickson (1998, 2004, 2009, 2013) has underlined the transformative character of hope, as one of the ten most frequently experienced positive emotions in daily life, with the effect of fostering personal growth and well-being. The effect of hope, as a positive emotion, is that it broadens the mindset, the scope of attention and the thought and action repertoire, nurturing the psychological, social, intellectual and even physical resources to cope with adversity. The second important effect of hope as a positive emotion is that it transforms the individual for the better. While certain emotions such as a good mood and pleasure nourish hedonic happiness, hope can be considered a part of the eudaemonic domain of flourishing that is connected to inner personal growth, meaning in life and in relation with others (Cohn & Fredrickson, 2009). Because of this broadening and growth effect, hopeful people tend to display a more altruistic and generative behavior by helping others, taking a long-term view of things, instead of satisfying short-term needs, thinking beyond the struggles of the present moment, and adopting moral values such as friendship, gratitude, generativity, selflessness, kindness and inclusiveness towards strangers (Cohn & Fredrickson, 2006). Apart from cognitive (analytical, planning, logical) skills, hope can be nourished by social, religious and spiritual practices such as meditation and prayer, creating a deeper connection to the inner self, to other people and to a higher spiritual power (Fredrickson, 2002, 2013).

Table 1.1 shows a brief summary of the main differences in the conceptualization of hope by the different theories presented until now.

Thanks to an increasing amount of empirical research and theory building efforts, many authors have come to the conclusion that hope is a multidimensional phenomenon and that the diverse and sometimes contradictory definitions and conceptualizations should ideally be integrated into more comprehensive theories and models (Dufault & Martocchio, 1985; Farran, Herth, & Popovich, 1995; Scioli, Ricci, Nyugen, & Scioli, 2011; Staats & Stassen, 1985). For example, hope cannot simply be reduced only to cognition or emotion, but includes rational, relational, existential and spiritual components, which all interact.

Another learning point has been, that even though hope is a universal human phenomenon, its concrete experience and expression are quite culture specific (Averill et al., 1990). Different cultures and even different groups within society can conceive of hope differently with fundamental implications for example with regard to the objects or events a person may hope for and the kind of actions taken to achieve them (Averill & Sundararajan, 2005). Among the many things a person may hope for are material goods (e.g. more money), personal achievement (e.g.

Table 1.1 Basic polarities in the conceptualization of hope

Personal	Interpersonal
Own capabilities/self-reliance	Trust in others
Cognition	Emotion
Value neutral	Moral values
Personal trait	Human virtue
Self-centered	Self-transcendent
Personal control	Little personal control
Achievement goals	Attachment goals
Universal	Culture specific
Material	Spiritual
Personal efficacy	Faith/beliefs
High probability of fulfilment	Low probability of fulfilment
All types of goals	Life meaning and purpose
Self-interest	Generativity/altruism
Everyday situations	Threatening situations

performance, success), hedonic experiences (e.g. fun, leisure time), interpersonal relationships (e.g. good friends), or altruistic motives (e.g. helping other people). Depending on the objects hoped-for, the activities and actions towards their achievement could also vary significantly: Working harder, becoming better organized, planning activities, being more creative, being more risk-taking, relating with others to get support, relying on faith, meditating, praying, etc. (Averill et al., 1990).

Measuring Hope

The empirical work on measuring hope can be seen in the context of a fundamental tension between the diverse understandings of the phenomenon that should be measured, the question as to whether people would be able to accurately describe their own level of hope at all and the necessity to develop valid instruments for a more comprehensive assessment of hope to improve scientifically sound explanations. The existing variety of hope concepts and theories have given rise to the development of different instruments for its measurement (for an overview see Farran et al., 1995; Lopez et al., 2003). Central questions that have been discussed when developing new measures of hope were their dimensionality and complexity (uni- or multidimensional), the method (qualitative or quantitative), the length and parsimony (short or long), the applicability (culture specific or universal), the concreteness (general trait or specific goals), the approach (direct or indirect) and the psychometric properties, fundamentally the convergent and discriminant validity vis-à-vis related constructs such as optimism and self-efficacy.

Especially in non-clinical settings, the measure of hope mostly used has been Snyder's Adult Dispositional Trait Hope Scale (Snyder et al., 1991), which includes

4 items to assess the motivational dimension called Agency, 4 items to assess the cognitive dimension called Pathways and 4 distractors. The Dispositional Hope Scale is relatively short, easy to use and has shown very good psychometric properties such as internal consistency, temporal stability, a good factor structure and good convergent and discriminant validity with other measures such as the Life Orientation Test of Scheier and Carver (1985) (Babyak, Snyder, & Yoshinobu, 1993; Carifio & Rhodes, 2002; Snyder et al., 1991). Despite its extensive use and its merits, Snyder's measure of hope has been questioned from many different standpoints: (1) It only assesses the rational and self-centered thought processes and neglects other dimensions like the relational and spiritual (Farran et al., 1995); (2) it only considers goals and aspects in life which one feels in control of, but is less applicable to situations considered to be out of one's direct control (Tong et al., 2010); (3) many items are nearly identical to items used to measure other constructs such as coping and self-efficacy (Tennen et al., 2002); and (4) Agency and Pathways thinking do not reflect how ordinary people define hope for themselves (Averill et al., 1990; Bruininks & Malle, 2005; Tong et al., 2010).

Relating to alternative conceptualizations of hope, other authors have developed multidimensional scales to assess the cognitive, relational, affective and/or spiritual elements included in their conceptualizations of hope. The instruments mostly used are the Hope Index Scale (Obayuwana et al., 1982) including 60 items and 5 sub-scales (ego-strength, religion, family support, education and economic assets), the Miller Hope Scale (Miller & Powers, 1988) with 40 items representing 3 sub-scales (satisfaction with self, others and life, avoidance of hope threats and anticipation of a future), the Nowotny Hope Scale (Nowotny, 1988) comprising 29 items and 6 sub-scales (confidence in outcome, relates to others, future is possible, spiritual beliefs, active involvement and inner readiness), the Herth Hope Scale (Herth, 1991) with 30 items covering 3 dimensions (cognitive-temporal, affective behavioral and affiliative-contextual), and the shorter Herth Hope Index (Herth, 1992). More recently, Scioli and his colleagues (2011, 2016) have developed the Comprehensive Trait Hope Scale including 56 items belonging to 4 sub-scales (mastery, attachment, survival and spirituality) and a shorter Comprehensive State Hope Scale with 40 items. In the psychiatric context, Schrank, Woppmann, Sibitz, and Lauber (2011) have integrated several dimensions of the Miller Hope Scale, the Herth Hope Index and Snyder's Dispositional Hope Scale into a 23-item long Integrative Hope Scale. All these measures have helped to gain differentiated insights into the various elements of hope. However, important concerns regarding the utilization of these measures relate to the length and complexity of the questionnaires, the possible overlap with associated and similar constructs such as spirituality, and the cultural bias of their implicit definitions (e.g. Tennen et al., 2002; Tong et al., 2010). Therefore, a need for measures still exists that assess hope in a simple and direct manner, and that could be used in several cultures and with different population subgroups. For this, certain authors have been using a one-item hope measure for a quick assessment, e.g. 'I feel hopeful about the future' (Tong et al., 2010).

Another approach trying to integrate quantitative methods and a more differentiated form to take into account the various targets of hope is the development of hope scales using specific future-oriented goal statements as items, and asking the participants to rate on a Likert scale the importance or desirability of each goal (affective component) on the one hand, and on the other hand the probability, expectancy or likelihood of its attainment (cognitive component) (Erickson, Post, & Paige, 1975; Stoner, 2004). For example, in her Hope Index, Staats (1989) uses 16 short goal statements, of which 8 are self-referenced (e.g. "To be happy", "To have money") and 8 refer to general goals (e.g. "Peace in the world", "The country to be more productive"). The main criticisms of these kinds of methods have been that several items are too specific to the western middle-class culture and probably not applicable to other cultures, that the length of the scales could be too demanding and the double rating for importance and likelihood too complex for certain individuals and finally that it is questionable if the sum of the hope-level in specific circumstances can be equated to a general level of hope (Farran et al., 1995).

A fundamentally different approach is the attempt to qualitatively understand how people implicitly perceive hope in everyday life, independent from the theoretical constructs defined by researchers (Averill et al., 1990; Gottschalk, 1974). The empirical studies using qualitative methods have shown for example that hope has different connotations in different cultures (Averill et al., 1990) and that hope is different from optimism and more similar to wishes in that it refers to situations in which one perceives to have less personal control and the likelihood of achievement is lower (Bruininks & Malle, 2005). These kinds of studies are very useful but they are also rather complex, time consuming and need several speech samples making it more difficult to target a large number of individuals in different places.

The many definitions and measures of hope have resulted in a multifaceted picture of the phenomenon under scrutiny but have also led to a certain confusion and ambiguity of the term (Lopez et al., 2003). To achieve a clearer demarcation and avoid content overlap or confounding, more empirical studies were needed to explore the nature of hope more thoroughly, including related constructs and empirically distinguishing hope from similar concepts such as self-efficacy, etc. (Rand & Cheavens, 2009; Tennen et al., 2002; Tong et al., 2010). There is still an open issue as to how to assess hope directly in order to gain access to individuals' own understanding and an unfiltered judgment of their own level of hopefulness but avoiding the bias of socially desirable or even faked answers (Lopez et al., 2003). Since hope has been regarded as a universal construct but with a variety of connotations and values across cultures, measures are needed that could be applicable in different countries and ethnic groups. For many years now there has been a call for new short, simple and psychometrically sound instruments to measure hope as perceived by ordinary people that can be used in different cultural environments and could be applied to larger demographic samples (Farran et al., 1995).

The Hope-Barometer Research Program

Background and Purpose

The public discourse regarding the future perspectives and societal changes in Europe has been largely dominated by the discussion of risks and crises. Although it is a main task of political and social institutions to recognize new opportunities and to support a positive development in society, the mass media and the general public have focused their attention primarily on the discussion of worries and concerns about the future. The attention on the negative aspects of life has a long tradition, especially in the German speaking countries. Since the early 1970s, the population has been largely surveyed with regard to their major concerns and anxieties e.g. unemployment, social security, retirement provision, health care, personal safety and to what extent they trust (or mistrust) political, economic and social institutions. The study of worries and fears may have a particular value, but it overlooks the phenomenon of self-fulfilling prophecies (Jones, 1977; Jussim, 1986). If we concentrate our attention on the negative side of life, we will start to see mainly negative developments, with the consequence of accentuating the negative even more, leading to a downward spiral, which affects the culture of an entire society. The result of such a self-fulfilling vicious circle was the emergence of a negative cultural bias known by the term "German Angst" (Bode, 2008), which describes the German propensity to see the world through glasses tainted by fears and worries.

For this reason, the Hope-Barometer research program was created in 2009 as a counter-initiative to the classical Worries- and Fears-Barometers with the purpose of explicitly focusing on the positive attitudes and expectations of the population towards the future (Walker & Mueller, 2010). Since then, the Hope-Barometer is a yearly cross-sectional survey with three major objectives: (1) to generate and support a public discourse focusing on positive thoughts and perspectives about the future; (2) to initiate a scientifically sound study of the phenomenon of hope, especially in Europe; and (3) to contribute to the general conceptualization of hope from a European and international perspective. In 2009–2011 the Hope-Barometer was limited to German speaking Switzerland. During recent years the survey was expanded to other countries (which will be presented later) with more than 10,000 people participating in the survey every year. The main results are published annually in several newspapers over Christmas and the New Year with the purpose of conveying good news at a particularly hopeful time of the year.

Definition and Conceptualization of Hope

Taking into account the many and sometimes contradictory definitions of hope, it was a special challenge within the framework of the Hope-Barometer program to find out which conceptualization of hope best suits the international and multicultural context of the survey. With Averill and Sundararajan (2005) as well as Eliott (2005) we maintain that the specific understanding of hope is related to the cultural tradition of the society or group of people under study. It is the task of science to investigate the similarities and differences in the interpretation of the phenomenon that should be explained. At the same time, there is also the need within a multinational research project, to come up with an understanding of the phenomenon under scrutiny that could serve as a common denominator to guide the basic structure and methodology of the research. Based on theoretical considerations and empirical findings, a working definition and conceptual framework of hope has been formulated over the years.

> We understand hope as the general belief, trust and confidence, that specific things, objectives and circumstances, which we desire because they are important to us and which we wish to attain, will develop the way which is right and good for us and for our social environment, regardless of the adversities and obstacles as well as possible negative expectancies and seemingly opposing objective facts, so that it remains worthwhile to persevere and keep involved.

With this conceptualization of hope we do not maintain that all people understand hope the same way. Some people may need objective facts and a high probability of success to keep hoping. Other people can only hope in relation to the fulfillment of their concrete desires and expectations. However, with this definition a clear distinction between hope and expectancies as well as between hope and desires has been drawn.

The following elements have been considered in our definition and conceptualization of hope:

1. Hope contains two spheres as proposed by Dufault and Martocchio (1985): A *generalized* and a *specific domain.*
2. One central element of hope is a sense of *belief.* This belief can be orientated to a spiritual or religious higher power or be grounded in a particular value system.
3. Hope entails a sort of *trust* in oneself, another person and / or a transcendent instance.
4. A positive view towards the future is based on the *confidence* in positive outcomes for oneself and others.

5. Hope can be a *general feeling* but often it refers to *concrete objectives* and circumstances that are considered possible to realize.
6. Hope as a *virtue* should be directed to things that are right and good for oneself and also for the larger (social) environment.
7. People hope for things that are *relevant, meaningful* und *important* to them and for which they have the will to commit themselves.
8. The fulfillment of one's own hopes is never certain, since there are always more or less *adverse conditions* and *barriers* to overcome.
9. Expectancies and objective facts sometimes seem to contradict the outcomes hoped-for. However, objective facts are never definitive and can also be interpreted in many ways.
10. Things and conditions are basically in flux, they evolve with time. Therefore, hoping can be considered a *process*.
11. To believe that things will develop in the best possible way, regardless of the fulfillment of certain concrete wishes, is a testimony of *absolute* or *fundamental hope* as philosophically defined by Marcel (1951) and Godfrey (1987).
12. Hope is often a *social phenomenon*, which does not only concern the individual person but the entire social environment.
13. To hope is not a passive stance, but an attitude that entails *motivation, involvement, action* and *perseverance* towards the attainment of something worthy and meaningful.
14. Not included in this definition and conceptualization of hope is the idea of probability, likelihood and feasibility of goal accomplishment.
15. Nor does this conceptualization of hope include certain dimensions such as the cognitive, affective or spiritual, since people in several cultures and with different backgrounds can perceive and experience hope in diverse ways.

Development and Description of Methods

Existing hope scales have been criticized for being confounded with items of other variables, for containing a theoretical or cultural bias of the researcher or for being too complex and too long for certain research settings and purposes. The first step of the Hope-Barometer research program was, therefore, to develop a short measure for targeting hope in a direct and explicit manner, allowing respondents to consider their own perceptions of hope. The contents for the Perceived Hope Scale (PHS) have been developed taking and reformulating the four items of hope and optimism from the English version of the WHOQOL-SRPB questionnaire (Skevington, Gunson, & O'connell, 2013) and adding two additional indicators (Krafft, Martin-Krumm, & Fenouillet, 2017).

Since the PHS does not address the question regarding the nature of hope and the different dimensions it may have, the next step was thus to develop instruments that allow the assessment of different elements and dimensions of hope, i.e. (1) the satisfaction and expectations with different domains, (2) targets of hope in form of personal objectives and wishes, (3) experiences that support the feeling of hope, (4) activities performed to attain the targets hoped-for, and (5) hope providers people turn to or count on. These scales have been conceived to assess the different aspects related to hope but it was not intended to develop scales with which an overall value or level of hope could be calculated. The instruments are especially valuable if we want to understand the different conceptualizations and implications of hope in different cultures and groups. The items of these scales were developed with a multidisciplinary group of scientists and practitioners invited to several workshops at the beginning and during the first phase of the research project. Some of these scales are used every year to allow a medium to long-term comparison of the results and other scales were only employed once or twice.

The Hope-Barometer starts with 5 items for the assessment of the satisfaction in different domains and the (optimistic or pessimistic) expectations people have with regard to these domains for the forthcoming year, including (1) their private life, (2) the national economy, (3) the national politics, (4) the climate and the environment, as well as (5) contemporary social issues.

A pool of 17 items then addresses the targets and objects hoped-for including similar indicators to those used in the Hope Index of Staats (1989) and Erickson's Hope Scale (Erickson et al., 1975) but with the following characteristics: We only included self-referenced targets and no general goals such as 'Peace in the world'. The items belong to aspects people hope-for in different domains of their lives, e.g. performance goals ('Success at the workplace, at school/university or in other activities'), relational goals ('Good and trustful relationships with other people'), material goals ('More money'), hedonistic goals ('More sex'), health related goals ('Personal health'), altruistic goals ('Helping other people'), spiritual goals ('Religious experiences, experience of God'), etc. We asked the participants to rate only the importance of the hopes for themselves but not the perceived likelihood of their attainment. This group of items has also been used to assess the satisfaction of people with these life domains.

The next pool of items consists of a list of 25 personal experiences people revert to in order to nourish their hopes. These items represent the religious dimension (e.g. 'I have felt God's closeness'), the social dimension (e.g. 'Good relations with friends'), the personal coping dimension (e.g. 'I came through an illness successfully'), the cognitive dimension (e.g. 'Successful completion of education or university'), the materialistic dimension (e.g. 'I earned a lot of money'), the hedonic dimension (e.g. 'I experienced great concerts and parties') and the altruistic dimension (e.g. 'Doing good for a meaningful purpose').

The objective of a further instrument was to gain a better knowledge of what kind of actions people undertake to see their hopes fulfilled, similarly done by Averill et al. (1990). Here again, several distinct areas of actions were considered using 13 items, i.e. cognitive ('I think a lot and analyze circumstances.'), spiritual ('I pray, meditate.'), relational ('I motivate my friends.'), religious ('I go to church/to the temple.') and motivational ('I take responsibility and engage myself.').

An additional instrument consists of a list of hope providers from whom people expect the transmission and spread of hope. One central theoretical question was, whether hope is an individual or rather a relational phenomenon. We developed 16 items with subjects from different social environments including the closer family members (e.g. 'Wife, husband, partner'), peers (e.g. 'Friends'), business (e.g. 'Colleagues/Business partners'), politics (e.g. 'Politicians, the government'), education (e.g. 'Teachers, educators, professors, coaches'), religion (e.g. 'God'), and included two special items that refer to oneself ('I give myself hope – It's the responsibility of every single person him-/herself') and to an abstract category formulated as 'The many ordinary people without great names that mastered their fate admirably'.

To be able to investigate hope in relation to other relevant constructs that have been connected to hope in the literature, the Hope-Barometer has included a set of different additional scales every year. For practical reasons, the aim was to employ short scales, but with sound psychometric properties. In those cases where no validated translations were available, members of the national teams of the research project translated the items and cross-checked them. In the course of the last 7 years the following scales have been used: Dispositional Hope (Snyder et al., 1991), Self-efficacy (Schwarzer & Jerusalem, 1999), Resilience (Smith et al., 2008), Positive Relations (Ryff & Keyes, 1995), Generativity (Schnell, 2009), Helping Others (Nickell, 1998), Gratitude (McCullough, Emmons, & Tsang, 2002), Spiritual Beliefs (Parsian & Dunning, 2009), Religious Faith (Plante & Boccaccini, 1997), Satisfaction with Life (Diener, Emmons, Larsen, & Griffin, 1985), Subjective Happiness (Lyubomirsky & Lepper, 1999), Depression and Anxiety (Kroenke, Spitzer, Williams, & Löwe, 2009), Physical Health (Ferring et al., 2004), Psychological Health (Ferring et al., 2004), Posttraumatic Growth (Joseph, Linley, Shevlin, Goodfellow, & Butler, 2006), Meaning in Life (Schnell, 2009; Steger, Frazier, Oishi, & Kaler, 2006), Optimism and Pessimism (LOT-R) (Scheier, Carver, & Bridges, 1994), Loneliness (Hughes, Waite, Hawkley, & Cacioppo, 2004), Positive and Negative Emotions (SPANE) (Diener et al., 2010), Compassion (Hwang, Plante, & Lackey, 2008), Harmonious and Obsessive Passion (Vallerand et al., 2003), and Harmony in Life (Kjell, Daukantaité, Hefferon, & Sikström, 2016).

General Procedure

The studies presented in this book are based on different samples of the Hope-Barometer, as a yearly cross-sectional survey that has been performed in Switzerland since 2009, in Germany and France since 2012, in the Czech Republic since 2013, in Malta since 2014, in Poland and India since 2015, and in Spain in 2016. In South Africa, the research team has used several scales (e.g. the Perceived Hope Scale) in 2016 and has joined the project in 2017, as did a research institute in Israel. Data collection was done by internet and via e-mails, social networks, and diverse websites. Thanks to the cooperation with several large national newspapers that draw great attention to the survey every year and link the respective questionnaire to their webpages during a period of 2–3 weeks during November, many samples include a considerable number of people of different ages, with different educational backgrounds, diverse family status as well as different religious and spiritual orientations. Basically, priority has been placed on reaching as many participants as possible, with the objective of promoting personal reflection and an extensive public discourse about the positive side of (future) life, instead of ensuring strict representativeness in terms of demographic structure.

Methods used for data analysis as well as the composition of the samples will be presented individually in the following chapters of the book.

References

Aristotle. (1962). *The Nichomachean ethics* (M. Oswald, Trans.). New York: The Bobs-Merrill Company.

Averill, J. R., Catlin, G., & Chon, K. K. (1990). *Rules of hope: Recent research in psychology.* New York: Springer.

Averill, J. R., & Sundararajan, L. (2005). Hope as rhetoric: Cultural narratives of wishing and coping. In J. Eliott (Ed.), *Interdisciplinary perspectives on hope* (pp. 133–165). New York: Nova Science Publication.

Babyak, M. A., Snyder, C. R., & Yoshinobu, L. (1993). Psychometric properties of the hope scale: A confirmatory factor analysis. *Journal of Research in Personality, 27*(2), 154–169.

Bandura, A. (1977). Self-efficacy: Toward a unifying theory of behavioral change. *Psychological Review, 84*(2), 191.

Bloch, E. (1959). Das Prinzip Hoffnung. In *fünf Teilen.* Frankfurt am Main, Germany: Suhrkamp Taschenbuch Verlag.

Bode, S. (2008). *Die deutsche Krankheit – German Angst.* München, Germany: Piper Verlag.

Bruininks, P., & Malle, B. F. (2005). Distinguishing hope from optimism and related affective states. *Motivation and Emotion, 29*(4), 324–352.

Carifio, J., & Rhodes, L. (2002). Construct validities and the empirical relationships between optimism, hope, self-efficacy, and locus of control. *Work, 19*(2), 125–136.

Cohn, M. A., & Fredrickson, B. L. (2006). Beyond the moment, beyond the self: Shared ground between selective investment theory and the broaden-and-build theory of positive emotions. *Psychological Inquiry, 17*(1), 39–44.

Cohn, M. A., & Fredrickson, B. L. (2009). Positive emotions. *Oxford Handbook of Positive Psychology, 2*, 13–24.

Diener, E. D., Emmons, R. A., Larsen, R. J., & Griffin, S. (1985). The satisfaction with life scale. *Journal of Personality Assessment, 49*(1), 71–75.

Diener, E. D., Wirtz, D., Tov, W., Kim-Prieto, C., Choi, D. W., Oishi, S., & Biswas-Diener, R. (2010). New well-being measures: Short scales to assess flourishing and positive and negative feelings. *Social Indicators Research, 97*(2), 143–156.

Dufault, K., & Martocchio, B. C. (1985). Symposium on compassionate care and the dying experience. Hope: Its spheres and dimensions. *The Nursing Clinics of North America, 20*(2), 379–391.

Eliott, J. A. (2005). What have we done with hope? A brief history. In J. A. Eliott (Ed.), *Interdisciplinary perspectives on hope* (pp. 3–45). New York: Nova Publishers.

Erickson, R. C., Post, R. D., & Paige, A. B. (1975). Hope as a psychiatric variable. *Journal of Clinical Psychology, 31*(2), 324–330.

Erikson, E. (1963). *Childhood and Society* (2nd ed. Rev. and enl). New York: W.W. Norton & Co.

Farran, C. J., Herth, K. A., & Popovich, J. M. (1995). *Hope and hopelessness: Critical clinical constructs.* Thousand Oaks, CA/London: Sage Publications, Inc.

Ferring, D., Balducci, C., Burholt, V., Wenger, C., Thissen, F., Weber, G., & Hallberg, I. (2004). Life satisfaction of older people in six European countries: Findings from the European study on adult well-being. *European Journal of Ageing, 1*(1), 15–25.

Frankl, V. E. (1959). The spiritual dimension in existential analysis and logotherapy. *Journal of Individual Psychology, 15*(2), 157–165.

Fredrickson, B. L. (1998). What good are positive emotions? *Review of General Psychology, 2*(3), 300–318.

Fredrickson, B. L. (2002). Positive emotions. In C. R. Snyder & S. J. Lopez (Eds.), *Handbook of positive psychology* (pp. 120–134). New York: Oxford University Press.

Fredrickson, B. L. (2004). The broaden-and-build theory of positive emotions. *Philosophical Transactions-Royal Society of London Series B Biological Sciences, 359*, 1367–1378.

Fredrickson, B. L. (2009). *Positivity: Groundbreaking research reveals how to embrace the hidden strengths of positive emotions, overcome negativity, and thrive.* New York: Crown.

Fredrickson, B. L. (2013). Positive emotions broaden and build. *Advances in Experimental Social Psychology, 47*, 1), 1–1),53.

Godfrey, J. J. (1987). *A philosophy of human hope.* Dordrecht, The Netherlands: Martinus Nijhoff.

Gottschalk, L. A. (1974). A hope scale applicable to verbal samples. *Archives of General Psychiatry, 30*(6), 779–785.

Herth, K. (1991). Development and refinement of an instrument to measure hope. *Scholarly Inquiry for Nursing Practice, 5*(1), 39–51.

Herth, K. (1992). Abbreviated instrument to measure hope: Development and psychometric evaluation. *Journal of Advanced Nursing, 17*(10), 1251–1259.

Hughes, M. E., Waite, L. J., Hawkley, L. C., & Cacioppo, J. T. (2004). A short scale for measuring loneliness in large surveys results from two population-based studies. *Research on Aging, 26*(6), 655–672.

Hwang, J. Y., Plante, T., & Lackey, K. (2008). The development of the Santa Clara brief compassion scale: An abbreviation of Sprecher and Fehr's compassionate love scale. *Pastoral Psychology, 56*(4), 421–428.

Jones, R. A. (1977). *Self-fulfilling prophecies: Social, psychological, and physiological effects of expectancies.* Hillsdale, MI: Lawrence Erlbaum Associates.

Joseph, S., Linley, P. A., Shevlin, M., Goodfellow, B., & Butler, L. D. (2006). Assessing positive and negative changes in the aftermath of adversity: A short form of the changes in outlook questionnaire. *Journal of Loss and Trauma, 11*(1), 85–99.

Jussim, L. (1986). Self-fulfilling prophecies: A theoretical and integrative review. *Psychological Review, 93*(4), 429.

Kjell, O., Daukantaité, D., Hefferon, K., & Sikström, S. (2016). Harmony in life scale complements the satisfaction with life scale: Expanding the conceptualization of the cognitive component of subjective well-being. *Social Indicators Research, 126*, 893–919.

Krafft, A. M., Martin-Krumm, C., & Fenouillet, F. (2017). Adaptation, further elaboration, and validation of a scale to measure hope as perceived by people: Discriminant value and predictive utility Vis-à-Vis dispositional hope. *Assessment.* https://doi.org/10.1177/1073191117700724.

Krafft, A. M., & Walker, A. M. (2018). *Positive Psychologie der Hoffnung - Grundlagen aus Psychologie, Philosophie, Theologie und Ergebnisse aktueller Forschung.* Berlin/Heidelberg: Springer.

Kroenke, K., Spitzer, R. L., Williams, J. B., & Löwe, B. (2009). An ultra-brief screening scale for anxiety and depression: The PHQ–4. *Psychosomatics, 50*(6), 613–621.

Lopez, S. J., Snyder, C. R., & Pedrotti, J. T. (2003). Hope: Many definitions, many measures. In S. J. Lopez & C. R. Snyder (Eds.), *Positive psychological assessment: A handbook of models and measures* (Vol. 1, pp. 91–107). Washington, DC: American Psychological Association.

Lyubomirsky, S., & Lepper, H. S. (1999). A measure of subjective happiness: Preliminary reliability and construct validation. *Social Indicators Research, 46*(2), 137–155.

Marcel, G. (1951). *Homo Viator: Introduction to a metaphysics of hope* (E. Crawfurd & P. Seaton, Trans.) (South Bend, IN: St. Augustine Press, 2010).

McCullough, M. E., Emmons, R. A., & Tsang, J. A. (2002). The grateful disposition: A conceptual and empirical topography. *Journal of Personality and Social Psychology, 82*(1), 112–127.

Michalson, G. E. (1999). *Kant and the problem of god*. Malden, MA: Blackwell Publishers.

Miller, J. F., & Powers, M. J. (1988). Development of an instrument to measure hope. *Nursing Research, 37*(1), 6–10.

Moltmann, J. (1968). *Theologie der Hoffnung*. München, Germany: Chr. Kaiser.

Nickell, G. S. (1998). *The helping attitude scale: A new measure of prosocial tendencies*. Paper presented at the American Psychological Association, San Francisco.

Nowotny, M. L. (1988). Assessment of hope in patients with cancer: Development of an instrument. *Oncology Nursing Forum, 16*(1), 57–61.

Obayuwana, A. O., Collins, J. L., Carter, A. L., Rao, M. S., Mathura, C. C., & Wilson, S. B. (1982). Hope index scale: An instrument for the objective assessment of hope. *Journal of the National Medical Association, 74*(8), 761–765.

Parsian, N., & Dunning, T. A. (2009). Developing and validating a questionnaire to measure spirituality: A psychometric process. *Global Journal of Health Science, 1*(1), 2–11.

Peterson, C., & Seligman, M. E. (2004). *Character strengths and virtues: A handbook and classification*. Oxford, UK: Oxford University Press.

Plante, T. G., & Boccaccini, M. T. (1997). The Santa Clara strength of religious faith questionnaire. *Pastoral Psychology, 45*(5), 375–387.

Pruyser, P. W. (1986). Maintaining hope in adversity. *Pastoral Psychology, 35*(2), 120–131.

Rand, K. L., & Cheavens, J. S. (2009). Hope theory. In S. J. Lopez (Ed.), *Oxford handbook of positive psychology* (pp. 323–333). Oxford, UK: Oxford University Press.

Ryff, C. D., & Keyes, C. L. M. (1995). The structure of psychological well-being revisited. *Journal of Personality and Social Psychology, 69*(4), 719–727.

Scheier, M. F., & Carver, C. S. (1985). Optimism, coping, and health: Assessment and implications of generalized outcome expectancies. *Health Psychology, 4*(3), 219.

Scheier, M. E., & Carver, C. S. (1987). Dispositional optimism and physical well-being: The influence of generalized outcome expectancies on health. *Journal of Personality, 55*(2), 169–210.

Scheier, M. F., Carver, C. S., & Bridges, M. W. (1994). Distinguishing optimism from neuroticism (and trait anxiety, self-mastery, and self-esteem): A reevaluation of the life orientation test. *Journal of Personality and Social Psychology, 67*(6), 1063.

Schnell, T. (2009). The sources of meaning and meaning in life questionnaire (SoMe): Relations to demographics and well-being. *The Journal of Positive Psychology, 4*(3), 483–499.

Schrank, B., Woppmann, A., Sibitz, I., & Lauber, C. (2011). Development and validation of an integrative scale to assess hope. *Health Expectations, 14*(4), 417–428.

Schwarzer, R., & Jerusalem, M. (1999). *Skalen zur Erfassung von Lehrer- und Schülermerkmalen*. Berlin, Germany: Freie Universität Berlin.

Scioli, A., & Biller, H. (2009). *Hope in the age of anxiety*. Oxford, UK: Oxford University Press.

Scioli, A., Chamberlin, C. M., Samor, C. M., Lapointe, A. B., Campbell, T. L., Macleod, A. R., & McLenon, J. (1997). A prospective study of hope, optimism, and health. *Psychological Reports, 81*(3), 723–733.

Scioli, A., Ricci, M., Nyugen, T., & Scioli, E. R. (2011). Hope: Its nature and measurement. *Psychology of Religion and Spirituality, 3*(2), 78–97.

Scioli, A., Scioli-Salter, E. R., Sykes, K., Anderson, C., & Fedele, M. (2016). The positive contributions of hope to maintaining and restoring health: An integrative, mixed-method approach. *The Journal of Positive Psychology, 11*(2), 135–148.

Skevington, S. M., Gunson, K. S., & O'connell, K. A. (2013). Introducing the WHOQOL-SRPB BREF: Developing a short-form instrument for assessing spiritual, religious and personal beliefs within quality of life. *Quality of Life Research, 22*(5), 1073–1083.

Slezáčková, A. (2017). *Hope and well-being: Psychosocial correlates and benefits of hope*. Msida, Malta: Centre for Resilience and Socio-Emotional Health, University of Malta.

Smith, B. W., Dalen, J., Wiggins, K., Tooley, E., Christopher, P., & Bernard, J. (2008). The brief resilience scale: Assessing the ability to bounce back. *International Journal of Behavioral Medicine, 15*(3), 194–200.

Snyder, C. R. (1994). *The psychology of hope: You can get there from here.* New York: Simon and Schuster.

Snyder, C. R. (2000). Hypothesis: There is hope. In C. R. Snyder (Ed.), *Handbook of hope: Theory, measures, and applications* (pp. 3–21). San Diego, CA: Academic press.

Snyder, C. R. (2002). Hope theory: Rainbows in the mind. *Psychological Inquiry, 13*(4), 249–275.

Snyder, C. R., Harris, C., Anderson, J. R., Holleran, S. A., Irving, L. M., Sigmon, S. T., & Harney, P. (1991). The will and the ways: Development and validation of an individual-differences measure of hope. *Journal of Personality and Social Psychology, 60*(4), 570–585.

Snyder, C. R., Sympson, S. C., Michael, S. T., & Cheavens, J. (2001). Optimism and hope constructs: Variants on a positive expectancy theme. In E. C. Chang (Ed.), *Optimism and pessimism: Implications for theory, research, and practice* (pp. 101–125). Washington, DC: American Psychological Association.

Staats, S. (1989). Hope: A comparison of two self-report measures for adults. *Journal of Personality Assessment, 53*(2), 366–375.

Staats, S. R., & Stassen, M. A. (1985). Hope: An affective cognition. *Social Indicators Research, 17*(3), 235–242.

Steger, M. F., Frazier, P., Oishi, S., & Kaler, M. (2006). The meaning in life questionnaire: Assessing the presence of and search for meaning in life. *Journal of Counseling Psychology, 53*(1), 80–93.

Stoner, M. H. (2004). Measuring hope. In M. Frank-Stromborg & S. Olsen (Eds.), *Instruments for clinical health-care research* (pp. 215–228). Sudbury, MA: Jones and Bartlett Publications.

Stotland, E. (1969). *The psychology of hope.* San Francisco: Jossey-Bass.

Tennen, H., Affleck, G., & Tennen, R. (2002). Clipped feathers: The theory and measurement of hope. *Psychological Inquiry, 13*(4), 311–317.

Tong, E. M., Fredrickson, B. L., Chang, W., & Lim, Z. X. (2010). Re-examining hope: The roles of agency thinking and pathways thinking. *Cognition and Emotion, 24*(7), 1207–1215.

Vallerand, R. J., Blanchard, C., Mageau, G. A., Koestner, R., Ratelle, C., Léonard, M., ... Marsolais, J. (2003). Les passions de l'ame: on obsessive and harmonious passion. *Journal of Personality and Social Psychology, 85*(4), 756.

Walker, A. M., & Mueller R. (2010). *Hoffnung.* swissfuture: Magazin für Zukunftsmonitoring 2010/1, Luzern.

Chapter 2
Exploring the Concept and Experience of Hope – Empirical Findings and the Virtuous Circle of Hope

Andreas M. Krafft and Andreas M. Walker

Introduction and Objectives

The purpose of this contribution is to give a first overview of the central results using the German speaking samples of the Hope-Barometer between 2011 and 2016. The main objective is to assess the character, the elements and levels of hope as reported by the German speaking population in Germany and Switzerland. Furthermore, we want to study the interrelations between the many different elements of hope and the general level of hope, satisfaction in life and happiness. Based on these results, many striking conclusions can be drawn about the characteristics and general nature of hope, at least from the perspective of the German speaking population. These conclusions will be interpreted in the light of the different definitions and conceptualizations of hope presented in Chap. 1 of this book.

Procedure and Samples

Data collection was done by internet, thanks to two of the largest and most popular German and Swiss newspapers drawing great attention to the survey every year and linking the questionnaires to their webpages every November (2011–2016) over a period of 2–3 weeks. The samples include a total of 37'913 participants of different age ranges, with different educational backgrounds and family status (see composition of the samples in Table 2.1). For data analysis we only used the fully answered

A. M. Krafft (✉)
Institute of Systemic Management and Public Governance, University of St. Gallen,
St. Gallen, Switzerland
e-mail: andreas.krafft@unisg.ch

A. M. Walker
Swissfuture, Lucerne, Switzerland

© Springer International Publishing AG, part of Springer Nature 2018   21
A. M. Krafft et al. (eds.), *Hope for a Good Life*, Social Indicators Research
Series 72, https://doi.org/10.1007/978-3-319-78470-0_2

Table 2.1 Demographic structure of the samples

	2011	2012	2013	2014	2015	2016
	N (%)	N (%)	N (%)	N (%)	N (%)	N (%)
Total	3134 (100)	10,633 (100)	4581 (100)	7997 (100)	7282 (100)	4286 (100)
Switzerland	3134 (100)	4185 (39.4)	2072 (45.2)	3836 (48.0)	6057 (83.2)	3272 (76.3)
Germany	–	6448 (60.6)	2509 (54.8)	4161 (52.0)	1225 (16.8)	1014 (23.7)
Gender						
Male	1474 (48.0)	6153 (57.9)	2212 (48.3)	3976 (49.7)	2847 (39.1)	1860 (43.4)
Female	1315 (52.0)	4479 (42.1)	2369 (51.7)	4021 (50.3)	4435 (60.9)	2426 (56.6)
Age						
18–29	1047 (33.4)	3979 (37.4)	1511 (33.0)	2647 (33.1)	2598 (35.7)	1150 (26.8)
30–39	547 (17.5	2097 (19.7)	854 (18.6)	1611 (20.1)	1458 (20.0)	914 (21.3)
40–49	1343 (42.9)	1830 (17.2)	810 (17.7)	1409 (17.6)	1175 (16.1)	723 (16.9)
50–59		1482 (13.9)	763 (16.7)	1277 (16.0)	1158 (15.9)	815 (19.0)
60–69	197 (6.3)	957 (9.0)	487 (10.6)	811 (10.1)	672 (9.2)	525 (12.2)
70–79		261 (2.5)	141 (3.1)	219 (2.7)	200 (2.7)	148 (3.5)
80+		27 (0.3	15 (0.3)	23 (0.3)	21 (0.3)	11 (0.3)
Highest levels of education						
Did not finish school	3 (0.1)	45 (0.4)	30 (0.7)	52 (0.7)	44 (0.6)	23 (0.5)
Primary school	117 (3.7)	629 (5.9)	214 (4.7)	556 (7.0)	419 (5.8)	217 (5.1)
Secondary school	188 (6.0)	616 (5.8)	277 (6.0)	711 (8.9)	368 (5.1)	230 (5.4)
College	1183 (37.7)	806 (7.6)	343 (7.5)	616 (7.7)	443 (6.1)	251 (5.9)
Professional education		2541 (23.9)	1964 (42.9)	3058 (38.2)	3148 (43.2)	1683 (39.3)
Higher professional education	790 (25.2)	3106 (29.2)	783 (17.1)	1348 (16.9)	1493 (20.5)	928 (21.7)
University	848 (27.1)	2890 (27.2)	970 (21.2)	1656 (20.7)	1367 (18.8)	954 (22.3)
Family status						
Living with parents	801 (25.6)	2836 (26.7)	452 (9.9)	700 (8.8)	894 (12.3)	352 (8.2)
Single			821 (17.9)	1485 (18.6)	1178 (16.2)	751 (17.5)
Living in a partnership	1168 (37.3)	4497 (42.3)	1244 (27.1)	2354 (29.5)	2082 (28.6)	1135 (26.5)

(continued)

Table 2.1 (continued)

	2011 N (%)	2012 N (%)	2013 N (%)	2014 N (%)	2015 N (%)	2016 N (%)
Married	841 (26.8)	2770 (26.1)	1644 (35.9)	2788 (34.9)	2554 (35.1)	1634 (38.1)
Separated/divorced	93 (3.0)	297 (2.8)	292 (6.4)	457 (5.7)	476 (6.5)	360 (8.4)
Widowed	47 (1.5)	132 (1.2)	67 (1.5)	125 (1.6)	98 (1.3)	54 (1.3)
Something different	184 (5.9)	101 (1.0)	61 (1.3)	88 (1.1)	–	–

questionnaires of participants aged 18 and above, and removed all those files with obviously incorrect answers, i.e. when a large number of questions were rated with only one option (0 or 1). The percentage of removed cases was between 4.7% and 6.7%. For the analysis, threshold values of skewness <2 and kurtosis <3 (West, Finch, & Curran, 1995) were used to assess data distribution. Since from 2014 on all the questions were defined as compulsory, there are no missing values between 2014 and 2016. Missing values in the other samples were listwise excluded from the analysis. All the studies were performed using SPSS (IBM, 2014) and AMOS 23 (Arbuckle, 2014) as software.

Methods

The Hope-Barometer consists of a variety of measures that aim to capture the different elements of hope (e.g. the level of hope, targets of hope, sources of hope, future expectations, places of hope, hope experiences, hope providers, etc.) and a set of standardized scales to assess related aspects such as satisfaction with life, subjective happiness, meaning in life, positive relations, positive feelings, self-efficacy, harmony in life, etc. While many scales are used every year to allow comparisons over time, other measures were only used once or twice following a concrete research question (see also Krafft & Walker, 2018).

Measures of Hope

To be able to assess the different elements and aspects of hope that the act of hoping might entail, a variety of new scales and pools of items have been developed and were included in the Hope-Barometer in different years.

Perceived Hope Scale (PHS) To be able to measure hope as perceived by people, we adapted and reformulated the four items of hope and optimism from the English version of the WHOQOL-SRPB questionnaire (Skevington, Gunson, & O'connell, 2013) and added two additional items with aspects of hope not covered by the WHOQOL-SRPB. This resulted in a unidimensional scale with six items called the

Perceived Hope Scale (PHS) (Krafft, Martin-Krumm, & Fenouillet, 2017). Two examples of these items are: "In my life, hope outweighs anxiety" and "I am hopeful with regard to my life". The items are rated on a 6-point Likert-scale from 0 (strongly disagree) to 5 (strongly agree). In the validation study, the PHS revealed good internal consistency with Cronbach alphas between .87 and .89.

Adult Dispositional Hope Scale (DHS) To assess the cognitive-rational concept of hope and compare it to perceived hope, Snyder's Adult Dispositional Hope Scale (Snyder et al., 1991) has been included in the survey. This scale (displaying alpha-values from .74 to .84 in the validation article) consists of four items to assess the motivational dimension of Agency (alphas from .71 to .76) and four items to assess the cognitive dimension of Pathways (alphas from .63 to .80). The items are scored on a 6-point scale from 0 (strongly disagree) to 5 (strongly agree).

Satisfaction and Future Expectations in Different Fields In general, hope has been understood as a positive expectancy towards the future. However, hope and expectations are not always identical (Cristea et al., 2011; David, Montgomery, & DiLorenzo, 2006; David, Montgomery, Stan, DiLorenzo, & Erblich, 2004; Montgomery, David, DiLorenzo, & Erblich, 2003). At the beginning of the questionnaire, participants are asked about their level of satisfaction as well as about their future expectations in five different fields: (1) Their private life, (2) the national economy, (3) the national politics, (4) the climate and environment, and (5) social issues. The five items are rated from 1 (very unsatisfied) to 5 (very satisfied) and from 1 (very pessimistic) to 5 (very optimistic). It is not the intention here to calculate an overall value for satisfaction and for future expectations but to compare the values of the five indicators and relate them to the general level of hope.

Personal Hopes for the Coming Year and Satisfaction with Several Life Domains Every year participants are asked to rate the importance they attribute to 17 life domains in terms of their hopes for the coming year. The 17 life domains belong to six basic dimensions: (1) Personal well-being (e.g. "personal health", "harmony in life"), (2) social relations (e.g. "good and trusting relations to other people"), (3) hedonic experiences (e.g. "more sex", "more spare time"), (4) work and material goods (e.g. "success at the workplace", "more money"), (5) religiosity/ spirituality (e.g. "religious and spiritual experiences") and (6) meaning and purpose (e.g. "meaningful and satisfying tasks", "helping other people"). The items are rated on a 4-point scale from 0 (not important) to 3 (very important). In accordance with our definition of hope, the participants are only asked to rate the importance but not the perceived probability of attainment of these life domains. Nor should an overall value composed of the sum of the 17 single ratings be calculated. The same 17 items were used to assess the level of satisfaction with the single life domains. The scoring scale goes from 0 (not at all satisfied) to 3 (very satisfied).

Hope Providers As stated in Chap. 1, having good relations to other people can be an important source of hope. Hence, the participants were asked every year to evaluate a list of 16 people or categories of people to assess to what extent these individuals are hope providers for them. The 16 items cover six basic dimensions: (1) The self-centered category of oneself, (2) the inner circle of people in the closer social environment (e.g. "wife, husband, partner"), (3) a group of people in the work environment (e.g. "colleagues, business partners"), (4) people in the wider social environment that are usually known personally (e.g. "physicians, therapists, etc."), (5) people in the general social environment (e.g. "experts, scientists, etc.") and (6) the transcendent environment ("God"). The single items are rated on a Likert scale from 0 (not at all) to 3 (yes, definitely), and, again, the single scores are not added to obtain a total value.

Activities to Fulfil One's Own Hopes To hope has been characterized as a disposition to act. Thus, one further question evaluates the activities people perform in order to fulfil their own hopes. This pool of items includes 13 activities belonging to four dimensions: (1) The cognitive-rational dimension (e.g. "I think a lot and analyze circumstances"), (2) the social-relational dimension (e.g. "I motivate my friends"), (3) the spiritual-religious dimension (e.g. "I pray, meditate"), and (4) the motivational/agency dimension (e.g. "I take responsibility and engage myself"). The Likert scale for rating the single items goes from 0 (not at all) to 3 (very often).

Experiences that Promote Hope In 2011 the participants received a list of 25 items to score different experiences supposed to help improving their feeling of hope. The 25 experiences fit into 6 categories: (1) Religious (e.g. "I have felt God's closeness"), (2) social-relational (e.g. "good relations to friends", (3) coping "e.g. I came through an illness successfully", (4) hedonic-experiential (e.g. "I experienced great concerts and parties"), (5) personal mastery (e.g. "I am proud of my professional success and performance", and (6) material-financial (e.g. "I earned a lot of money"). The items were defined as dummy variables with the possibility either to agree or disagree with them.

Places of Hope Also in 2011 we presented to the participants a list of 17 contexts, asking which of them were related to a feeling of hope. The 15 items represent the following categories: (1) In nature (e.g. "at the top of a mountain"), (2) leisure (e.g. "on a sports field"), (3) intellectual (e.g. "in the library"), and (4) religious (e.g. "in a church or temple"). These items were also used as dummy variables to agree or disagree with.

Other Measures

In addition to the newly developed scales and sets of items, the Hope-Barometer yearly includes different standardized scales, in order to be able to perform a series of comparative analyses. Here is a brief description of selected measures that have been used for the studies presented in this paper.

Satisfaction with Life The Satisfaction with Life Scale (SLS) was designed to assess global life satisfaction, defined as the comparison of life circumstances to one's expectations. The SLS consists of 5 items scored on a 7-point scale from 1 (strongly disagree) to 7 (strongly agree). Diener, Emmons, Larsen, and Griffin (1985) reported a coefficient alpha of .87.

Happiness The Subjective Happiness Scale (SHS) assesses happiness from the respondent's own perspective. The 4 items represent a subjective and global judgment about the extent to which people feel happy or unhappy (Lyubomirsky & Lepper, 1999). The possible scores go from 1 to 7. The reported Cronbach alphas ranged from .79 to .94.

Optimism Optimism has been measured by using the revisited version of the Life Orientation Test (LOT-R) developed by Scheier, Carver, and Bridges (1994). With 6 items, the LOT-R assesses the generalized expectations for positive (3 items) and for negative (3 items) outcomes, using a 5-point response scale ranging from 1 (strongly disagree) to 6 (strongly agree). A total optimism score is achieved by reversing the negative items and calculating a total value for all items. Cronbach's alpha for the entire six items was .78.

Harmony in Life Kjell, Daukantaité, Hefferon, and Sikström (2016) have recently developed the Harmony in Life Scale to measure psychological experiences of inner balance, peace of mind, calm and unity. The five items ($\alpha = .89$) are scored on a 7-point scale from 1 (strongly disagree) to 7 (strongly agree). From a psychological perspective, the authors highlight the concept of harmony in life as being related to a holistic world-view that incorporates a more balanced and flexible approach to personal well-being.

Meaning in Life Meaning in Life was measured with two different scales in 2013 and 2015. In 2013 we used the meaningfulness sub-scale of the Sources of Meaning and Meaning in Life Questionnaire of Schnell (2009) with five items scored on a 6-point scale from 0 (strongly disagree) to 5 (strongly agree) ($\alpha = .74$) which measures the degree of subjectively experienced sense of meaning, based on an appraisal of one's life as coherent, significant, directed and with a sense of belonging. In 2015 the five items measuring the presence of meaning in life from the Meaning in Life Questionnaire (Steger, Frazier, Oishi, & Kaler, 2006) were used. The authors reported a good internal consistency of the subscale with Cronbach alphas between .82 and .86. The items were scored on a 7-point Likert scale from 1 (strongly disagree) to 7 (strongly agree).

Resilience We used the 6 items' Brief Resilience Scale (BRS) scored on a 5-point Likert scale from 1 to 5 (Smith et al., 2008). In past studies, the BRS showed good internal consistency with Cronbach alpha values ranging from .80 to .91. The BRS has been positively correlated with optimism, active coping, social support and purpose in life, and negatively correlated with pessimism, anxiety, depression and negative interactions.

Self-Efficacy To measure self-efficacy, we utilized the German version of the General Self-Efficacy Scale (GSES) with 10 items developed by Schwarzer and Jerusalem (1999), using a 4-point Likert scale from 0 to 3. In past research projects, the GSES yielded internal consistency alpha-values between .75 and .91. Self-efficacy has shown moderate correlations to other constructs, such as optimism and proactive coping, as well as to Agency.

Positive Feelings To measure positive feelings the six items designed by Diener et al. (2010) to assess pleasant emotional experiences and feelings were applied ($\alpha = .87$ was reported). The participants were asked to think about what they have been doing and experiencing during the past 4 weeks and to score feelings such as "good", "pleasant" and "joyful" on a 5-point scale from 1 (very rarely or never) to 5 (very often or always).

Attachment The Attachment subscale of Scioli's Comprehensive Trait Hope Scale (Scioli, Ricci, Nyugen, & Scioli, 2011) measures the degree of interpersonal bonds, openness and basic trust towards other people. Individuals with high attachment scores are more likely to trust people and to disclose private thoughts and feelings. They also believe their friends and loved ones would, if need be, drop whatever they were doing to help them. In the validation paper the internal consistency was good ($\alpha = 84$). The possible scores go from 0 (not me) to 3 (exactly like me).

Positive Relations The Positive Relations sub-scale from Ryff and Keyes' (1995) Psychological Well-being Scale has shown very good internal consistency ($\alpha = 91$) with 9 items to be rated on a 6-point scale from 1 (strongly disagree) to 6 (strongly agree). Positive relations are characterized by warm, satisfying and trusting relationships with others and are based on strong empathy, affection and intimacy.

Spiritual Beliefs We employed the 4 items of the Importance of Spiritual Beliefs in Life, a subscale of the Spirituality Questionnaire (Parsian & Dunning, 2009) which is rated on a 4-point scale (1–4). The scale revealed a very good internal consistency of $\alpha = .91$.

Religious Faith The Santa Clara Strength of Religious Faith Questionnaire (SCSRFQ) evidenced significant positive correlations to adaptive coping and to dispositional hope (Plante & Boccaccini, 1997). The short-form of the SCSRFQ (Storch, Roberti, Bravata, & Storch, 2004) reduced to 5 items and scored on a 4-point scale (1–4) has reached excellent internal consistency ($\alpha = .95$).

Gratitude Gratitude was measured with a 6-item questionnaire developed by McCullogh, Emmons and Tsang (2002), to be rated on a 7-point scale (1–7). The authors reported a good reliability alpha-coefficient of .82 and positive correlations with Agency (r = .67) and Pathways (r = .42).

Helping Others Helping others is a pro-social attitude and behavior that positively correlates with empathy, social responsibility and altruism, and negatively correlates with selfishness. We measured this attitude with a short-form of the Helping Attitude Scale (Nickel, 1998), employing 7 items with a 5-point scale from 1 to 5. Cronbach alpha reliability was reported to be .86.

Compassion The Brief Santa Clara Compassion Scale with five items was developed by Hwang, Plante, and Lackey (2008) as a short version of the Compassionate Love Scale from Sprecher and Fehr (2005). Compassion has been defined as an attitude toward others, containing feelings, cognition, and behavior that are focused on caring, concern, tenderness, and a pro-social orientation toward supporting, helping, and understanding others. The five items, scored on a Likert scale from 1 (not at all true for me) to 7 (very true for me), revealed a very good internal consistency ($\alpha = .90$).

Depression and Anxiety The ultra-brief Patient Health Questionnaire for Depression and Anxiety (PHQ–4) is a composite four-item scale for measuring both phenomena (Kroenke, Spitzer, Williams, & Löwe, 2009). Since the questionnaire asks the participants to assess how often they are bothered by certain negative feelings, responses are scored from 0 (not at all), 1 (several days), 2 (more than half the days) to 3 (nearly every day). The alpha-coefficient reported in the validation study was .85.

Physical and Psychological Health A subjective rating of physical and psychological health was obtained by asking "How would you assess the level of your physical / psychological or emotional health?", with responses on a 6-point scale ranging from 1 (I am seriously ill) to 6 (I am perfectly healthy) (Ferring et al., 2004).

Data Analyses

Relating to the theoretical and methodological foundations (see Chap. 1), selected results of 6 years of Hope-Barometer in German speaking Europe are presented in seven steps. A summary of the objectives and data analysis techniques is displayed in Table 2.2.

In a first step, we explored how general hope – perceived and dispositional – is related to demographic variables and to other hope related constructs of well-being, such as self-efficacy, resilience, spirituality, altruism and health. The second step focuses on the level of satisfaction and future expectations in different life and social domains – private life, the economy, politics, the environment and social issues – and evaluates these fields in relation to the generally perceived level of hope. In keeping with our definition of hope presented in Chap. 1, which differentiates between gen-

Table 2.2 Outline of our analyses

Steps	Objectives	Data analysis
1. Nature and levels of hope	Evaluate the level of hope in different demographic groups Explore the concepts of perceived and dispositional hope	Answer tree methodology Group comparisons Bivariate correlation and correlation comparisons
2. Satisfaction and future expectations	Evaluate the satisfaction and future expectations in central life and social domains Assess the relations of these five fields with the general perceived hope	Answer distributions Multiple regression analysis
3. Personal hopes and satisfaction	Assess the importance of personal hopes and satisfaction in different individual life domains Relate the importance of personal hopes with satisfaction Evaluate personal hopes and satisfaction in relation to perceived hope	Comparison of mean values Bivariate correlations Multiple regression analysis
4. Sources of hope	Evaluate the sources of hope such as hope experiences, places of hope, hope providers and hope related activities Explore the relation of specific sources of hope with general perceived hope	Comparison of mean values Multiple regression analysis
5. Positive relations, feelings and hope	Evaluate the relation between attachment, positive feelings and perceived hope Evaluate the relation between positive feelings, harmony in life and perceived hope	Partial mediation modelling
6. Hope and health	Evaluate the predictors of psychological health Evaluate the relation between resilience, hope and psychological health Evaluate the relation between hope and posttraumatic growth Explore the relation between physical health, perceived hope and depression/anxiety	Partial mediation modelling Univariate analysis of variance (ANOVA)
7. Hope, happiness and meaning in life	Assess the relation of satisfaction in different life domains and of hope related activities with happiness and meaning in life Evaluate the relation between meaning in life, positive relations, hope and happiness Explore the relation between physical health, perceived hope and happiness	Multiple regression analysis Partial mediation modelling Univariate analysis of variance (ANOVA)

eral hope and particular hopes, the third step contains results about the importance of specific personal hopes and the levels of satisfaction in a series of individual life domains and relates these results to the general level of perceived hope. The next step reports the roots and sources of hope as perceived by the population including personal experiences that foster hope, places of hope, hope providers and activities to fulfil one's own hopes and explores their relation to perceived hope. The further steps deal with different aspects of a good life and present several models to explore the role of hope. We start with the interaction of hope and positive relations, positive feelings and harmony in life. The next analysis examines the role of hope in the context of psychological and physical health as well as posttraumatic growth. The last analysis is dedicated to the factors that might be related to the highest goods of happiness and meaning in life and the relationship to hope.

Results

Structure and Levels of Perceived and Dispositional Hope

Against the background of the many definitions of hope as presented in Chap. 1 and taking into account the serious concerns regarding the concept of dispositional hope, the purpose of this study is to explore the nature and level of hope, focusing on the two concepts of perceived and dispositional hope. This study encompasses two objectives: (1) Investigate the levels of hope in relation to different demographic groups and (2) explore the nature of hope based on the correlations with other constructs of well-being, personal mastery and coping, spirituality, altruism and health.

Perceived and Dispositional Hope Among Demographic Groups

The Hope-Barometer includes a series of demographic variables to be specified by the participants of the survey: Gender, age, education, family status, main activity (e.g. household, part or full time job, etc.) and professional status (e.g. staff member, middle management, upper management, etc.). To analyze the relation of these demographic variables and the level of perceived and dispositional hope, the answer tree classification technique was used. Answer trees are based on an exploratory technique to study the relationship between a dependent variable and a set of categorical predictor variables which themselves may interact. The mostly used approach is the Chi-square Automatic Interaction Detector (CHAID) (Hartigan, 1975; Kass, 1980). Following a step-by-step hierarchical regression analysis, the most important factors are identified (reduction of variables at $p < .001$). The resulting diagram should be understood as a classification tree with progressive splits into smaller and smaller groups that shows how major "types" formed from the independent (predictor or splitter) variables differentially predict the dependent variable. It is worth mentioning for those unfamiliar with the answer tree methodology that the basic technique is analogous to a "forward" step by step regression analysis, with similar high statistical standards.

For the first analysis, using the sample of 2015 (N = 7282), perceived hope was entered as the dependent variable and all the previously mentioned demographic variables as predictors. The most interesting result to be reported here is that the family status was the main predictor of perceived hope. The tree split the sample into three groups ($p < .001$): Married people achieved the highest mean value regarding perceived hope ($M = 3.59$, $SD = 0.82$), followed by a second group of people with a partner, divorced, separated or widowed people ($M = 3.46$, $SD = 0.85$) and finally by singles and people still living with their parents ($M = 3.16$; $SD = 0.96$). When entering dispositional hope as the dependent variable, the main predictor was not the family status anymore, but the professional status. Again three groups were discerned by the tree ($p < .001$): The results of the respondents in upper management positions, board members, entrepreneurs and business owners had the highest mean values of dispositional hope ($M = 4.02$, $SD = 0.63$). The second group is composed of people in junior and middle management functions and freelancers ($M = 3.80$, $SD = 0.69$). Finally, the third group with the lowest dispositional hope values ($M = 3.46$, $SD = 0.78$) includes employees, people doing housekeeping, unemployed and those still in education or training. The conclusion of these two analyses reveals a first difference between the nature of perceived and dispositional hope. While perceived hope is much more related to a social (and emotional) dimension of life (family status), dispositional hope is primarily related to a cognitive dimension (professional status).

Looking at the other demographic variables, the following interesting findings can be reported: Women are slightly but significantly higher in perceived hope than men ($M = 3.50$, $SD = 0.88$ for women and $M = 3.40$, $SD = 0.99$ for men, $p < .001$), an effect, which still remains after controlling for the professional status. The opposite is the case for dispositional hope ($M = 3.72$, $SD = 0.76$ for men and $M = 3.67$, $SD = .73$ for women, $p < .05$), but in this case the reason is the professional status of the person (in higher positions there are more men than women). The level of both perceived and dispositional hope rises with the degree of education. Regarding age, the level of perceived hope continually increases until the eighties and older, but the level of dispositional hope rises until the age of 60 to 69 and decreases then during the seventies and later (Fig. 2.1).

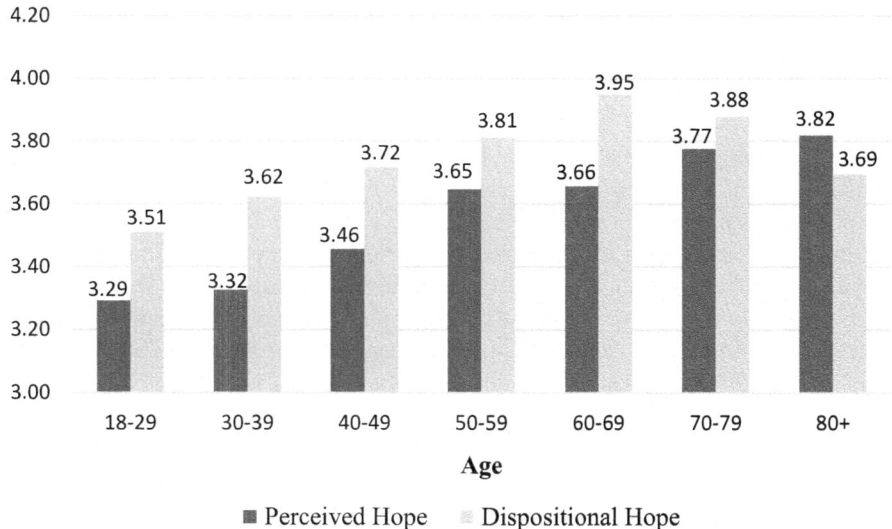

Fig. 2.1 Mean values of perceived hope and dispositional hope by age (year 2016)

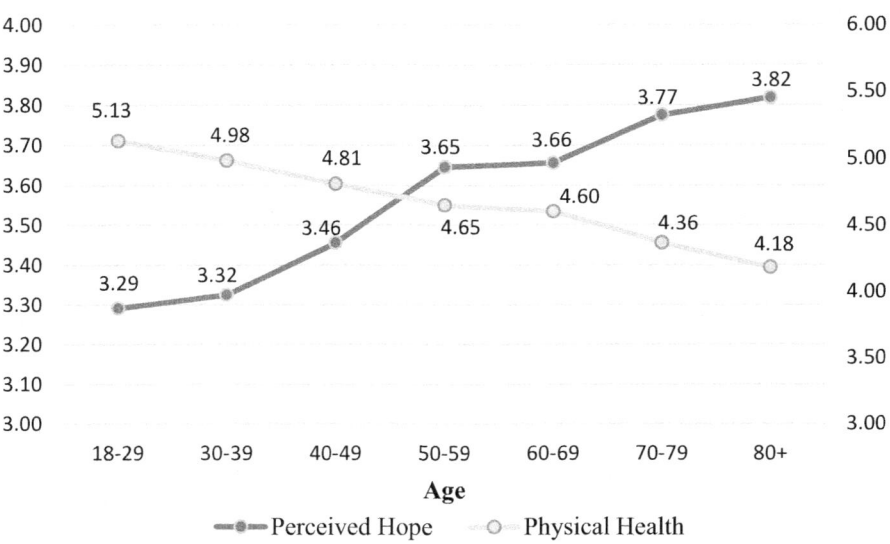

Fig. 2.2 Mean values of perceived hope and subjective physical health by age (year 2016)

Figure 2.2 exhibits the mean values of perceived hope as well as of the self-reported level of subjective physical health for different age groups. Interestingly, while the health level tends to decrease with the years, the level of hope continually goes up. These results are in line with the findings reported by Baltes, Staudinger, and Lindenberger (1999) and by Carstensen et al. (2011), who demonstrated that with the years the emotional well-being of people rises, despite the decline of body functions and the increase of health problems.

The Relation of Perceived and Dispositional Hope to Other Variables

The objectives of the next analysis are to investigate the relation of hope with other related psychological constructs described in Chap. 1 and to compare correlation values in order to assess the main commonalities and differences between perceived and dispositional hope. To examine the significance of the difference between correlation coefficients, we used Fischer's correlation comparison procedure. As explained in Chap. 1, many authors have started to question if the Dispositional Hope Scale, based on Snyder's cognitive conceptualization of hope, really measures what it intends to measure, and that hope as perceived by the general public is something different to just the estimation of one's own will- and way-power.

Table 2.3 shows the reliability Cronbach alpha coefficients, the mean values and the standard deviations of the constructs. Looking at the correlation values, the following findings become evident: All correlation values are highly significant. Strong correlation values could be partly an effect of the large size of the sample. The highest correlation coefficient is that between dispositional hope and self-effi-

Table 2.3 Central constructs: Cronbach alphas, Mean values, Standard deviations, Pearson correlations, and Correlation comparisons

	α-value	M	SD	PHS, r	DHS, r	z	p
Self-efficacy	.89	2.04	0.49	.49	.74	−17.94	.000
Resilience	.85	3.45	0.80	.41	.49	−4.59	.000
Optimism (LOT-R)	.79	4.17	0.88	.69	.62	7.42	.000
Satisfaction with life	.89	5.01	1.25	.60	.59	.93	.352
Happiness	.82	4.95	1.29	.63	.58	4.76	.000
Meaning in life	.90	5.07	1.38	.56	.57	−.89	.374
Harmony in life	.90	4.92	1.22	.63	.62	.76	.447
Positive relations	.82	4.53	0.87	.46	.45	.58	.562
Attachment	.79	2.20	0.57	.47	.47	0	1.00
Positive feelings	.92	3.72	0.78	.61	.49	8.00	.000
Spiritual beliefs	.97	1.91	0.98	.24	.13	6.44	.000
Religious faith	.92	1.76	0.85	.21	.07	8.08	.000
Gratitude	.76	5.51	1.02	.51	.42	5.26	.000
Helping others	.89	4.05	0.70	.22	.15	4.09	.000
Compassion	.89	4.67	1.39	.20	.08	5.67	.000
Depression/anxiety	.85	0.58	0.64	−.51	−.47	2.97	.003
Physical health	–	4.83	1.02	.21	.19	1.32	.187
Psychological health	–	4.89	1.08	.47	.43	3.17	.001
Perceived hope	.91	3.46	0.93	–	.64	–	–
Dispositional hope	.88	3.69	0.74	–	–	–	–

Note. *PHS* Perceived Hope Scale, *DHS* Dispositional Hope Scale, *LOT-R* Life Orientation Test Revised. All correlations significant at p < .001

cacy, which is significantly higher than the correlation value between self-efficacy and perceived hope. The DHS exhibits also a significantly higher correlation value with resilience than the PHS. The PHS correlated the most with optimism, happiness, harmony in life and positive feelings. With optimism, happiness and positive feelings, the PHS displayed a significantly higher correlation value compared to the DHS. Although on a lower level, the PHS also revealed significantly higher correlation values with gratitude, spiritual beliefs, helping others, religious faith, compassion, depression/anxiety (with negative sign), and psychological health. Similar moderate correlation coefficients with the PHS and the DHS resulted from the analysis with satisfaction with life, meaning in life, harmony in life, positive relations, attachment and physical health.

Firstly, these results underline the self-centered and cognitive nature of the dispositional hope concept, based on its similarity to self-efficacy. Compared with the DHS, the significantly lower correlation value of perceived hope with resilience, gives support to the argument that hope becomes especially relevant in situations where people feel less able to cope by means of their own resources alone. On the other hand, perceived hope is more clearly associated than dispositional hope to constructs related to a sense of transcendence and altruism, such as spiritual beliefs, religious faith, helping others and compassion. However, for the German speaking population, hope is still more closely related to the cognitive dimension in comparison to spiritual, religious, and altruistic factors. Nevertheless, perceived hope reveals a stronger connection to positive feelings and subjective happiness compared with the DHS, emphasizing the emotional nature of hope. The relational dimension, however, has a similar moderate relationship to both, perceived and dispositional hope, suggesting that good social relations are relevant for the cognitive-rational as well as for the emotional component of hope.

Satisfaction and Future Expectations

In this study, a broad evaluation of the satisfaction and the future expectations of the public in five general fields takes place. The objective is to assess the importance of the levels of satisfaction and future expectations in these fields with regard to their relation to the overall level of hope of the population.

Satisfaction with Central Life and Social Domains

The first question of the Hope-Barometer is to what extent people are satisfied with respect to their private life, the national economy, national politics, the climate and environment and the major social issues in their country. The distribution of answers illustrated in Fig. 2.3 indicates that 54.4% of the respondents are satisfied with their private life, but only 28% are satisfied with the national economy and less than 15% are satisfied with the national politics and the situation concerning social issues.

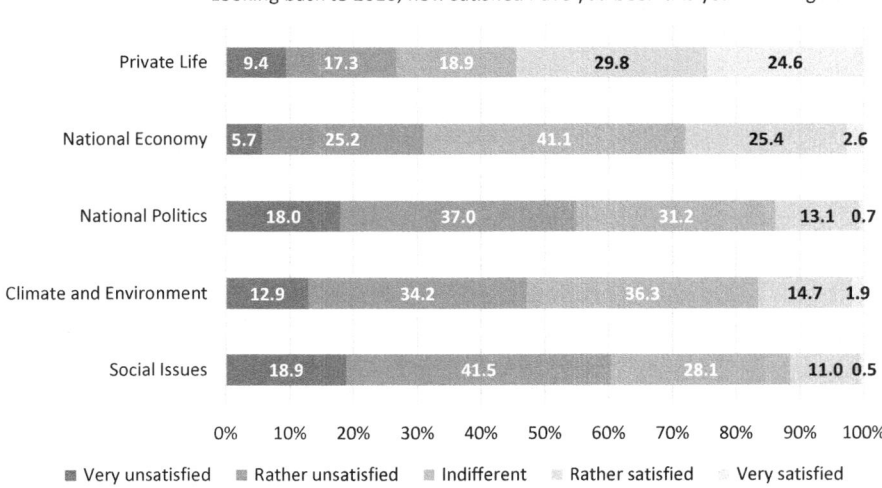

Fig. 2.3 Satisfaction during 2016 – distribution of values in percentage

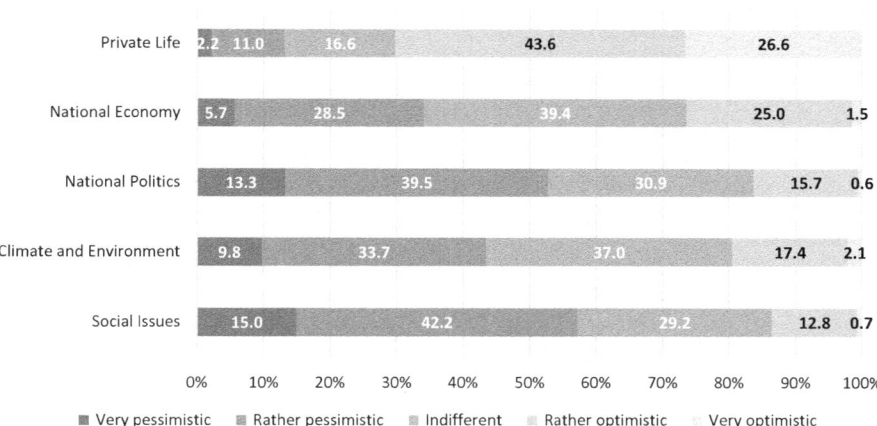

Fig. 2.4 Expectations for 2017 in five areas – distribution of values in percentage

This means that for many people satisfaction with their private life seems to have a different character from the satisfaction in the other areas. Over recent years, these results have been almost identical.

Future Expectations in Central Life and Social Domains

A similar picture emerges when people are asked about their pessimistic or optimistic expectations for the next year (Fig. 2.4). More than 70% of the respondents are rather or very optimistic regarding their private life and only 13.2% are pessimistic, even though only 26.5% are optimistic in relation to the economy and less than 20% with the political, environmental and social developments. The results over the last years have always been very similar. This could have two basic explanations: On the one hand, it could be an effect of the so-called optimistic bias described by Weinstein (1980, 1989). According to this author, most people tend to believe that their own future will be brighter than the future of other people and that more good instead of bad things will happen to them in comparison to the average population. On the other hand, these results suggest that the expectations concerning a person's own private life depend on aspects other than the vicissitudes of the economy and the society at large.

Future Expectations as Predictors of Hope

Based on these results, we wanted to know to what extent expectations about the future in different fields are related to the general level of hope of the people. In a multiple hierarchical regression analysis, the expectations in the five fields

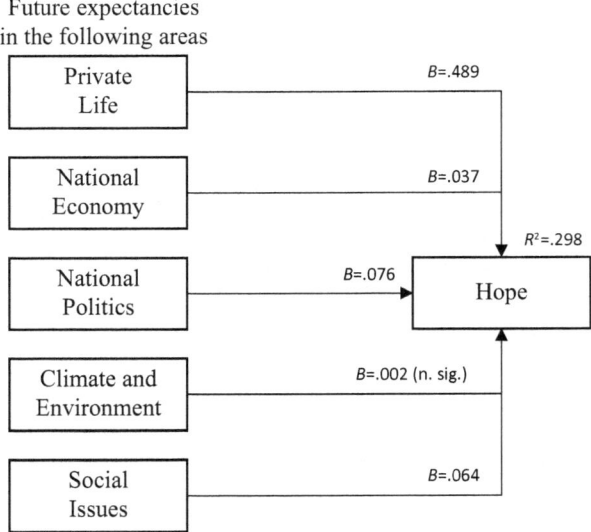

Future expectancies
in the following areas

Fig. 2.5 Future expectations as predictors of Perceived Hope (all standardized coefficients sig. at p < .01) (year 2016)

presented above were defined as independent and perceived hope as dependent variable, entering gender, age and education as control variables. The resulting model was significant at $F(7, 4278) = 315.81$; $p < .001$. Two striking results arise from the analysis (Fig. 2.5): (1) The major predictor of perceived hope is the level of expectation about one's private life. The economic, political, environmental and social issues are of much lower relevance. (2) The future expectations about one's private life explain only 24% of the variance of perceived hope (and the bivariate correlation between both was moderate $r = .53$; $p < .001$). This means that the rest of the variance might be explained by other factors rather than future expectations, supporting the hypothesis that people often distinguish between hopes and expectations (Cristea et al., 2011; David, Montgomery, & DiLorenzo, 2004; David, Montgomery, Stan et al., 2006; Montgomery et al., 2003).

Personal Hopes and Satisfaction in Different Life Domains

The next question in the Hope-Barometer is directed to finding out the principle hope targets of the population. Averill and his colleagues (Averill, Catlin, & Chon, 1990; Averill & Sundararajan, 2005) have distinguished different kinds of events and objects for which a person may hope, e.g. materialistic hope outcomes (material goods, money, etc.), personal achievements (performance, success, career, etc.), hedonistic pursuits (fun, sexuality, spare time, etc.), interpersonal relationships (romantic relations, friends, etc.), altruistic motives (to help other people), etc.

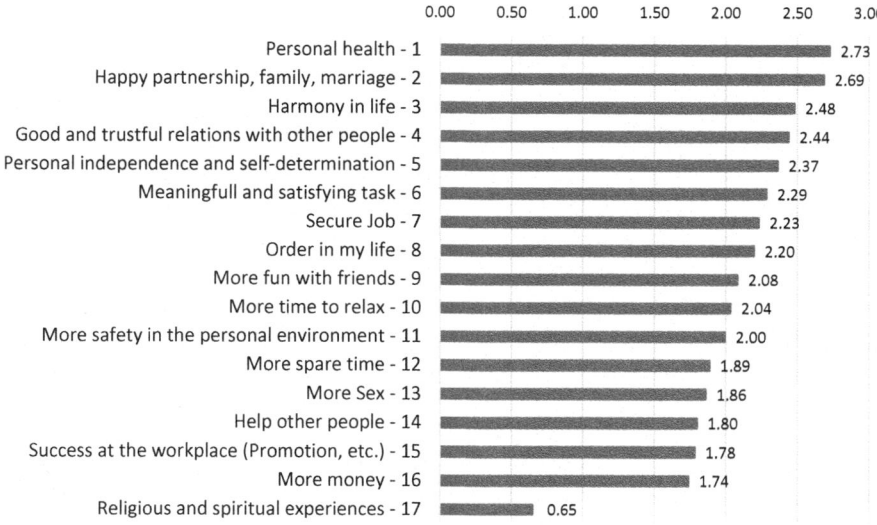

Fig. 2.6 Personal hopes in terms of their importance – mean values (year 2014)

The objectives of study three are to assess the importance of personal hopes and the level of satisfaction in different life domains, to correlate the importance of personal hopes and the level of satisfaction with each other and to evaluate the personal hopes and satisfaction in relation to perceived hope.

Personal Hopes in Different Life Domains

The Hope-Barometer includes every year 17 items representing possible personal hope targets. In accordance with our working definition of hope presented in Chap. 1 and in contrast to the similar Hope Index of Staats (1989), only the importance (but not the probability) of fulfilment of the several hope domains have to be scored. Figure 2.6 presents the mean values of the 17 items in a decreasing rank order. The top six personal hopes refer to central domains of people's well-being (personal health, family bonds, harmony in life, good social relations, personal independence and a meaningful task) that have been denominated as eudaimonic in the happiness literature (Delle Fave, Brdar, Freire, Vella-Brodrick, & Wissing, 2011). These domains stay in contrast to the much lower scored hedonic aspects such as more time to relax, more spare time, more sex and more money, emphasizing the greater importance for most people of eudaimonic life domains in comparison to hedonic experiences.

Satisfaction in Different Life Domains and Its Relation to Hope

In 2014, participants were additionally asked to rate their satisfaction in these 17 life domains. We then correlated the mean ratings with their specific hope values. The purpose was to explore to what extent the personal value of individual hopes is related to a sense of deficit and a lack of satisfaction or vice-versa if higher satisfaction corresponds with higher levels of hope. Results from bivariate correlation analyses reveal for all 17 domains significant relations between hope values and satisfaction ($p < .01$). Two findings shall be noted: Firstly, the correlation coefficients of the eudaimonic domains such as a happy partnership, family, marriage ($r = .28$), good and trusting relations to other people ($r = .20$) and meaningful and satisfying tasks ($r = .18$) are positive, whereas those of the materialistic and hedonic items, for instance more money ($r = -.36$), more time to relax ($r = -.18$) and more sex ($r = -.05$), are negative. This means, that the higher the satisfaction with eudaimonic life domains, the higher are also the levels of hope, whereas the lower the satisfaction with the hedonic life domains, the higher is the importance of the related hopes.

The second finding relates to the magnitude of the correlation coefficients. In some cases, e.g. personal health ($r = .02$) and success at the workplace ($r = .01$), the correlation coefficient is close to zero, suggesting that the degree of hope is almost independent from the level of satisfaction. Regardless of whether somebody feels healthy or ill, the hope for personal health is important for nearly everyone. In other cases, the correlation coefficient is significant and of moderate magnitude, for example for religious and spiritual experiences ($r = .37$), a happy partnership, family, marriage ($r = .28$) and helping other people ($r = .26$). This means that an increase in satisfaction is related to an increase in hope.

The two highest correlation values underscore the two extreme poles of different life domains, the religious (with positive sign; $r = .37$) and the materialistic 'more money' (with negative sign; $r = -.36$), which at the same time are the two domains with the lowest importance in terms of hope (see Fig. 2.6). In particular, a majority of participants has scored the item religious and spiritual experiences very low, regarding both, its importance and satisfaction. However, those people with higher levels of satisfaction with religious and spiritual experiences also evaluate these experiences as more important in terms of personal hope. The opposite happens in the case of more money. The higher the satisfaction with it, the lower the importance of the related hope and the lower the satisfaction, the higher its importance.

Life Domains as Predictors of Hope

The next analyses have the purpose of identifying which life domains predict the level of general perceived hope more strongly than others do. Two multiple linear regression analyses were performed defining perceived hope as dependent variable and the 17 items (once in terms of satisfaction and once in terms of importance) as predictors. Starting with the 17 items of satisfaction, 32.3% of the variance of perceived hope was explained ($p < .001$). The general model was significant at $F(11,$

7380) = 320.96 ($p < .001$). The main predictors at a significance level of $p < .001$ are (1) harmony in life ($\beta = .142$), (2) meaningful and satisfying task ($\beta = .138$), (3) good and trustful relations to other people ($\beta = .100$), (4) happy partnership, family, marriage ($\beta = .116$), (5) personal health ($\beta = .098$), and (6) religious and spiritual experiences ($\beta = .08$), all items belonging to the eudaimonic dimension of well-being.

When entering the 17 hope importance items, the adjusted R^2 was .19 ($p < .001$) [$F(14, 7668) = 93.57$; $p < .001$] and the best predictors at $p < .001$ turned out again to be related to the eudaimonic dimension, i.e. (1) helping other people ($\beta = .16$), (2) religious and spiritual experiences ($\beta = .15$), (3) a happy partnership, family and marriage ($\beta = .13$), (4) meaningful and satisfying tasks ($\beta = .13$), and (5) personal health ($\beta = .11$). Hedonic oriented hopes like more time to relax, more spare time, more sex, and more fun with friends were not significant. These analyses suggest that there are certain life domains, namely those belonging to the edaimonic dimension (social relations, spirituality, altruism, meaning), which both, in terms of satisfaction and importance, can nurture the general level of hope, and that other life domains, specifically those related to hedonic experiences, seem to have a much lower or no relation at all with the perception of hope.

These findings are congruent with the classification of goals and motivations in two categories as proposed by Ryan and Deci (2000) following the philosophical foundations of Aristotle: (1) First-order or intrinsic goals and values are those pursued for their own sake, linked to personal growth, a sense of community and health, which are oriented to satisfy the basic psychological needs of feeling autonomous, competent and related to others. Ryan and Deci connect this category to the eudaimonic concept of living well (Ryan, Huta, & Deci, 2013). (2) Second-order or extrinsic goals and values, such as wealth and hedonic entertainments, create good feelings but are not connected to what is intrinsically worthwhile to human beings. In the same manner, the results of the Hope-Barometer suggest that there are two kinds of hope targets: (1) First-order targets of hope have an intrinsic value to pursue a good (eudaimonic) life. These hopes are connected to family bonds, personal health, a sense of purpose and meaning, a prosocial attitude, as well as psychological and social well-being. (2) Second-order hope targets are of subordinate value and are related to domains resulting in momentary good feelings, but contribute only little to long-lasting flourishing and personal development.

Sources of Hope

The next set of questions from study four pertain to the roots and sources of hope, i.e. the personal experiences, places, people and activities that foster hope as subjectively reported by the respondents. Considering that the appraisal of certain people as hope providers and the expressed hope related activities are supposed to be connected to higher levels of general perceived hope, additional analyses were performed in order to identify the main hope providers and activities that predict hope.

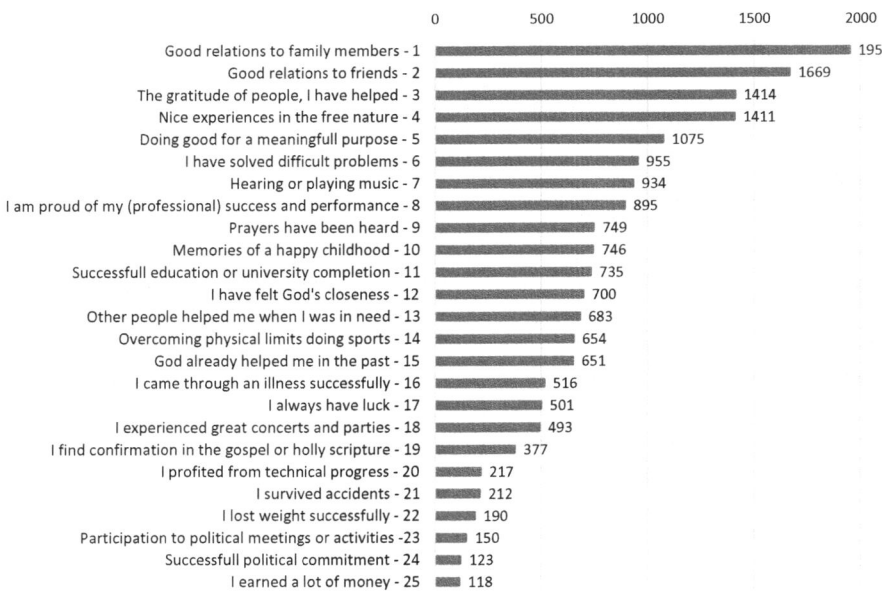

Fig. 2.7 Experiences that enhance hope – number of positive answers (year 2011)

Experiences that Foster Hope

In 2011, the Hope-Barometer included a set of 25 items representing experiences supposed to strengthen people's level of hope. Figure 2.7 shows the number of answers for each experience, listing the items in decreasing order. The five most agreed items concern social (family relations), experiential (experiences in nature) and altruistic issues (helping others), followed by several instances of mastery (solving problems) and next by religious and spiritual occurrences (prayers that have been heard). Least relevant are coping, materialistic and hedonic matters such as having earned a lot of money, profiting from technical progress, recovering from illness or having experienced great concerts and parties.

Places of Hope

In the same year, 2011, the participants of the Hope-Barometer were asked to select from a list of 17 places those in which they believe to feel more hopeful (Fig. 2.8). At top of the list are three items related to the connection with nature (besides at home). Peterson and Seligman (2004) included hope in their catalogue of character strengths common across cultures as belonging to the virtue of transcendence, which implies feeling oneself connected to a bigger whole. Hope is linked to other character strengths of transcendence such as appreciation of beauty and excellence as well as spirituality. Less relevant as places of hope seem to be one's own

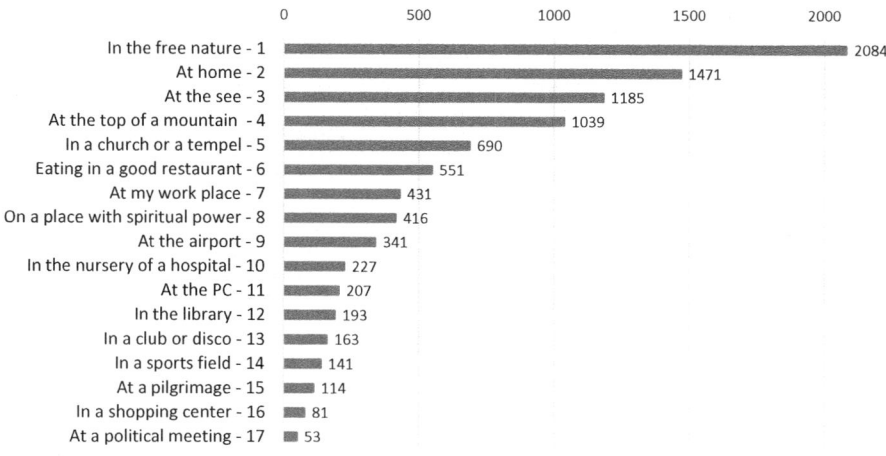

Fig. 2.8 Places of hope – number of positive answers (year 2011)

workplace, at the PC and the libraries, all places with a more cognitive character. Religious places like churches and spiritual places are of intermediate relevance. Of little value are clubs, discos and shopping centers, commonly known as places for consumption and recreation.

Hope Providers

According to Erikson (1963) hope is the first human virtue acquired during the early stages of childhood, which comes with the resolution of the fundamental conflict between basic trust and basic anxiety and mistrust. Hope is related to a feeling of familiarity and inner goodness in association with people (principally family members) the person feels connected to. Thus, hope is based on feelings of trust, confidence, faith, love and care within a robust social network. Nowadays, several authors have also highlighted the importance of the social dimension of hope. Other people can influence a person's hope through their encouragement, support or by simply being present (Farran, Herth, & Popovich, 1995). Scioli and Biller (2009) refer to the existence of hope providers, such as parents, friends but also a larger spiritual force, who offer availability, presence and contact to the person who is hoping and inspire trust, safety and openness.

To be able to investigate the social bonding dimension of hope, the Hope-Barometer includes a list of 16 potential hope providers, asking the participants to score to what extent they expect from them the transmission and spread of hope. The first six outstanding items of the ranking in Fig. 2.9 represent two clearly delineated categories. On the one hand, family members and closer friends are seen as very strong hope providers. On the other hand, many people believe that every person must rely on him- or herself and that hope is one's own responsibility in mastering one's own fate. An exploratory factor analysis supported the existence of these

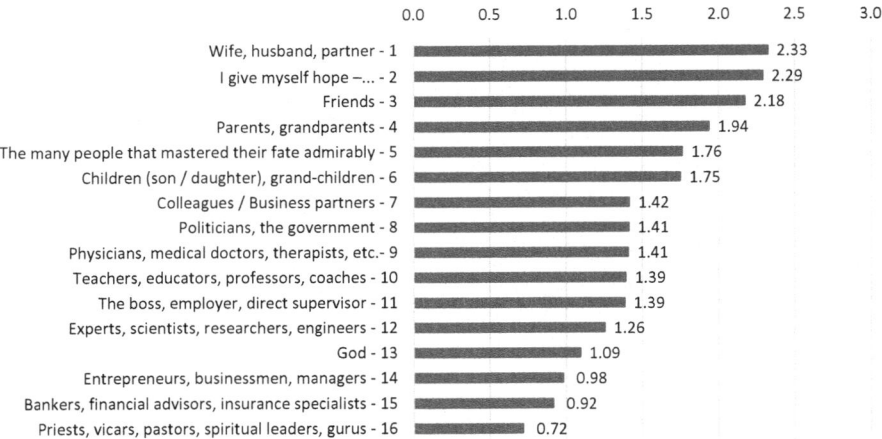

Fig. 2.9 Hope providers – mean values (year 2016)

two categories. A third group of hope providers with moderate scores consists of people in the direct social and professional environment (colleagues, physicians, teachers, and the boss). Even though politicians generally do not belong to the direct personal social environment, most people are regularly in touch with them via the mass media. The last group of hope providers from whom the average population barely expects the transmission and reinforcement of hope, is composed of people in the wider social environment such as experts, scientists, entrepreneurs, bankers, etc. For many people, also God and especially religious leaders seem to be very far from their daily lives.

These results of the Hope-Barometer confirm the idea of Feudtner (2005) about the existence of a social and cultural ecology of hope, consisting of a social network of relationships, hierarchically structured in different layers according to their relevance and closeness to the person with hope.

The level of trust and connection to other people should result in a higher level of general hope. In a multiple linear regression analysis, we tested which categories of people best predict the level of perceived hope. Using the 16 hope providers as predictors, 21% of the variance of perceived hope could be explained ($p < .001$). The general model was significant at $F(11, 4274) = 106.02; p < .001$. The four most predictive (p < .001) items are: (1) I give myself hope, it's the responsibility of the person him−/herself ($\beta = .28$); (2) God ($\beta = .18$); (3) Wife, husband, partner ($\beta = .11$); and (4) Teachers, educators, professors, coaches ($\beta = .10$). These four items represent different dimensions of hope, which could be demonstrated by an exploratory factor analysis: The self-centered, the transcendent, the inner family circle and the direct social environment. All other items were of little or no significance (including friends). These findings underline the fact that individuals place their trust in different people in order to enhance their level of hope. Furthermore, that relying on oneself is a strong booster of hope, but that faith in God, although scarcely valued by most participants, also has a significant connection to hope.

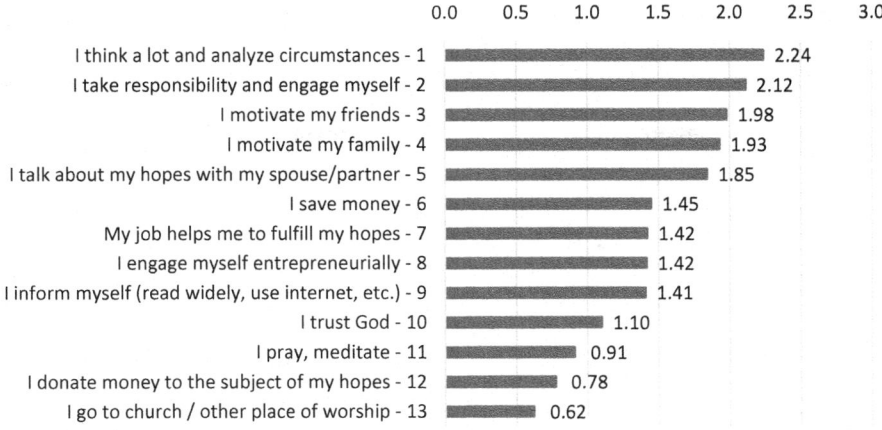

Fig. 2.10 Activities to fulfil one's own hopes – mean values (year 2016)

Activities to Fulfil One's Own Hopes

The structure and quality of hope of different people do not only differ with regard to the kind of the desired outcomes hoped-for, but also regarding the actions performed to achieve these outcomes. Averill and Sundararajan (2005) distinguish between two categories of hope: (1) A primary kind of hope focuses on mastery and the act of coping to overcome difficulties and obstacles. In this cognitive understanding of hope, the emphasis is put on personal control, on ambition, effort and pursuit, and consequently, on actions to achieve the outcome hoped-for, e.g. working harder, thinking more creatively, assessing the situation accurately, planning actions or taking risks. (2) Another type of hope is characterized by a sense of deep personal desire but with little personal control over the outcome. In this case, to hope is to rely on other people or a spiritual higher power, believing that things will turn out well, despite negative facts. Typical actions are to seek support from other people, to pray or to meditate, or just to trust. Faith comes particularly into play when people keep hoping in adverse conditions and in seemingly hopeless situations.

Figure 2.10 presents a list of 13 activities people perform to a greater or lesser extent in order to attain their personal hopes. Two self-centered items, a cognitive (to think and analyze) and a motivational one (personal engagement), are at the top of the list, followed by three items representing the relational dimension of hoping (friends, family and partner). On the other hand, religious and spiritual activities are situated at the end of the list.

It can be assumed, that the activities pursued to fulfil one's own hopes, might have an impact on the general level of hope. Whatever a person does to attain a certain goal, this activity will in general be accompanied by the expectation of a positive effect. By performing a multiple linear regression analysis, our purpose was to explore the connection between the hope related activities (entered as predictors) and the general level of perceived hope (entered as dependent variable). The 13 items helped to explain 28% of the variance of perceived hope. The general model was significant at $F(9, 4276) = 187.14$; $p < .001$. Five activities had the strongest predictive power regarding hope (at $p < .001$): (1) I take responsibility and engage myself ($\beta = .19$); (2) I talk about my hopes with my spouse/partner ($\beta = .14$); (3) I motivate my family ($\beta = .14$); (4) I trust God ($\beta = .12$); and (5) I motivate my friends ($\beta = .09$). These activities represent the motivational, relational and religious/spiritual dimensions of hope. Not significant at all are the cognitive activities (I inform myself, I think a lot and analyze circumstances, and I save money), as well as the religious activity of going to church. Of less predictive capacity but still significant, is the activity of praying or meditating ($\beta = .04$; $p = .05$).

This analysis allows to highlight the following three findings: (1) Activities which stand for the motivational and relational dimensions of hope are highly valued by people and also resulted to have a strong predictive power in relation to a higher level of hope. (2) Religious and spiritual activities have the least priority in the consciousness of people, however, to trust God (and to a lesser extent to pray or meditate), has a comparable predictive value regarding hope compared to the social activities. (3) The cognitive activities, although they are very attractive to many people, did not have any predictive effect on the level of hope. These findings tell us, that thinking a lot, analyzing circumstances and informing oneself about how to attain one's own personal hopes, is less effective than we generally consider it to be. On the other hand, to believe in and to trust God seems to be much more helpful than usually deemed.

Positive Relations, Feelings, Harmony in Life and Hope

In this and the next sections, a series of analyses will be presented, with the objective of deepening the understanding of the most salient topics resulting from the former analyses and findings. Following the results presented until now, good family and social relations are an important factor, both in terms of personal hopes as well as of sources of sustaining hope. Additionally, harmony in life belongs to the very dominant personal hopes and is furthermore the most relevant predictor of perceived hope. Against this background, we analyzed the relationship between attachment, positive feelings and hope as well as between positive feelings, harmony in life and hope by partial mediation modelling, arriving at the following results.

Attachment, Positive Feelings and Hope

The model in Fig. 2.11 demonstrates the role of good and positive feelings, such as joy and happiness, as partial mediator between attachment and perceived hope. This means, that to have family members and good friends, to whom one feels close, is a

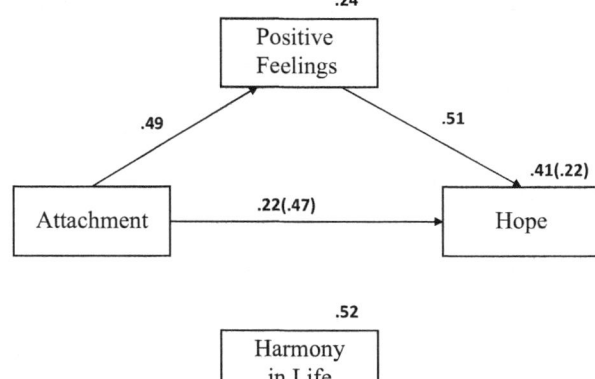

Fig. 2.11 Positive Feelings as partial mediator between Attachment and Perceived Hope (all standardized coefficients sig. at $p < .001$) (year 2016)

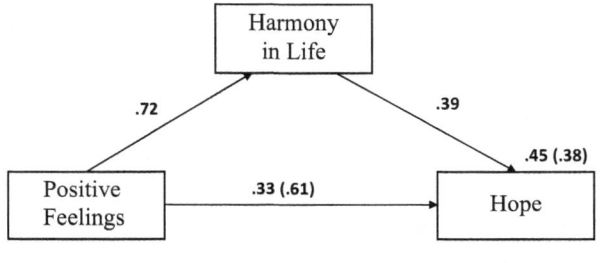

Fig. 2.12 Harmony in Life as partial mediator between Positive Feelings and Perceived Hope (all standardized coefficients sig. at $p < .001$) (year 2016)

good predictor of the level of hope, but largely, because these good and trustful relations are related to good and positive feelings, which in turn show a strong connection to hope.

Positive Feelings, Harmony in Life and Hope

Going one step further, the next question is how positive feelings relate to harmony in life. The Greek philosopher Aristotle, as well as differentiating between the eudaimonic and hedonic ways of life, also distinguished between two kinds of pleasures: The sensual pleasure and the pleasure arising from performing activities in accordance with human virtues. Eudaimonia is the result of a virtuous life, which the person perceives as joyful and pleasant. People can achieve eudaimonia, authentic happiness as Seligman (2004) put it, because behaving in agreement with non-egoistic and self-transcendent human values such as generosity, gentleness, friendliness and temperance, generates positive feelings. In psychology, while satisfaction with life only represents the cognitive side of well-being based on the fulfilment of self-centered expectations, harmony in life takes into account a more holistic view of well-being that also acknowledges the social and environmental life domains (Kjell et al., 2016).

Figure 2.12 exhibits the partial mediation model in which positive feelings predict hope, but largely via the partial effect of harmony in life. This reveals that not all types of positive feelings (e.g. sensual pleasures) are related to hope, but mainly those feelings, which relate to a sense of harmony in our lives, essentially to be found in harmonious social relations, in the performance of a meaningful and satisfying task (e.g. helping others) and/or in the perception of spiritual union with a larger whole.

Hope and Health

The immense value of hope in preserving and restoring health and well-being has been the focus of psychological and nursing research for decades (Eliott, 2005; Farran et al., 1995). Personal health turned out to be the mostly valued personal hope in our Hope-Barometer survey (Fig. 2.6) as well as one of the main predictors of perceived hope. In recent years, new studies have demonstrated the positive mechanisms of resilience and posttraumatic growth to reestablish and increase optimal functioning, besides the already known aspects of self-efficacy, meaning in life and positive relations. The focus of this analysis is to evaluate the role of hope with regard to subjective psychological health, especially in relation to the afore mentioned phenomena.

Predictors of Psychological Health

Instead of focusing only on positive feelings as an indicator of subjective well-being, several authors started to study the experience of flourishing, including in their conceptualization of psychological well-being dimensions such as self-competence, optimism, meaning and positive relations, amongst others (Huppert & So, 2013; Ryff & Keyes, 1995). In 2014, the Hope-Barometer besides asking the participants about their general level of perceived hope also collected people's self-evaluation regarding their degree of self-efficacy, meaning in life, positive relations and psychological health. In a multiple linear regression analysis defining psychological health as dependent variable, perceived hope was the main predictor of psychological health, followed by self-efficacy, meaning in life and positive relations (Fig. 2.13) $[F(4, 7993) = 977.64; p < .001]$. This means that psychological health is strongly related to a positive and confident view of one's own future.

Hope, Resilience and Psychological Health

The remarkable role of hope in maintaining or regaining psychological health can be assumed by relating it to resilience, the capacity to recover after setbacks and difficult times in life. Masten, Cutuli, Herbers, and Reed (2009) counted a positive view towards the future as an important factor of resilience. Being aware that measuring resilience in a cross-sectional study with a self-reported method without a concrete challenging life situation is of limited value, we nevertheless included a scale in the Hope-Barometer of 2014 to evaluate the resilience capacity as perceived by the participants. Figure 2.14 exposes the role of perceived hope as partial

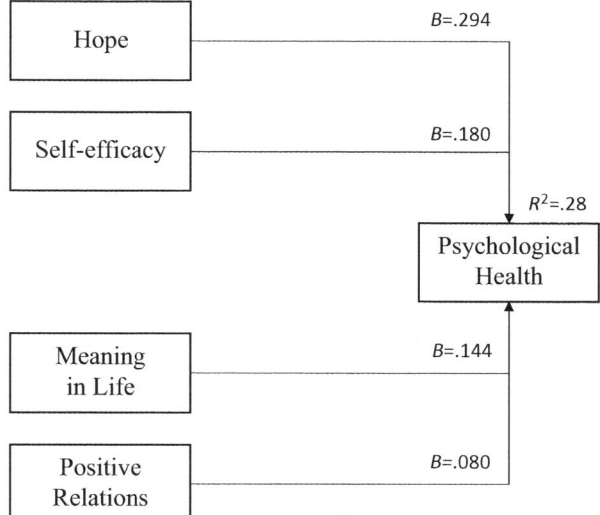

Fig. 2.13 Predictors of Psychological Health (all standardized coefficients sig. at *p* < .001) (year 2014)

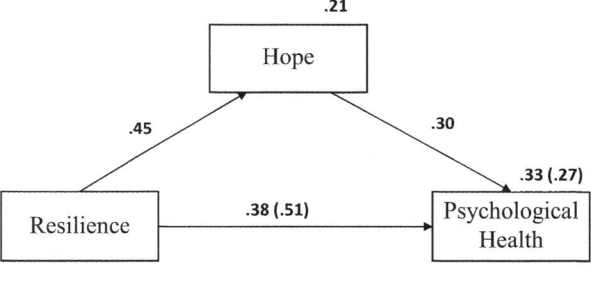

Fig. 2.14 Perceived Hope as partial mediator between Resilience and Psychological Health (all standardized coefficients sig. at *p* < .001) (year 2014)

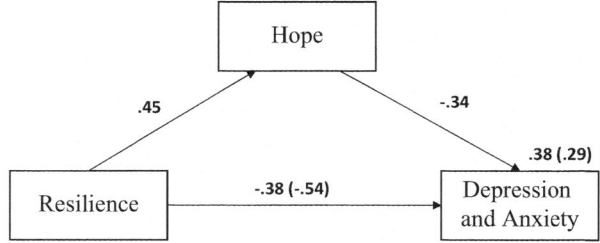

Fig. 2.15 Perceived Hope as partial mediator between Resilience and Depression/ Anxiety (all standardized coefficients sig. at *p* < .001) (year 2014)

mediator between resilience and psychological health. The model suggests that the positive effect of resilience on psychological health takes place partly because of its strong connection to hope. Individuals that rated themselves as resilient feel more hopeful and enjoy a better psychological health.

A similar effect can be observed between resilience, depression/anxiety and perceived hope (Fig. 2.15). The compelling (negative) effect of resilience on symptoms of depression and anxiety can partly be explained by the mediation role of perceived hope.

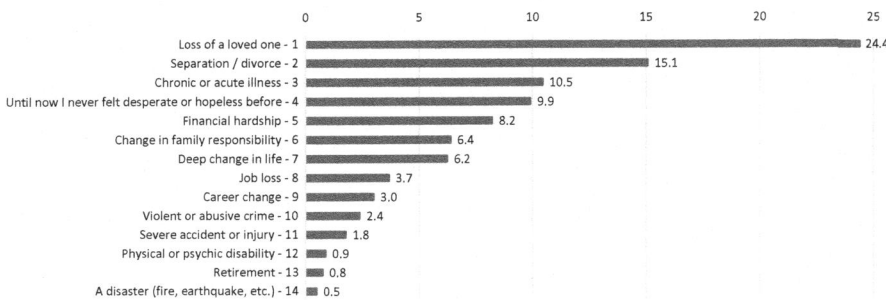

Fig. 2.16 Situations of Hopelessness in % of the total Sample (year 2013)

Situations of Hopelessness and Posttraumatic Growth

In 2013, one major focus of the Hope-Barometer was on the topic of posttraumatic growth. Several authors demonstrated that after critical life situations many people report not only a recovery to normal levels of functioning, but, furthermore, also positive changes for the better, such as closer relationships, a more positive view on life and enhanced self-esteem, reducing also the symptoms of depression and anxiety (Linley, Joseph, & Goodfellow, 2008; Tedeschi & Calhoun, 2004). Linley and Joseph (2011) revealed that finding meaning in a new life situation after a traumatic event is consistently associated with greater positive psychological changes. Using the short form of the Changes in Outlook questionnaire (Joseph, Linley, Shevlin, Goodfellow, & Butler, 2006), participants of the Hope-Barometer could choose one major experience among a list of 14 distressing events when they felt particularly hopeless. Based on that experience, the respondents could assess 10 items from which five reflect a positive posttraumatic growth (e.g. "I value my relationships much more now") and the other five express a negative impact (e.g. "I have very little trust in myself now"). Joseph et al. (2006) explained that posttraumatic growth and posttraumatic distress are not just the two poles of a continuum but, rather, represent separate dimensions of experience. Thus, the reduction of posttraumatic stress will not automatically lead to enhanced posttraumatic growth.

The distressing events causing a feeling of hopelessness more often reported, were the loss of a loved one, the experience of separation or divorce from one's partner and a chronic or acute illness (Fig. 2.16). These results, underline again the central role of intimate relationships and of personal health in relation with the phenomenon of hope.

Defining meaning in life as the predictor of both, positive and negative growth and entering later perceived hope as mediator variable, revealed following (Fig. 2.17): Meaning in life displayed a medium predictive effect on positive growth ($\beta = .30$; $R^2 = .09$; $p < .001$) and a higher effect on negative growth ($\beta = -.38$; $R^2 = .14$; $p < .001$). When entering perceived hope in the model, the partial mediation effect in relation to positive growth was significant ($p < .001$) but rather modest ($\Delta R^2 = .01$). On the other hand, the partial mediation result with respect to negative

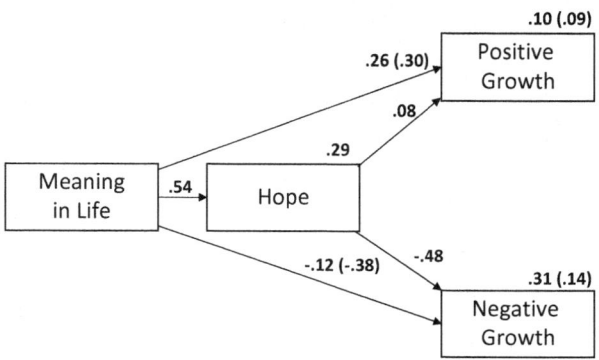

Fig. 2.17 Perceived Hope as partial mediator between Meaning in Life and Positive and Negative Posttraumatic Growth (all standardized coefficients sig. at $p < .001$) (year 2013)

growth was significant and considerably higher ($\Delta R^2 = .17$). These results suggest that meaning in life in association with perceived hope could be considered an important protective factor in alleviating the negative effects of distressing events. Regarding the development of positive outcomes, the role of perceived hope seems to be less apparent. For a more conclusive analysis, a longitudinal study to measure hope before and during the distressing experience would be of great value.

Hope, Physical Health and Depression/Anxiety

Since a chronic and acute illness was one of the major distressing experiences for more than 10% of the sample (Fig. 2.16), and taking into account that a physical illness can lead to symptoms of depression and anxiety, a further analysis was performed in 2014. Using univariate analysis of variance (ANOVA), the sample was divided into nine groups with regard to physical health and perceived hope (factors) and depression and anxiety as dependent variables. The sample was categorized into three health related groups, one group of healthy people (n = 5797), one with moderate health problems (n = 1882), and one containing people with a serious physical illness (n = 318). Also three groups of people with high (n = 1155), moderate (n = 5753) and low (n = 1089) levels of hope were created, calculating one standard deviation above and below the mean value of the whole sample.

The profile plot exhibited in Fig. 2.18 contains a group A with healthy and highly hopeful people that enjoys the lowest level of depression and anxiety ($M = 0.22$, $SD = 0.35$) and another group B of healthy people with low levels of hope and with moderate values of Depression and Anxiety ($M = 1.04$, $SD = 0.78$). The highest values of depression and anxiety ($M = 1.88$, $SD = 0.91$) are displayed by group C, seriously ill people with low levels of hope. Especially remarkable are the results of group D, people with a serious illness but with high levels of hope, who possess the second lowest value of depression and anxiety ($M = .40$, $SD = 0.53$). Although, there

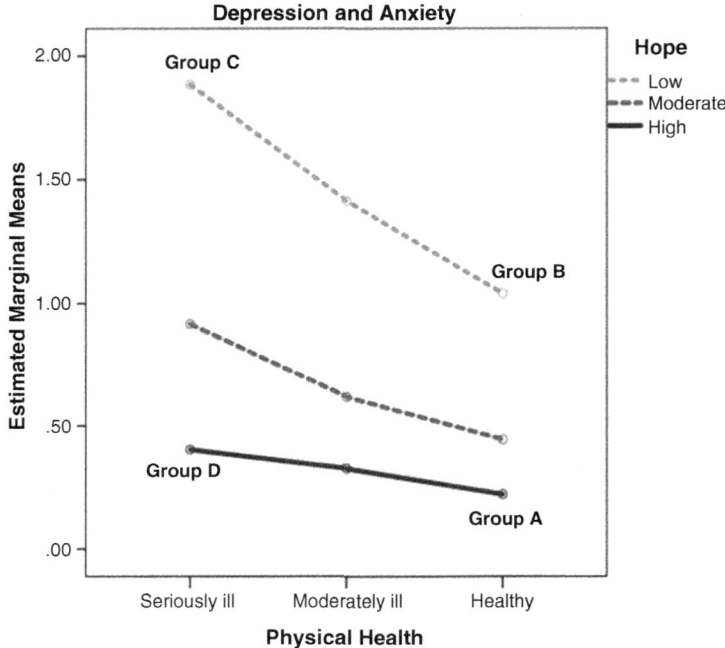

Fig. 2.18 ANOVA with the dependent variable Depression/Anxiety and the factors Physical Health and Perceived Hope (year 2014)

could be differences in how painful and how severe the prognosis of an illness could be, it is nevertheless noteworthy, that people who could retain a high sense of hope despite a serious physical illness display relatively low symptoms of depression and anxiety, nearly comparable to both groups of people with moderate and no health burdens.

Hope, Happiness and Meaning in Life

The last analysis is dedicated to explore the relation between hope and happiness. While satisfaction with life tends to represent the cognitive dimension of well-being, happiness has often been conceptualized as the affective side that is also nourished by hope (Lyubomirsky, Sheldon, & Schkade, 2005). The Subjective Happiness Scale describes a global judgment about the extent to which people feel happy (or unhappy) and enjoy life regardless of what is going on, getting the most out of everything (as one item formulates it).

Predictors of Happiness and Meaning in Life

Reverting to the life domains which people estimate as more or less important in terms of their personal hopes (see Fig. 2.6) and taking the level of satisfaction reported with these domains as predictors, two multiple linear regression analyses were performed defining subjective happiness and meaning in life as dependent variables. The 17 items explain 49% of the variance of happiness [$F(14, 7377) = 481.47$; $p < .001$] and 32% of meaning in life [$F(12, 7379) = 292.71$; $p < .001$]. The four main predictors of happiness with β-values $>.10$ ($p < .001$) are represented by the satisfaction with (1) harmony in life ($\beta = .21$), (2) partnership, family, marriage ($\beta = .16$), (3) meaningful and satisfying task ($\beta = .11$), and (4) personal health ($\beta = .11$). These four (eudaimonic) life domains are among the most valued personal hopes (see Fig. 2.6), belong to the most relevant predictors of perceived hope and additionally to the principle experiences connected to a happy life. Moreover, a meaningful and satisfying task ($\beta = .21$), partnership, family marriage ($\beta = .14$), harmony in life ($\beta = .11$) in addition to religious experiences ($\beta = .08$) are the main predictors of meaning in life ($p < .001$).

Further multiple regression analyses were run with the 13 predictor variables describing the activities people accomplish to fulfil their personal hopes (see Fig. 2.10) and happiness [adj. $R^2 = .16$; $F(11, 7270) = 128.08$; $p < .001$] as well as meaning in life [adj. $R^2 = .23$; $F(11, 7270) = 196.98$; $p < .001$] as dependent variables. The three striking activities predicting both, happiness and meaning in life are (1) talking with the spouse or partner ($\beta = .17$ and $\beta = .17$), (2) motivating the family ($\beta = .14$ and $\beta = .15$) and (3) taking responsibility and engaging oneself ($\beta = .13$ and $\beta = .15$) (all at $p < .001$). These results suggest that activities sustaining and promoting good relations to one's own partner and family members along with a personal sense of responsibility have the strongest connection to the highest goods of happiness and meaningfulness.

Meaning in Life, Positive Relations, Hope and Happiness

Based on these findings we tested a model where meaning in life (Steger et al., 2006) and positive relations (Ryff & Keyes, 1995) are partially mediated by perceived hope to predict happiness. As can be observed in Fig. 2.19, meaning in life and positive relations are moderately correlated and together explain 41% of the variance of happiness. Both variables also explain 37% of the variance of perceived hope, which functions as partial mediator, raising the variance explained of happiness to 51% (by reducing the effects of the other two variables). These findings suggest that people who report having a meaning and purpose in life and maintain positive relations to other people experience happiness in their life, not only because they experience pleasant thoughts and emotions in the present, but also because they hold a positive and confident view of the future.

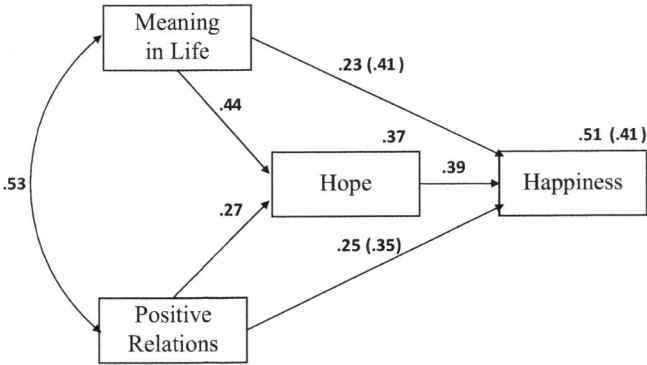

Fig. 2.19 Perceived Hope as partial mediator between Meaning in Life, Positive Relations and Subjective Happiness (all standardized coefficients sig. at $p < .001$) (year 2015)

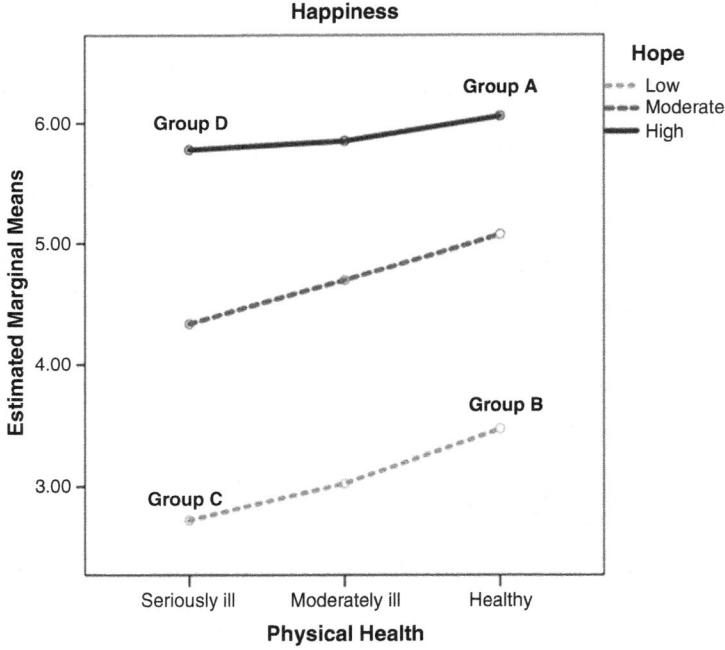

Fig. 2.20 ANOVA with the dependent variable Subjective Happiness and the factors Physical Health and Perceived Hope (year 2014)

Hope, Physical Health and Happiness

That hope cannot only serve to foster happiness in good times and to mitigate negative consequences such as depression and anxiety in bad times, can be confirmed by the results shown in Fig. 2.20. The profile plot exhibited is the result of a similar analysis of variance as presented in Fig. 2.18, but defining happiness as dependent variable instead of depression and anxiety. Again, the noticeable finding is the existence of a group of people (group D), who reported being seriously ill but at the same time highly hopeful, and declaring to be very happy ($M = 5.78$, $SD = 1.08$), close to the levels of happiness reported by completely healthy people (group A; $M = 6.06$, $SD = 0.81$). This means that in painful situations, hope cannot only lead people to feel less sad and depressed, but it also can foster happiness and permit people to flourish, despite the adversities and sufferings of life.

General Findings

The purpose of this chapter is to present the results of the Hope-Barometer between 2011 and 2016 among the German speaking population, in order to give an overview of the variety of topics and findings, which will be addressed more in detail in the following contributions to this book. The concrete objectives are threefold: (1) to assess the characteristics of hope by comparing the two concepts of perceived and dispositional hope with regard to demographic variables and related constructs such as self-efficacy, spirituality, social relations, altruism, and health; (2) to explore the different aspects and elements of hope as perceived by the German speaking sample, in terms of e.g. targets hoped-for, hope enhancing experiences and activities, hope sources; and (3) to assess the predictive value of hope in relation to various dimensions for a good life such as life satisfaction, positive relations, positive feelings, personal health and well-being, meaning in life and happiness.

The first findings are associated with the characteristics of hope. The main demographic predictor of perceived hope is the family status, which evidences the social and emotional character of hope. Married individuals express higher levels of hope than separated, divorced and widowed people, as well as people living with a partner. Singles exhibit the lowest levels of hope. On the other hand, the strongest demographic predictor of dispositional hope is the professional status. People in higher professional positions possess greater levels of hope. Furthermore, while in general terms women demonstrate slightly but significantly higher values of perceived hope than men do, the opposite is the case with regard to dispositional hope. Perceived hope rises continuously with age, almost until very old age, despite one's health condition worsening with time. Dispositional hope, instead, reaches its peak in a person's 60s and then declines, probably together with physical and cognitive capabilities in older age. Finally, perceived hope is closely related to well-being, emotional, altruistic and (on a lower scale) the spiritual-religious dimensions of life, more than dispositional hope, which is very closely connected to self-centered and cognitive domains such as self-efficacy and resilience. However, among the German speaking population, the spiritual-religious dimension is in general terms less pronounced than the cognitive domain.

With regard to the level of satisfaction and hope in five major domains of general concern, the majority of the sample stated they were rather or very satisfied with their private life and even more people declared they were optimistic with regard to their own future for the coming year. This despite the fact that only few people are satisfied with and hardly optimistic about the state and progress of the national economy, the national politics, the climate and environment and the current social issues in their country. Moreover, the level of general perceived hope is mainly connected to the experiences in one's own private life and largely independent from the realities of the economy, the politics, the environment and the social issues. These results suggest that the worries regarding the general economic, political and social developments have a much smaller impact on the life and well-being of people than frequently believed.

These findings invite us to explore which life domains are especially important to people in terms of their personal hopes and their feelings of satisfaction. The principal personal hopes refer to central life domains of people's eudaimonic well-being, namely family bonds, harmony in life, good social relations, personal independence and a meaningful task. Hedonic aspects such as more time to relax, more spare time, more sex and more money are of much smaller importance, as well as religious and spiritual experiences. It is also worth noting, that higher levels of satisfaction with the eudaimonic oriented life domains are associated with higher scores of hope (in terms of the significance of the respective life domain). On the contrary, the lower the level of satisfaction with hedonic life domains, the higher the importance of the related hope, or, to put it the other way round, the higher the satisfaction with a hedonic domain, the lower the relevance of the respective hope. Particularly striking extremes are the spiritual-religious dimension on the one hand and the materialistic dimension on the other. Higher satisfaction with religious experiences correspond to a decidedly higher importance of the corresponding hope, whereas higher satisfaction with material possessions is associated negatively with the respective hope. This would mean that the levels of satisfaction and hope of the eudaimonic domains seem to have a mutually reinforcing character, whereas the hedonic and materialistic domains seem to be of importance especially when people experience a deficit or feeling of lack, losing their importance when the respective desires or wishes have been satisfied.

These conclusions could be substantiated by observing that eudaimonic life domains, such as good social relations, altruism (helping other people), meaning and also religious beliefs, turn out to be strong predictors of the general perception of hope, whereas the hedonic domains almost not at all. In analogy to Ryan and Deci's (2000) first- and second-order goals, we suggest differentiating between first- and second-order targets of hope. First-order targets of hope, such as good family relations, personal health, a sense of purpose and meaning, an altruistic attitude and religious experiences, have an intrinsic value for a good life. Second-order targets of hope are of subordinate value and relate to domains that display a momentary good feeling, with less importance for long-lasting personal development.

These findings have been complemented by exploring the sources of individuals' perceived hope. The mostly agreed on experiences that foster a sense of hope are good family relations, nice experiences out in nature and instances of having helped other people, followed by the mastery of difficult problems, personal success and to a lesser extent religious-spiritual experiences. Of considerably less relevance are coping, materialistic and hedonic affairs (e.g. "I earned a lot of money"). Besides one's own home, several places out in nature were rated as the most prominent places of hope, suggesting that the appreciation of beauty and the transcendent or spiritual feeling of connection to a bigger whole are precious sources that nourish hope. Less valued are places of consumption and recreation.

When reflecting on the people considered as hope providers, the key role of trust in another loved or valued person as a vital source of hope becomes evident. In principle, one's own relatives and closer friends are the most valued hope providers. However, many people choose the self-centered approach to give oneself hope, i.e. the belief that hope is an individual's own responsibility. God and religious leaders (likewise businesspeople and bankers) are considered the least hope providers by a majority of people. However, an interesting finding is that God, together with one-self and one's own partner, is one of the main hope providers in terms of a signifi-cant predictor of generally perceived hope.

A similar picture emerges when looking at the activities people declare to per-form in order to fulfil their own hopes. The mostly reported activities are of a ratio-nal (thinking and analyzing), a motivational (engaging oneself) and a relational (motivating friends and talking to family members) nature. Religiously motivated activities such as trusting God, praying or going to church, are considered the least performed by a majority of people. In spite of these preferences, the motivational, relational and religious activities are the most likely to predict the general level of perceived hope. In conclusion, three categories of activities could be identified when considering people's preferences and their effect on hope: (1) motivational and relational activities are highly valued by people and show a strong predictive effect on general hope; (2) religious activities (particularly trusting in God) are barely considered but demonstrate a significant effect on hope; (3) rational-cognitive activities (analyzing, informing oneself) are highly preferred but show a lower or even no effect on the degree of hope as generally perceived.

Based on these findings, a series of further analyses were performed so as to bet-ter understand the role and the value of hope for a healthy, fulfilling and happy life. Considering the importance of positive relations, good feelings and harmony in life as targets and sources of hope, and looking at the relation between them, the follow-ing conclusions can be drawn: People that experience positive relations in terms of close attachments to others, possess remarkably higher levels of hope, particularly because positive relations are connected to positive emotions, which in turn are tightly linked to hope. It is worth observing, that especially those emotions associ-ated with a feeling of harmony in life – i.e. in harmony with oneself, with others and with a larger whole – are relevant in terms of hope.

With regard to the relation of hope to psychological health and personal growth after traumatic events, perceived hope turned out to be the main predictor of psycho-logical health followed by other central aspects of psychological well-being, such as self-efficacy, meaning in life and positive relations. Furthermore, hope displayed an important partial mediation role between resilience and psychological health, revealing that people who feel resilient, enjoy better psychological health partly because they hold a more positive and confident view about their future. Similarly, hope seems to be an important protective factor together with the phenomenon of sense making in cases of distressing events, such as the loss of a loved one, separation, divorce or an acute illness, being associated with significantly less negative effects. Another remarkable result refers to the fact, that some people with a serious physical illness can retain high levels of hope and that these people state they have very few symptoms of depression and anxiety, comparable with healthy people and in contrast to seriously ill people with moderate or low levels of hope.

Happiness and meaning in life are among the highest goods to be achieved for most people. In a last series of analyses, we aimed at exploring the relationship between general hope as well as the particular targets of hope and reported happiness and meaning. Results reveal that the level of satisfaction with the aspects in life mostly hoped-for, namely a harmonious life, a happy partnership, family, marriage, a meaningful and satisfying task as well as personal health, turned out to be the main predictors of happiness and meaning as well as of perceived hope. Satisfaction with these (eudaimonic) life domains explains 45% of the variance of happiness, 32% of meaning in life and 29% of perceived hope. Especially talking with one's spouse or partner about one's own hopes has, above all other activities, the strongest relation to happiness and meaning in life. Furthermore, meaning in life together with positive relations in the present have a strong connection to happiness, but largely because both experiences are related to a hopeful outlook for the future. The crucial role of hope with regard to happiness becomes evident when observing the results of seriously ill people, who participated to the Hope-Barometer. Those who retained high levels of hope stated they enjoyed as high levels of happiness as completely healthy people, whereas those with low levels of hope were the most unhappy of the sample.

Conclusion: The Virtuous Circle of Hope

Our findings so far converge into one common overall conclusion: The existence of a general phenomenon we would like to describe as the virtuous circle of hope (Fig. 2.21). The fundamental conclusion to be drawn out from the results of the Hope-Barometer in German speaking Europe is that the main eudaimonic aspects in life – namely a happy partnership, family and marriage, harmony in life, good relations to other people, a meaningful task and an attitude of helpfulness – together with personal health are the main sources of hope and at the same time the life domains on which people focus their most important hopes. These dimensions in life are intrinsically and mutually reinforcing, whereas other aspects such as personal success, more money and sensual pleasures are neither central sources nor important targets of hope.

A particular finding is related to the spiritual-religious dimension. On the one hand, for a majority of people the spiritual and religious domains of life – e.g. trusting in God, praying or meditating, visiting a church – are neither important targets

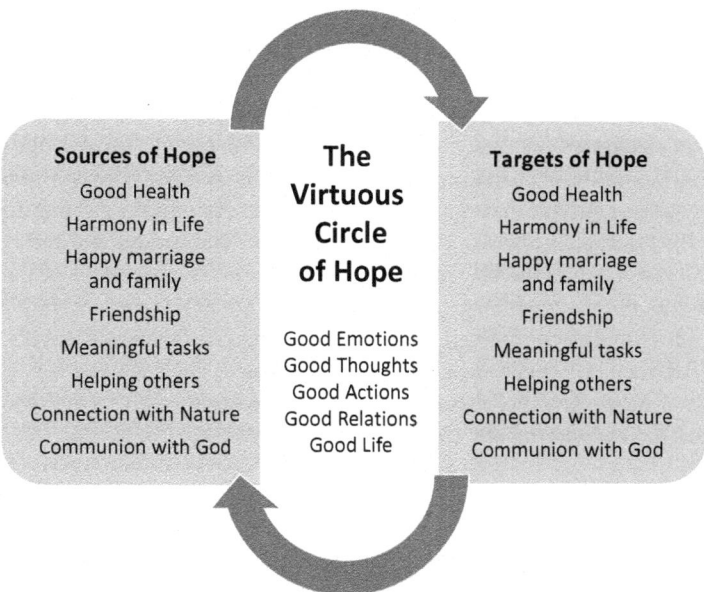

Fig. 2.21 The virtuous circle of hope

nor valued sources of hope. On the other hand, when looking more closely, there is a group of people, for whom spiritual and religious experiences are both important targets as well as valuable sources of hope. Moreover, to believe in and trust in God proved to be one of the major significant factors for a hopeful and meaningful life. If to believe in God proves to be as important as other sources for a harmonious, meaningful and happy life together with our loved ones and other people, then it is worthwhile including this self-transcendent component in the virtuous circle of hope.

To sum up, hope needs personal involvement and commitment, it is centered on a meaningful task or experience in life, and what is more, it requires harmonious and caring relations to other people, especially to one's own family and to a transcendent higher power to be found in nature and in God. The virtuous circle of hope is finally characterized by good feelings and emotions, positive thoughts, well meant actions, loving relations, and, overall, by a good and fulfilling life.

Limitations

The first limitation relates to the fact that the Hope-Barometer is a cross-sectional survey, making it impossible to derive causal explanations. In future research, it would be of value to include the Perceived Hope Scale in longitudinal studies in order to evaluate reciprocal effects with variables such as happiness, posttraumatic growth, resilience, health, spirituality and meaning in life. Another limitation is the self-report character of the questionnaire. For example, phenomena such as physical and psychological health should be assessed using medical data to be able to have standardized criteria allowing better comparisons. A further limitation is that, although our analyses are based on large and differentiated samples, these are not strictly representative of the German and the German-speaking Swiss population, in terms of gender, age, familial status, occupation, etc., but they are rather focused on people with Internet literacy and access. However, web-based research possesses clear advantages, since the size and the heterogeneous composition of the samples are better than other convenience samples often obtained by researchers. Finally, the findings and conclusions gained from our analyses are restricted to the German-speaking participants, making it necessary to explore and evaluate the generalizability of our results to other nations and cultures. Several chapters in this book have the purpose to compare results from different countries.

References

Arbuckle, J. (2014). *IBM® SPSS® Amos™ 23 user's guide*. Chicago, IL: IBM.

Averill, J. R., Catlin, G., & Chon, K. K. (1990). *Rules of hope: Recent research in psychology*. New York: Springer.

Averill, J. R., & Sundararajan, L. (2005). Hope as rhetoric: Cultural narratives of wishing and coping. In J. Eliott (Ed.), *Interdisciplinary perspectives on hope* (pp. 133–165). New York: Nova Science Publishers.

Baltes, P. B., Staudinger, U. M., & Lindenberger, U. (1999). Lifespan psychology: Theory and application to intellectual functioning. *Annual Review of Psychology, 50*(1), 471–507.

Carstensen, L. L., Turan, B., Scheibe, S., Ram, N., Ersner-Hershfield, H., Samanez-Larkin, G. R., et al. (2011). Emotional experience improves with age: Evidence based on over 10 years of experience sampling. *Psychology and Aging, 26*(1), 21–33.

Cristea, I. A., Sucala, M., Stefan, S., Igua, R., David, D., & Tatar, A. (2011). Positive and negative emotions in cardiac patients: The contributions of trait optimism, expectancies and hopes. *Cognition, Brain, Behaviour, 15*(3), 317–329.

David, D., Montgomery, G., & DiLorenzo, T. (2006). Response expectancy versus response hope in predicting distress. *A brief research report Erdelyi Pszichologiai Szemle, 1*, 1–13.

David, D., Montgomery, G. H., Stan, R., DiLorenzo, T., & Erblich, J. (2004). Discrimination between hopes and expectancies for nonvolitional outcomes: Psychological phenomenon or artifact? *Personality and Individual Differences, 36*(8), 1945–1952.

Delle Fave, A., Brdar, I., Freire, T., Vella-Brodrick, D., & Wissing, M. P. (2011). The eudaimonic and hedonic components of happiness: Qualitative and quantitative findings. *Social Indicators Research, 100*(2), 185–207.

Diener, E. D., Emmons, R. A., Larsen, R. J., & Griffin, S. (1985). The satisfaction with life scale. *Journal of Personality Assessment, 49*(1), 71–75.

Diener, E. D., Wirtz, D., Tov, W., Kim-Prieto, C., Choi, D. W., Oishi, S., & Biswas-Diener, R. (2010). New well-being measures: Short scales to assess flourishing and positive and negative feelings. *Social Indicators Research, 97*(2), 143–156.

Eliott, J. A. (2005). What have we done with hope? A brief history. In J. A. Eliott (Ed.), *Interdisciplinary perspectives on hope* (pp. 3–45). New York: Nova Science Publishers.

Erikson, E. (1963) *Childhood and society* (2nd ed., rev. and enl.). New York: W.W. Norton & Co.

Farran, C. J., Herth, K. A., & Popovich, J. M. (1995). *Hope and hopelessness: Critical clinical constructs*. Thousand Oaks, CA: Sage.

Ferring, D., Balducci, C., Burholt, V., Wenger, C., Thissen, F., Weber, G., et al. (2004). Life satisfaction of older people in six European countries: Findings from the European study on adult well-being. *European Journal of Ageing, 1*(1), 15–25.

Feudtner, C. (2005). Hope and the prospects of healing at the end of life. *The Journal of Alternative and Complementary Medicine, 11*(supplement 1), 23–30.

Hartigan, J. A. (1975). *Clustering algorithms*. New York: Wiley.

Huppert, F. A., & So, T. T. (2013). Flourishing across Europe: Application of a new conceptual framework for defining well-being. *Social Indicators Research, 110*(3), 837–861.

Hwang, J. Y., Plante, T., & Lackey, K. (2008). The development of the Santa Clara brief compassion scale: An abbreviation of Sprecher and Fehr's compassionate love scale. *Pastoral Psychology, 56*(4), 421–428.

IBM. (2014). *IBM SPSS advanced statistics 23*. Chicago: Author.

Joseph, S., Linley, P. A., Shevlin, M., Goodfellow, B., & Butler, L. D. (2006). Assessing positive and negative changes in the aftermath of adversity: A short form of the changes in outlook questionnaire. *Journal of Loss and Trauma, 11*(1), 85–99.

Kass, G. V. (1980). An exploratory technique for investigating large quantities of categorical data. *Applied Statistics, 29*(2), 119–127.

Kjell, O., Daukantaité, D., Hefferon, K., & Sikström, S. (2016). Harmony in life scale complements the satisfaction with life scale: Expanding the conceptualization of the cognitive component of subjective well-being. *Social Indicators Research, 126*, 893–919.

Krafft, A. M., Martin-Krumm, C., & Fenouillet, F. (2017). Adaptation, further elaboration, and validation of a scale to measure hope as perceived by people: Discriminant value and predictive utility vis-à-vis dispositional hope. *Assessment*, 1073191117700724.

Krafft, A. M., & Walker, A. M. (2018). *Positive Psychologie der Hoffnung. Grundlagen aus Psychologie, Philosophie, Theologie und Ergebnisse aktueller Forschung*. Berlin/Heidelberg: Springer.

Kroenke, K., Spitzer, R. L., Williams, J. B., & Löwe, B. (2009). An ultra-brief screening scale for anxiety and depression: The PHQ–4. *Psychosomatics, 50*(6), 613–621.

Linley, P. A., & Joseph, S. (2011). Meaning in life and posttraumatic growth. *Journal of Loss and Trauma, 16*(2), 150–159.

Linley, P. A., Joseph, S., & Goodfellow, B. (2008). Positive changes in outlook following trauma and their relationship to subsequent posttraumatic stress, depression, and anxiety. *Journal of Social and Clinical Psychology, 27*(8), 877–891.

Lyubomirsky, S., & Lepper, H. S. (1999). A measure of subjective happiness: Preliminary reliability and construct validation. *Social Indicators Research, 46*(2), 137–155.

Lyubomirsky, S., Sheldon, K. M., & Schkade, D. (2005). Pursuing happiness: The architecture of sustainable change. *Review of General Psychology, 9*(2), 111.

Masten, A. S., Cutuli, J. J., Herbers, J. E., & Reed, M. G. (2009). Resilience in development. In S. J. Lopez & C. R. Snyder (Eds.), *The Oxford handbook of positive psychology* (pp. 117–131). New York: Oxford University Press.

McCullough, M. E., Emmons, R. A., & Tsang, J. A. (2002). The grateful disposition: A conceptual and empirical topography. *Journal of Personality and Social Psychology, 82*(1), 112–127.

Montgomery, G. H., David, D., DiLorenzo, T., & Erblich, J. (2003). Is hoping the same as expecting? Discrimination between hopes and response expectancies for nonvolitional outcomes. *Personality and Individual Differences, 35*(2), 399–409.

Nickell, G. S. (1998) *The helping attitude scale: A new measure of prosocial tendencies*. Paper presented at the American Psychological Association, San Francisco.

Parsian, N., & Dunning, T. A. (2009). Developing and validating a questionnaire to measure spirituality: A psychometric process. *Global Journal of Health Science, 1*(1), 2–11.

Peterson, C., & Seligman, M. E. (2004). *Character strengths and virtues: A handbook and classification*. New York: Oxford University Press.

Plante, T. G., & Boccaccini, M. T. (1997). The Santa Clara strength of religious faith questionnaire. *Pastoral Psychology, 45*(5), 375–387.

Ryan, R. M., & Deci, E. L. (2000). Self-determination theory and the facilitation of intrinsic motivation, social development, and well-being. *American Psychologist, 55*(1), 68–78.

Ryan, R. M., Huta, V., & Deci, E. L. (2013). Living well: A self-determination theory perspective on eudaimonia. In D. Favè (Ed.), *The exploration of happiness: Present and future perspectives* (pp. 117–139). New York: Springer.

Ryff, C. D., & Keyes, C. L. M. (1995). The structure of psychological well-being revisited. *Journal of Personality and Social Psychology, 69*(4), 719–727.

Scheier, M. F., Carver, C. S., & Bridges, M. W. (1994). Distinguishing optimism from neuroticism (and trait anxiety, self-mastery, and self-esteem): A reevaluation of the Life Orientation Test. *Journal of Personality and Social Psychology, 67*(6), 1063.

Schnell, T. (2009). The Sources of Meaning and Meaning in Life Questionnaire (SoMe): Relations to demographics and well-being. *The Journal of Positive Psychology, 4*(3), 483–499.

Schwarzer, R., & Jerusalem, M. (1999). *Skalen zur Erfassung von Lehrer- und Schülermerkmalen.* Berlin, Germany: Freie Universität Berlin.

Scioli, A., & Biller, H. (2009). *Hope in the age of anxiety.* Oxford, MS: Oxford University Press.

Scioli, A., Ricci, M., Nyugen, T., & Scioli, E. R. (2011). Hope: Its nature and measurement. *Psychology of Religion and Spirituality, 3*(2), 78–97.

Seligman, M. E. (2004). *Authentic happiness: Using the new positive psychology to realize your potential for lasting fulfillment.* New York: Simon and Schuster.

Skevington, S. M., Gunson, K. S., & O'connell, K. A. (2013). Introducing the WHOQOL-SRPB BREF: Developing a short-form instrument for assessing spiritual, religious and personal beliefs within quality of life. *Quality of Life Research, 22*(5), 1073–1083.

Smith, B. W., Dalen, J., Wiggins, K., Tooley, E., Christopher, P., & Bernard, J. (2008). The brief resilience scale: Assessing the ability to bounce back. *International Journal of Behavioral Medicine, 15*(3), 194–200.

Snyder, C. R., Harris, C., Anderson, J. R., Holleran, S. A., Irving, L. M., Sigmon, S. T., & Harney, P. (1991). The will and the ways: Development and validation of an individual-differences measure of hope. *Journal of personality and social psychology, 60*(4), 570–585.

Sprecher, S., & Fehr, B. (2005). Compassionate love for close others and humanity. *Journal of Social and Personal Relationships, 22*(5), 629–651.

Staats, S. (1989). Hope: A comparison of two self-report measures for adults. *Journal of Personality Assessment, 53*(2), 366–375.

Steger, M. F., Frazier, P., Oishi, S., & Kaler, M. (2006). The meaning in life questionnaire: Assessing the presence of and search for meaning in life. *Journal of Counseling Psychology, 53*(1), 80–93.

Storch, E. A., Roberti, J. W., Bravata, E., & Storch, J. B. (2004). Psychometric investigation of the Santa Clara strength of religious faith questionnaire—Short-form. *Pastoral Psychology, 52*(6), 479–483.

Tedeschi, R. G., & Calhoun, L. G. (2004). Posttraumatic growth: Conceptual foundations and empirical evidence. *Psychological Inquiry, 15*(1), 1–18.

Weinstein, N. D. (1980). Unrealistic optimism about future life events. *Journal of Personality and Social Psychology, 39*(5), 806–820.

Weinstein, N. D. (1989). Optimistic biases about personal risks. *Science, 246*(4935), 1232–1234.

West, S. G., Finch, J. F., & Curran, P. J. (1995). Structural equation models with nonnormal variables: Problems and remedies. In R. H. Hoyle (Ed.), *Structural equation modeling: Concepts, issues, and applications.* Thousand Oaks, CA: Sage Publications.

Part II
Levels, Relationships and Variations of Hope

Chapter 3
Hope, Meaning in Life and Well-Being Among a Group of Young Adults

Tharina Guse and Monique Shaw

Introduction

Investigating factors which could contribute to optimal functioning across the lifespan is an important goal in positive psychology research. Life transitions provide the opportunity to develop psychosocial skills and resources needed to successfully navigate towards subsequent life stages. This is specifically important for young (or emerging) adults at university, who are engaged in several psychosocial developmental tasks in preparation for adulthood, whilst also negotiating challenges and opportunities associated with the university context. Understanding and promoting factors which may enhance positive psychological functioning, including well-being, of these young adults is central to their future positive development. Hope and meaning in life are two factors which have consistently been associated with well-being. In this study, we report on the dynamics between these factors in their relationship with well-being among a group of South African university students.

Well-Being Among University Students

The period of emerging adulthood, referring to individuals aged 18–25, can be viewed as a unique developmental life stage (Arnett, 2000), characterized by opportunities for psychological growth and increased well-being (Arnett, 2007; Galambos, Barker, & Krahn, 2006). It has also been described as a turning point (Schwartz, 2016), where individuals can redirect their life course for better (for example, attaining further education) or worse (for example, engaging in risky behavior). Further, young adulthood is a stage associated with several risk factors which may decrease

T. Guse (✉) · M. Shaw
Department of Psychology, University of Johannesburg, Auckland Park, South Africa
e-mail: tguse@uj.ac.za

© Springer International Publishing AG, part of Springer Nature 2018
A. M. Krafft et al. (eds.), *Hope for a Good Life*, Social Indicators Research Series 72, https://doi.org/10.1007/978-3-319-78470-0_3

63

well-being (Newcomb-Anjo, Barker, & Howard, 2017). Since higher levels of well-being have consistently been associated with positive outcomes in life domains such as relationships, work, and health, including a lowered likelihood to develop life-style diseases and addictions (Diener & Ryan, 2009; Lyubomirsky, King, & Diener, 2005), it is important to examine factors which could promote well-being in this developmental stage.

Two perspectives on well-being have been widely discussed in positive psychology literature. The first views well-being as *feeling good* (hedonic well-being) while the second has a focus on *functioning well* (eudaimonic well-being) (Keyes & Annas, 2009). It is now generally accepted that well-being is multifaceted, and includes dimensions of both hedonic and eudaimonic perspectives (Kashdan, Biswas-Diener, & King, 2008; Keyes, 2013). Recently Disabato, Goodman, Kashdan, Short, and Jarden (2016) provided evidence that hedonic and eudaimonic well-being may form part of a higher order well-being construct. Additionally, some studies (e.g., Dambrun et al., 2012; Delle Fave, Brdar, Freire, Vella-Brodrick, & Wissing, 2011) reported that eudaimonic well-being is linked to hedonic well-being, supporting the importance of considering both concepts in understanding optimal functioning. This combined conceptualization of eudaimonic and hedonic well-being can also be referred to as psychosocial well-being or flourishing (Keyes, 2005). Accordingly, we operationalized well-being in this broad sense in our study.

While several personal characteristics and dispositional traits have been examined in relation to well-being, this study is concerned with hope and meaning in life. These aspects may be particularly important in the transition to adulthood. Hope entails thoughts about the future and can be a valuable psychological resource during challenging times (Snyder, 2000). Further, cultivating an enduring sense of meaning in life is an important developmental task during emerging adulthood (Arnett, 2000), associated with psychological, vocational and physical well-being among university students (Shin & Steger, 2016).

Hope

Most research on hope defined it as a cognitive-motivational construct and a dispositional trait, which plays a significant role in mental health in general (Peterson & Seligman, 2004; Snyder, 2000). It has also been linked to positive psychological functioning in adolescents (e.g. Chiarrochi, Parker, Kashdan, Heaven, & Barkus, 2015; Valle, Huebner, & Suldo, 2006) and university students (e.g. Gallagher, Marquez, & Lopez, 2017; Satici, 2016). This cognitive conceptualization of hope, put forward by Snyder (2000, 2002), described hope as two-dimensional, consisting of an individual's motivation to reach meaningful goals (i.e. agency) and the ability to reach these goals (i.e. pathways). However, other researchers have criticized this view of hope for not taking into account how individuals define hope in their own lives, for being too similar to optimism and self-efficacy, and for neglecting spiritual aspects of hope (Bruininks & Malle, 2005; Krafft, Martin-Krumm, & Fenouillet,

2017; Tong, Fredrickson, Chang, & Lim, 2010). Consequently, Krafft and his colleagues (Krafft, 2014; Krafft et al., 2017) developed and validated a measure of hope as experienced by ordinary people, referred to as perceived hope.

Perceived hope seems to be broader than dispositional hope, and may flow from self-transcendent sources such as spirituality or a connection with something higher than the self. Whereas dispositional hope is more self-centered in nature, focusing on self-efficacy in reaching goals, perceived hope seems to relate stronger to spiritual and transcendent aspects of hope (Krafft et al., 2017). Research on perceived hope is still in its early stages, but existing studies showed that it is related to life satisfaction and positive affect (Krafft, 2014), which have also been found to be indicators of well-being in the South African context (Wissing & Van Eeden, 2002). Recent research among Czech samples further reported positive associations between perceived hope, life satisfaction and meaning in life (Slezáčková & Krafft, 2016). To date, there have been no studies on perceived hope in the African context. As Kraftt et al. (2017) pointed to the need for extending research on perceived hope across cultures, our study was a first step in that direction.

Meaning in Life

The concept of meaning in life remains complex and various theoretical models have been put forward (e.g. Schnell, Höge, & Pollet, 2013: Steger, 2012; Wong, 2012). Meaning in life is generally viewed as a positive variable (Steger, Frazier, Oishi, & Kaler, 2006), showing a strong association with general psychological well-being (Ryff & Singer, 2008). Recent models on meaning in life include three core facets, i.e. a cognitive component (e.g., an understanding of who we are), a motivational component (e.g., pursuit and identification of purpose), and affective elements (e.g., feeling that life makes sense) (see Wissing, Khumalo, & Chigeza, 2014 for a summary).

Of interest to the current study is Steger et al.' (2006) conceptualization of meaning in life as a sense of coherence or understanding regarding the nature of one's being, as well as feelings of significance and attachment to something larger than the self. According Steger (2012), meaning in life further consists of two distinct constructs: the presence of meaning in life (PMIL) and the search for meaning in life (SMIL). Whereas presence of meaning in life refer to a quality that individuals may possess, the search for meaning in life involves a process (Trevisan, Bass, Powell, & Eckerd, 2017). More specifically, the presence of meaning in life is determined by the understanding of one's self and the world, one's fit in the larger context, as well as having an understanding of the purpose one is pursuing (Steger, 2012). Presence of meaning in life has consistently been associated with well-being, including life satisfaction and positive affect (Dezutter et al., 2014; Steger, Oishi, & Kesebir, 2011). Recent studies among South African samples similarly reported positive correlations between the presence of meaning in life, life satisfaction and hope (Nell, 2014, 2016). On the other hand, searching for meaning in life denotes the aspiration to ascertain or expand one's sense of meaning, but is associated with lower levels of well-being (Nell, 2014; Steger, Kashdan, Sullivan, & Lorentz, 2008; Trevisan et al., 2017).

Meaning in life is an important variable in the life of emerging adults. Forming a coherent comprehension of one's life, the world, and how one fits within this world, are critical to optimal psychological development during this period (Arnett, 2000), including identity development (Dezutter et al., 2014). Additionally, having a sense of meaning in life seems to be important to developing a meaningful career (Zhang, Hirsch, Hermann, Wei, & Zhang, 2017) and can support students in dealing with the challenges of obtaining an university education (Garrosa, Blanco-Donoso, Carmona-Cobo, & Moreno-Jiménez, 2017; Mason & Nel, 2011; Nell, 2014). Studies suggest that sense of meaning predicts students' academic performance (Mason, 2017), adjustment to university life (Makola & Van der Berg, 2010), task perseverance and completion of studies (Makola, 2014). This is particularly relevant in the South African context, where higher education is viewed as the pathway to a better future, but many students experience financial hardship and other challenges during this life trajectory (Mason, 2013).

Meaning in Life as Link Between Hope and Well-Being

Different facets of hope may lead to different paths to well-being. Dispositional hope, being a cognitive-motivational construct, has been associated with the presence of meaning in life, which also has a cognitive dimension (Nell, 2014). Existing research suggests that meaning in life leads to increased well-being because of hope (Dogra, Basu, & Das, 2011; Yalçın & Malkoç, 2015) but the influence may be bidirectional. Increased hope may also lead to increased meaning in life, and consequently increase well-being because hope makes it possible for individuals to set and reach meaningful goals (Snyder, 2000). This is particularly important in supporting the implementation of hope-enhancing interventions among participants in life stages where meaning in life may still be developing, such as early adulthood (Steger et al., 2009). Further, since perceived hope seems to be related to transcendent and spiritual dimensions of hope (Krafft et al., 2017), it is also possible that perceived hope may lead to an increased sense of having a purpose in life and being connected to something larger than the self (presence of meaning in life) and thus well-being. These dynamics of hope, meaning in life and well-being therefore needs further empirical clarification.

The Current Study

Tertiary education has become increasingly important in determining an individual's adult life course (Arnett, 2016). With more and more young adults entering university in South Africa, in a milieu of limited financial support and low completion rates (Habib, 2016; Walton, Bowman & Osman, 2015), it is important to examine factors which may support well-being, and accordingly, university success. In the long run, these factors may also play a part in obtaining employment, gaining financial security and maintaining positive psychological functioning (Howard, Galambos, & Krahn, 2010).

Hope and the presence of meaning in life have both been associated with student well-being (Gallagher et al., 2017; Nell, 2016; Trevisan et al., 2017) but most studies have focused only on hedonic aspects of well-being, including life satisfaction and affect. Further, up to the present, published research on perceived hope have not included broader measures of well-being. There also is an absence of research on perceived hope in the South African context.

Additionally, the dynamics of perceived hope and meaning in life, in its relationship with well-being, still need theoretical clarification. In particular, we intended to better understand the relationship between hope and well-being through examining meaning in life as a possible mechanism in this relationship. A mediating variable explains the relationship between two variables, and can act as a potential mechanism by which an independent variable (in this case, hope) can produce changes in a dependent variable (in this study, psychological well-being). Should the effect of the mediator (meaning in life) be removed, the relationship between hope and well-being may no longer be present. Put differently, mediating variables explain how or why one variable predicts another (Frazier, Tix, & Barron, 2004). Accordingly, we expected that higher levels of hope may be associated with psychological well-being because it strengthens a sense of meaning in life.

Against this backdrop, this study aimed to examine (a) levels of hope, meaning in life and well-being among a group of South African university students; (b) the possible mediating effect of presence of meaning in life in the relationship between dispositional hope and well-being and (c) the possible mediating effect of presence of meaning in life in the relationship between perceived hope and well-being. We expected that meaning in life would mediate the relationship between both dispositional and perceived hope and well-being.

Method

Participants

Students (n = 252) at the University of Johannesburg completed the measuring instruments by means of an online survey. There were 171 (68.1%) females and 81(31.9%) males. The majority were between 18 and 21 years old, with a mean age of 20.55 (SD = 1.95). Most (77.7%) of the participants self-identified as Black African, followed by White (Caucasian) (12%), Indian (7.2%) and Coloured (mixed ethnicity) (2.4%). The majority of the participants spoke an African language as first language (67.9%), followed by English (26.4%) and Afrikaans (5.7%), which is a language derived from Dutch.

Measuring Instruments

The participants completed the following measures in English, which is the medium of instruction at the university:

The Mental Health Continuum Short Form (MHC-SF; Keyes, 2009) This scale consists of 14 items and establishes an overall score of well-being. It also measures three subcomponents of well-being: emotional well-being, social well-being, and psychological well-being (Lamers, Westerhof, Bohlmeijer, ten Klooster, & Keyes, 2011). Participants reported on their experiences of well-being over the previous 4 weeks using a Likert-type scale ranging from "Never" to "Every day". There is extensive evidence of the reliability of the scale in various contexts, including South Africa (de Bruin & du Plessis, 2015; Keyes et al., 2008), with alpha coefficients ranging from .74 to .87. Our study yielded a Cronbach's alpha coefficient of .92 for the total score of the MHC-SF. For purpose of mediational analyses only the total score was used as measure of well-being, informed by recent findings on the factor structure of the MHC-SF (de Bruin & du Plessis, 2015; Jovanivić, 2015; Schutte & Wissing, 2017) which suggest that the scale measures a higher order well-being factor and that the total score should be used in regression analyses.

The Adult Hope Scale (AHS) (Snyder et al., 1991) This scale measures and conceptualizes hope as a cognitive-motivational construct. It contains 12 items, of which four measure the pathways (cognitive) construct of hope, four measure the agency (motivational) construct, and four serve as distracters. In particular, the scale is divided into two subscales that comprise Snyder's (2002) model of hope: (a) agency (i.e., goal-directed energy) and (b) pathways (i.e., planning involved in attaining goals). Participants respond to each item using an 8-point scale ranging from "Definitely False" to "Definitely True". The results can either be examined at the subscale level or the two subscales can be combined to create a total hope score. Higher scores reflect higher levels of hope. For the purposes of this study the total hope score was used. Snyder (2002) reported several studies reflecting adequate internal consistency (α ranging from .74 to .84) and reported extensive construct validation proving reliability and validity. The scale also showed a high level of internal consistency ($\alpha = .83$) in a South African study (Boyce & Harris, 2013). Our study found a Cronbach's alpha coefficient of .89 for the total scale.

The Perceived Hope Scale (PHS) (Krafft et al., 2017) The PHS measures hope as perceived by individuals and also taps into self-transcendent, spiritual, and religious elements of hope. Krafft et al. (2017) also suggested that perceived hope might be seen as self-transcendent hope. The six-item measure is scored on a six point Likert-type scale ranging from "Strongly Disagree" to "Strongly Agree". A higher score on the PHS indicates the presence of perceived hope. The PHS yielded satisfactory psychometric properties in Swiss and Czech samples, as evident by Cronbach's alphas ranging between .87 and .89 (Krafft et al., 2017). There is an absence of research on the PHS in South Africa, but we found a satisfactory alpha coefficient of .92.

The Meaning in Life Questionnaire (MLQ) (Steger et al., 2006) The MLQ is a 10-item, self-report questionnaire measuring perceived meaning in life. It comprises both presence (MLQ-P) and search (MLQ-S) for meaning in life as independent dimensions. The MLQ-P subscale (5 items) measures to what extent participants feel their lives are full of meaning, while the MLQ-S subscale (5 items) measures respondents' engagement and motivation to find meaning or develop their understanding of meaning in their lives. The scale is scored on a 7-point Likert type scale, ranging from "Strongly agree" to "Strongly disagree". Higher scores reflect higher levels of either PMIL or SMIL. Steger et al. (2006) reported satisfactory psychometric data for these scales, with Cronbach's alpha coefficients ranging between .86 and .88, good convergent and discriminant validity, as well as excellent factor structure and stability. A South African study by Temane, Khumalo, and Wissing (2014) found Cronbach's alpha coefficients of .85 for MLQ-P and .84 for MLQ-S, while we found coefficients of .87 for MLQ-S and .91 for MLQ-P respectively. In this study we only included the MLQ-P in the analyses, based on its established positive association with well-being.

Procedure

Prior to commencement of the study, the Faculty of Humanities Research Ethics Committee provided ethical approval to conduct the research. Participants responded online to a secure survey at a time that was convenient for them, but the survey was only available for a limited time period. Participation was voluntary and anonymous.

Data Analysis

IBM SPSS Version 23 was utilized to gather descriptive statistics and to determine correlations between hope, meaning in life and well-being. To test the prediction that meaning in life mediates the relationship between hope and well-being, we computed standard regression analyses of direct effect (c'), and bootstrapped bias-corrected 95% confidence intervals of the indirect effect (ab) using the PROCESS macro (Hayes, 2013), with 1000 bootstrapped samples. A significant indirect effect (mediation) is indicated by confidence intervals that do not contain zero.

Table 3.1 Descriptive statistics, reliabilities and correlations between well-being, dispositional hope, perceived hope and meaning in life

Measure	M	SD	α	1	2	3	4
1.Well-being	2.94	1.02	.92	1			
2. Dispositional hope	6.18	2.14	.88	.658	1		
3. Perceived hope	3.71	1.01	.92	.656	.668	1	
4. Meaning	4.92	1.48	.91	.647	.673	.684	1

Note: All correlations are significant at 0.01 level (two tailed)

Results

Sample descriptive statistics and zero-order correlations are reflected in Table 3.1. As expected, there were statistically significant positive correlations between well-being, hope and meaning in life.

We implemented a standard regression analysis to examine the mediating role of MIL in the relationship between dispositional hope and well-being. As reflected in Fig. 3.1, dispositional hope was associated with well-being, and this relationship was mediated by meaning in life. Dispositional hope had a significant indirect effect on well-being through the relationship of meaning in life, $\beta = 36$, CI [.4289, .7790]. It represents a large effect, $K^2 = .2391$ CI [.1547, .3349]. Almost 51% of the variance in well-being was accounted for by the predictors, dispositional hope and meaning in life ($R^2 = .51$).

Similarly, as seen in Fig. 3.2, perceived hope was associated with well-being, and the relationship was mediated by meaning in life. Perceived hope had a significant indirect effect on well-being through the relationship with meaning in life, $\beta = .60$, CI [.378, .823]. This represents a large effect, $K^2 = .2459$ CI [.1569, .3255]. Almost 44% of the variance in well-being was accounted for by the predictors, perceived hope and meaning in life ($R^2 = .44$).

Discussion

The aim of this study was to examine the levels of well-being, hope and meaning in life among a group of university students, and to investigate the possible mediating role of meaning in life in the relationship between dispositional hope as well as perceived hope and well-being. The results revealed relatively high scores on all variables, as well as statistically significant positive relationships between them. Meaning in life mediated the relationship between both dimensions of hope and well-being.

Mean scores for well-being, hope and meaning in life were above midpoint. The mean value for total well-being was similar to that reported in an earlier study among South African adults ($M = 2.8$, $SD = 0.69$, Keyes et al., 2008) but slightly lower than American college students ($M = 3.18$, $SD = 1.11$, Mitchell, Reason,

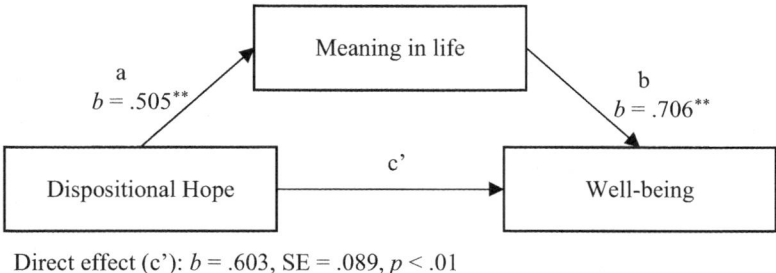

Direct effect (c'): $b = .603$, SE $= .089$, $p < .01$
Indirect effect (ab): $b = .357$, SE Boot $= .068$, CI $_{95} = 0.429\text{-}0.779$
Note: $^{**}p < .01$

Fig. 3.1 Mediation model of dispositional hope and well-being by meaning in life

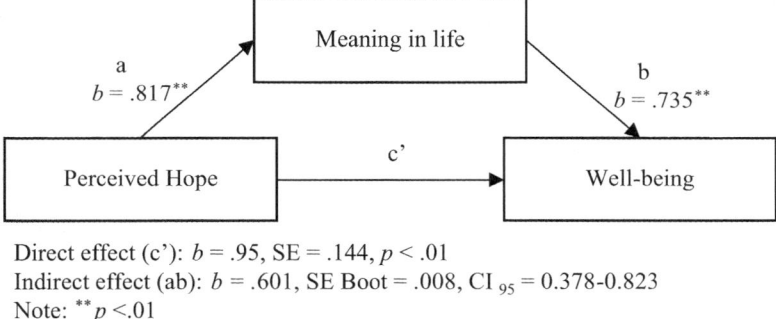

Direct effect (c'): $b = .95$, SE $= .144$, $p < .01$
Indirect effect (ab): $b = .601$, SE Boot $= .008$, CI $_{95} = 0.378\text{-}0.823$
Note: $^{**}p < .01$

Fig. 3.2 Mediation model of perceived hope and well-being by meaning in life

Hemer, & Finley, 2016). Nonetheless, overall the young adults in our sample still seemed to experience positive mental health. Concerning dispositional hope, the mean total score obtained for this study ($M = 48.41$, $SD = 9.94$), was higher than reported by Snyder et al. (1991) in a sample of American college students ($M = 25.24$, $SD = 2.81$). However, a more recent study among emerging adults in Hong Kong indicated similar levels of hope ($M = 41.28$; $SD = 13.45$) (Yuen, Ho, & Chan, 2014). Further, a South African study among a large sample of adults, reported mean scores of $M = 44.38$ (SD $= 0.67$) (Boyce & Harris, 2013). Levels of dispositional hope, in our sample of university students therefore seems high, similar to most other studies.

As this was the first study to investigate perceived hope in the South African context, the mean value of responses to the scale can only be interpreted by considering existing international studies. It appears that the participants in our study experienced similar levels of perceived hope, compared to those reported for Swiss ($M = 3.42$, $SD = .90$, Krafft et al., 2017), Maltese ($M = 3.12$, $SD = 1.03$, Dvorská, 2016) and Czech samples ($M = 3.73$, $SD = .88$) (Dvorská, 2016). Considering that the PHS measures hope as perceived by ordinary people (Krafft et al., 2017), we can infer that the young adults in our sample experienced relatively high levels of this transcendent dimension of hope.

The mean value for meaning in life was above midpoint, and the mean score for the scale measuring presence of meaning in life ($M = 24.77$, $SD = 7.25$) was similar to Khumalo, Wissing, and Schutte (2014) findings among a group of South African university students ($M = 25.9$, $SD = 6.10$) as well as s Woo and Brown's (2013) study ($M = 23.5$; $SD = 8.1$) with an American sample of emerging adults. However, Yalcin and Malkoc (2015) reported higher scores for Turkish university students ($M = 29.39$; $SD = 4.89$). Still, we can infer that this sample of young adults had an understanding of one's self and the world, one's fit in the larger context, as well as having an understanding of the purpose in life.

In terms of the association between well-being, hope and meaning in life, our results support previous studies which reported a positive relationship between dispositional hope and well-being among university students (Şahin, Aydın, Sarı, Kaya, & Pala, 2012), adolescents (Guse & Vermaak, 2011; Valle et al., 2006) and adults (Park, Peterson, & Seligman, 2004). A Czech study among university students also found perceived hope to be related to well-being (Slezáčková & Krafft, 2016). Similarly, our results evidenced support for the positive association between presence of meaning and life and well-being among university students (Khumalo et al., 2014; Yalçin & Malkoç, 2015). The findings are also in line with those from Slezáčková and Krafft (2016) who reported positive associations between dispositional hope, perceived hope, life satisfaction and meaning. In sum, our results then support existing research on the strong positive relationships between hope, meaning and well-being.

Our study indicated that meaning in life mediated the relationship between dispositional hope and well-being. While hope is driven by goals, meaning in life determines the importance of these goals and is also the source of life goals (Michael & Snyder, 2005). Meaning in life allows individuals to select appropriate and satisfactory goals. Through hopeful thinking an individual is able to utilize agency and pathways thinking to achieve these meaningful goals (Dogra et al., 2011). Perceiving goals as achievable and in line with personal values also directly influences well-being (McGregor & Little, 1998; Snyder, 2000). Thus, in addition to previous research which found that hope mediates the relationship between meaning in life and well-being, our findings suggest that this effect may be bidirectional, or at least, could also be understood from the other direction.

There is limited research on the relationship between perceived hope and well-being in the broader sense, thus the findings of our study adds to the understanding of the dynamics of this association. The results indicated that perceived hope is associated with well-being, but that meaning in life mediates this relationship. Similar to our findings, research conducted among a Czech sample found significant correlations between hope, MIL and well-being (conceptualized as life satisfaction and positive affect) (Slezáčková & Krafft, 2016). Both perceived hope and meaning in life have strong links to self-transcendence and spirituality (Atchley, 2009; Buck, 2006; Krafft, 2014; Steger et al., 2006), which may be the common denominator that increases well-being. It is thus plausible that, through experiencing a sense of purpose and a connection with something greater than the self, perceived hope provides meaning in life. People who are more hopeful tend to find their lives more meaningful (Slezáčková & Krafft, 2016), thus possibly positively influencing their well-being.

We are aware that our study had some limitations. It utilized a sample derived from a student population, which may limit the generalization of the outcomes to the larger population. It will be useful to implement a similar study among a more representative sample of the South African population. It may also be worthwhile to examine the dynamics of hope, meaning in life and well-being, taking into account gender, socioeconomic status, age and culture. Another limitation is that PHS has not yet been validated in the South African context, which may lead to questionable validity. Therefore, it is imperative to examine the psychometric properties of the PHS for use in the South African population. It is also important to keep in mind that the self-report questionnaires were administered in English and this may have limited the understanding of questions for participants whose first language is not English.

Conclusion

This study supported existing research which reported relatively high levels of well-being, hope and meaning in life among South African university students. Thus, despite developmental challenges associated emerging adulthood, and the South African university context in particular, the participants on our sample seem to have the needed psychological resources to meet these challenges on their way to adulthood. It is also evident that meaning in life is central to the relationship between hope and well-being. This study further adds to knowledge on the relatively new construct of perceived hope, opening up further avenues for research on hope as perceived by ordinary South Africans.

References

Arnett, J. J. (2000). Emerging adulthood: A theory of development from the late teens through the twenties. *American Psychologist, 55*(5), 469–480.

Arnett, J. J. (2007). Suffering, selfish, slackers? Myth and reality on emerging adults. *Journal of Youth and Adolescence, 36*, 23–29.

Arnett, J. J. (2016). Does emerging adulthood theory apply across social classes? National data on a persistent question. *Emerging Adulthood, 4*(4), 227–235.

Atchley, R. C. (2009). Spirituality, meaning, and the experience of aging. *American Society on Aging, 32*(2), 12–16.

Boyce, G., & Harris, G. (2013). Hope the beloved country: Hope levels in the new South Africa. *Social Indicators Research, 113*, 583–597. https://doi.org/10.1007/s11205-012-0112-y

Bruininks, P., & Malle, B. F. (2005). Distinguishing hope from optimism and related affective states. *Motivation and Emotion, 29*, 324–352.

Buck, H. (2006). Spirituality: Concept analysis and model development. *Holistic Nurse Practitioners, 20*(6), 288–292.

Chiarrochi, J., Parker, P., Kashdan, T. B., Heaven, P. C., & Barkus, E. (2015). Hope and emotional well-being: A six-year study to distinguish antecedents, correlates, and consequences. *The Journal of Positive Psychology, 10*(6), 520–532.

Dambrun, M., Ricard, M., Despres, G., Drelon, E., Gibelin, E., Gibelin, M., et al. (2012). Measuring happiness: From fluctuating happiness to authentic-durable happiness. Frontiers in Psychology. https://doi.org/10.3897fpsyg.2012.00016

de Bruin, G. P., & du Plessis, G. A. (2015). Bifactor analysis of the Mental Health Continuum-Short Form (MHC-SF). *Psychological Reports, 116*, 1–9.

Delle Fave, A., Brdar, I., Freire, T., Vella-Brodrick, D., & Wissing, M. P. (2011). The eudaimonic and hedonic component of happiness. *Social Indicators Research, 100*(2), 158–207.

Dezutter, J., Waterman, A. S., Schwartz, S. J., Luyckx, K., Beyers, W., Meca, A., et al. (2014). Meaning in life in emerging adulthood: A person-oriented approach. *Journal of Personality, 82*(1), 57–68.

Diener, E., & Ryan, K. (2009). Subjective well-being: A general overview. *South African Journal of Psychology, 39*, 391–406.

Disabato, D. J., Goodman, F. R., Kashdan, T. B., Short, J. L., & Jarden, A. (2016). Different types of well-being? A cross-cultural examination of hedonic and eudaimonic well-being. *Psychological Assessment, 28*(5), 471–4821.

Dogra, A. K., Basu, S., & Das, S. (2011). Impact of meaning in life and reasons for living to hope and suicidal ideation: A study among college students. *SIS Journal of Projective Psychology & Mental Health, 18*, 89–102.

Dvorská, P. (2016). *Deprese ve vztahu k naději, smysluplnosti života, generativitě a religiozitě: srovnání českého a maltského souboru* (Unpublished Doctoral theses), Mazaryk University. Retrieved from https://is.muni.cz/th/361648/ff_m?info=1;zpet=%2Fvyhledavani%2F%3Fsearch%3Dperceived%20hope%26start%3D1, September 2017

Frazier, P. A., Tix, A. P., & Barron, K. E. (2004). Testing moderator and mediator effects in counseling psychology research. *Journal of Counseling Psychology, 51*(1), 115.

Galambos, N. L., Barker, E. T., & Krahn, H. J. (2006). Depression, self-esteem, and anger in emerging adulthood: Seven-year trajectories. *Developmental Psychology, 42*(2), 350–365.

Gallagher, M. W., Marques, S. C., & Lopez, S. J. (2017). Hope and the academic trajectory of college students. *Journal of Happiness Studies, 18*(2), 341–352.

Garrosa, E., Blanco-Donoso, L. M., Carmona-Cobo, I., & Moreno-Jiménez, B. (2017). How do curiosity, meaning in life, and search for meaning predict college students' daily emotional exhaustion and engagement? *Journal of Happiness Studies, 18*(1), 17–40.

Guse, T., & Vermaak, Y. (2011). Hope, psychosocial well-being and socioeconomic status among a group of South African adolescents. *Journal of Psychology in Africa, 21*(4), 527–534.

Habib, A. (2016). Transcending the past and reimagining the future of the South African University. *Journal of Southern African Studies, 42*(1), 35–48. https://doi.org/10.1080/03057070.2016.1121716

Hayes, A. F. (2013). *Introduction to mediation, moderation, and conditional process analysis: A regression-based approach*. New York: The Guilford Press.

Howard, A. L., Galambos, N. L., & Krahn, H. (2010). Paths to success in young adulthood from mental health and life transitions in emerging adulthood. *International Journal of Behavioral Development, 34*(6), 538–546.

Jovanović, V. (2015). Structural validity of the Mental Health Continuum-Short Form: The bifactor model of emotional, social and psychological well-being. *Personality and Individual Differences, 75*, 154–159.

Kashdan, T. B., Biswas-Diener, R., & King, L. A. (2008). Reconsidering happiness: The costs of distinguishing between hedonics and eudaimonia. *Journal of Positive Psychology, 3*, 219–233.

Keyes, C. L., & Annas, J. (2009). Feeling good and functioning well: Distinctive concepts in ancient philosophy and contemporary science. *The Journal of Positive Psychology, 4*(3), 197–201.

Keyes, C. L. M. (2005). Mental illness and/or mental health? Investigating the axioms of the complete state of mental health. *Journal of Consulting and Clinical Psychology, 73*, 539–548.

Keyes, C. L. M. (2009). *Brief description of the Mental Health Continuum Short Form (MHC-SF).* Retrieved from http://www.sociology.emory.edu/ckeyes/

Keyes, C. L. M. (2013). Promoting and protecting positive mental health: Early and often throughout the lifespan. In C. L. M. Keyes (Ed.), *Mental well-being: International contributions to the study of positive mental health* (pp. 3–28). Atlanta, GA: Springer.

Keyes, C. L. M., Wissing, M., Potgieter, J. P., Temane, M., Kruger, A., & van Rooy, S. (2008). Evaluation of the Mental Health Continuum Short Form (MHC-SF) in Setswana speaking South Africans. *Clinical Psychology and Psychotherapy, 15*, 181–192.

Khumalo, I. P., Wissing, M. P., & Schutte, L. (2014). Presence of meaning and search for meaning as mediators between spirituality and psychological well-being in a South African sample. *Journal of Psychology in Africa, 24*(1), 61–72.

Krafft, A. M. (2014, June). *Distinguishing hope measures: Manifold determinants and predictors in the German and Swiss sample.* Paper delivered at The 7th European Conference of Positive Psychology, Amsterdam, The Netherlands.

Krafft, A. M., Martin-Krumm, C., & Fenouillet, F. (2017). Adaptation, further elaboration, and validation of a scale to measure hope as perceived by people: Discriminant value and predictive utility vis-à-vis dispositional hope. *Assessment,* 1073191117700724. https://doi.org/10.1177/1073191117700724

Lamers, S. M. A., Westerhof, G. J., Bohlmeijer, E. T., ten Klooster, P. M., & Keyes, C. L. M. (2011). Evaluating the properties of the Mental Health Continuum-Short Form (MHC-SF). *Journal of Clinical Psychology, 67*, 99–110.

Lyubomirsky, S., King, L., & Diener, E. (2005). The benefits of frequent positive affect: Does happiness lead to success? *Psychological Bulletin, 131*, 803.

Makola, S. (2014). Sense of meaning and study perseverance and completion: A brief report. *Journal of Psychology in Africa, 24*(3), 285–287.

Makola, S., & Van der Berg, H. (2010). A study on logotheory and adjustment in first-year university students. *International Forum for Logotherapy, 33*(2), 87–94.

Mason, H. D. (2013). Meaning in life within an African context: A mixed method study. *Journal of Psychology in Africa, 23*(4), 635–638.

Mason, H. D. (2017). Sense of meaning and academic performance: A brief report. *Journal of Psychology in Africa, 27*(3), 282–285.

Mason, H. D., & Nel, J. A. (2011). Student development and support using a logotherapeutic approach. *Journal of Psychology in Africa, 21*(3), 473–476.

McGregor, I., & Little, B. R. (1998). Personal objects, happiness, and meaning: On doing well and being yourself. *Journal of Personality and Social Psychology, 74*(2), 494–512.

Michael, S. T., & Snyder, C. R. (2005). Getting unstuck: The roles of hope, finding meaning, and rumination in the adjustment to bereavement among college students. *Death Studies, 29*, 435–458. https://doi.org/10.1080/07481180590932544

Mitchell, J. J., Reason, R. D., Hemer, K. M., & Finley, A. (2016). Perceptions of campus climates for civic learning as predictors of college students' mental health. *Journal of College and Character, 17*(1), 40–52.

Nell, W. (2014). Exploring the relationship between religious fundamentalism, life satisfaction, and meaning in life. *Journal of Psychology in Africa, 24*(2), 159–166.

Nell, W. (2016). Mindfulness and psychological well-being among black South African university students and their relatives. *Journal of Psychology in Africa, 26*(6), 485–490.

Newcomb-Anjo, S. E., Barker, E. T., & Howard, A. L. (2017). A person-centered analysis of risk factors that compromise wellbeing in emerging adulthood. *Journal of Youth and Adolescence, 46*(4), 867–883.

Park, N., Peterson, C., & Seligman, M. E. P. (2004). Strengths of character and well–being. *Journal of Social and Clinical Psychology, 23*(5), 603–619.

Peterson, C., & Seligman, M. E. (2004). *Character strengths and virtues: A handbook and classification.* New York: Oxford University Press.

Ryff, C. D., & Singer, B. H. (2008). Know thyself and become what you are: A eudaimonic approach to psychological well-being. *Journal of Happiness Studies, 9*(1), 13–39. https://doi.org/10.1007/s10902-006-9019-0

Şahin, M., Aydın, B., Sarı, S. V., Kaya, S., & Pala, H. (2012). Öznel iyi oluşu açıklamada umut ve yaşamda anlamın rolü [The role of hope and the meaning in life in explaining subjective well-being]. *Kastamonu Education Journal, 20*(3), 827–836.

Satici, S. A. (2016). Psychological vulnerability, resilience, and subjective well-being: The mediating role of hope. *Personality and Individual Differences, 102,* 68–73.

Schnell, T., Höge, T., & Pollet, E. (2013). Predicting meaning in work: Theory, data, implications. *The Journal of Positive Psychology, 8*(6), 543–554.

Schutte, L., & Wissing, M. P. (2017). Clarifying the factor structure of the mental health continuum short form in three languages: A Bifactor exploratory structural equation modeling approach. *Society and Mental Health*, Article first published online: May 23, 2017 https://doi.org/10.1177/2156869317707793.

Schwartz, S. J. (2016). Turning point for a turning point: Advancing emerging adulthood theory and research. *Emerging Adulthood, 4*(5), 307–317.

Shin, J. Y., & Steger, M. F. (2016). Supportive college environment for meaning searching and meaning in life among American college students. *Journal of College Student Development, 57*(1), 18–31.

Slezáčková, A., & Krafft, A. (2016). Hope – A driving force of optimal human development. In J. Mohan & M. Sehgal (Eds.), *Idea of excellence: Multiple perspectives* (pp. 1–12). Chandigarh, PB: Panjab University.

Snyder, C. R. (2000). Hypothesis: There is hope. In C. R. Snyder (Ed.), *Handbook of hope: Theory, measures, and applications* (pp. 3–21). San Diego, CA: Academic Press.

Snyder, C. R. (2002). Hope theories: Rainbows in the mind. *Psychological Inquiry, 13*(4), 249–275.

Snyder, C. R., Harris, C., Anderson, J., Holleran, S., Irving, L., Sigmon, S., et al. (1991). The will and the ways: Development and validation of an individual-differences measure of hope. *Journal of Personality and Social Psychology, 60,* 570–585.

Steger, M., Oishi, S., & Kesebir, S. (2011). Is a life without meaning satisfying? The moderating role of the search for meaning in satisfaction with life judgments. *Journal of Positive Psychology, 6,* 173–180.

Steger, M. F. (2012). Experiencing meaning in life: Optimal functioning at the nexus of well-being, psychopathology, and spirituality. In P. T. P. Wong (Ed.), *The human quest for meaning* (2nd ed., pp. 165–184). New York: Taylor & Francis.

Steger, M. F., Frazier, P., Oishi, S., & Kaler, M. (2006). The Meaning in Life Questionnaire: Assessing the presence of and search for meaning in life. *Journal of Counseling Psychology, 53,* 80–93.

Steger, M. F., Oishi, S., & Kashdan, T. B. (2009). Meaning in life across the life span: Levels and correlates of meaning in life from emerging adulthood to older adulthood. *The Journal of Positive Psychology, 4*(1), 43–52.

Steger, M. F., Kashdan, T. B., Sullivan, B. A., & Lorentz, D. (2008). Understanding the search for meaning in life: Personality, cognitive style, and the dynamic between seeking and experiencing meaning. *Journal of Personality, 76*(2), 199–228.

Temane, L., Khumalo, I. P., & Wissing, M. P. (2014). Validation of the Meaning in Life Questionnaire in an African context. *Journal of Psychology in Africa, 24*(1), 81–95.

Tong, E., Fredrickson, B., Chang, W., & Lim, Z. (2010). Re-examining hope: The roles of agency thinking and pathways thinking. *Cognition and Emotion, 24,* 1207–1215.

Trevisan, D. A., Bass, E., Powell, K., & Eckerd, L. M. (2017). Meaning in life in college students: Implications for college counselors. *Journal of College Counseling, 20*(1), 37–51.

Valle, M. F., Huebner, E. S., & Suldo, S. M. (2006). An analysis of hope as a psychological strength. *Journal of School Psychology, 44*, 393–406.

Walton, E., Bowman, B., & Osman, R. (2015). Promoting access to higher education in an unequal society: Part 2-leading article. *South African Journal of Higher Education, 29*(1), 262–269.

Wissing, M. P., Khumalo, I. P., & Chigeza, S. C. (2014). Meaning as perceived and experienced by an African student group. *Journal of Psychology in Africa, 24*(1), 92–101.

Wissing, M. P., & Van Eeden, C. (2002). Empirical classification of the nature of psychological well-being. *South African Journal of Psychology, 32*, 32–44.

Wong, P. T. P. (2012). Toward a dual-systems model of what makes life worth living. In P. T. P. Wong (Ed.), *The human quest for meaning: Theories, research, and applications* (pp. 3–22). New York: Taylor & Francis.

Woo, C. R. S., & Brown, E. J. (2013). Role of meaning in the prediction of depressive symptoms among trauma-exposed and nontrauma-exposed emerging adult. *Journal of Clinical Psychology, 69*(12), 1269–1283. https://doi.org/10.1002/jclp.22002

Yalçin, I., & Malkoç, A. (2015). The relationship between meaning in life and subjective well-being: Forgiveness and hope as mediators. *Journal of Happiness Studies, 16*, 915–929.

Yuen, A. N. Y., Ho, S. M. A., & Chan, C. K. Y. (2014). The mediating roles of cancer related rumination in the relationship between dispositional hope and psychological outcome among childhood cancer survivors. *Psycho-Oncology, 23*, 412–419. https://doi.org/10.1002/pon.3433

Zhang, C., Hirschi, A., Herrmann, A., Wei, J., & Zhang, J. (2017). The future work self and calling: The mediational role of life meaning. *Journal of Happiness Studies, 18*(4), 977–991.

Chapter 4
The Older, the Better? The Role of Hope for the Regulation of Subjective Well-Being Over Life-Span

Pasqualina Perrig-Chiello, Stefanie Spahni, and Katja Margelisch

Introduction

Subjective well-being is an ubiquitous concept in science as well as in everyday life. Feeling well and being happy have become highly valued individual life goals, if not even perceived as personal rights. Yet, the inflationary use of this concept is far more than a passing fad. It rather mirrors the changed social reality, namely an individualized world with new personal values and needs. As in other disciplines well-being has long been a marginal topic in psychology. However, during the last two decades there has been an impressive increase of theoretical and empirical work, mainly emerging from positive and life-span developmental psychology (Ehrler et al., 2016). After a long research tradition around the question, what makes people sick, these approaches have initiated a paradigmatic change focussing on determinants of well-being and happiness. Contextual determinants (social contexts, political systems, financial resources, etc.) were studied as well as social (being in a relationship, having children, friends, etc.) and personal ones (biographical and personality variables). Interestingly enough, personality variables deriving from the positive psychology approach such as character strengths were much less studied from a life-span perspective. This is especially true for hope and its relation to older age. In this contribution, we want to close some research gaps by focussing on the question of how hope, well-being and age are related. Particularly, we want to shed light on how dispositional hope (pathways and agency) can predict three major indicators of well-being (i.e. life satisfaction, happiness and meaning in life) and explain their variance. We first clarify the central concepts well-being and hope, and then give a literature review on the relation of hope, well-being and age. In the

P. Perrig-Chiello (✉) · S. Spahni · K. Margelisch
Institute of Psychology, Developmental Psychology,
University of Bern, Bern, Switzerland
e-mail: pasqualina.perrigchiello@psy.unibe.ch

© Springer International Publishing AG, part of Springer Nature 2018
A. M. Krafft et al. (eds.), *Hope for a Good Life*, Social Indicators Research
Series 72, https://doi.org/10.1007/978-3-319-78470-0_4

subsequent empirical part we present original data based on the Hope-Barometer 2015 addressing some of the above-mentioned research gaps.

Conceptual Considerations

Well-Being: Happy or Satisfied – What's the Difference?

Although in everyday discourse these concepts are often used as synonyms, they refer to different psychological states. There is however broad scientific consent, that both terms are elements of subjective well-being. In fact, subjective well-being is a multidimensional construct which can be subdivided in a more rational-cognitive component, such as life satisfaction, and in a more emotional one like happiness or psychological well-being (Luhmann, Hofmann, Eid, & Lucas, 2012).

1. *The rational-cognitive component* refers to a subjective appraisal of satisfaction with life in general or with specific domains of life. It is primarily a rational process, which is based e.g. on social comparisons or on a willingly adaptation of the individual's aspiration level.
2. *The emotional component* in turn can refer either to *hedonic well-being* or to *eudemonic well-being*. *Hedonic well-being (positive feelings)* results from search and maximizing happiness, pleasure and zest and from avoiding displeasure. Individual differences in the baseline of hedonic well-being are explained primarily by stable personal characteristics such as personality, in second line with social contexts. In contrast, *eudemonic well-being* (also called *psychological well-being*) is not characterized by the search of a positive pleasure-displeasure-balance, but by the pursuit of a good and meaningful life. Psychological well-being is understood as a multidimensional construct, which is based on personal strengths such as self-acceptance, personal growth, meaning of life, positive relations, mastery and autonomy (Ryff, 1995, 2014).

To summarize, we can say that a central characteristic of well-being regulation is the pursuit of a good life, be it by adapting life goals to needs and available resources, be it by maximizing pleasure or seeking meaningful tasks. The realization of these goals depends on multiple conditions, particularly from personal characteristics and attitudes – one of them being primarily having hope and trust.

Hope: Dispositional Hope – Domain Specific Hope

Hope is an important variable in the pursuit and achievement of life goals and hence for well-being. Hope has been conceptualized as a positive motivational state consisting of two distinct elements, which refer to the will and determination to pursuit life goals and to have the belief of being able to reach them. Accordingly, Snyder,

Irving, and Anderson (1991) distinguish between *Pathways thinking*, i.e. the perception of personal abilities to identify routes to desired goals, and *Agency thinking*, i.e. the perception of one's ability to initiate and pursue these routes. These two ways of thinking reinforce each other during the goal attainment process (Snyder, 2002). Besides these dimensions of general hope there are specific domains of hope related to various life concerns such as personal, familial, societal issues.

Independent of being general or domain specific, the concept of hope has become a central focus of positive psychology, where it has been related to various benefits such as positive emotions and subjective well-being (Boehm & Kubzansky, 2012). In positive psychology, hope is defined as character strength (McGrath, Rashid, Park, & Peterson, 2010). An important specification shall be noted here: Hope should not be confounded with optimism. Although both constructs reflect positive expectations about one's future, both are empirically distinguishable from each other (Alarcon, Bowling, & Khazon, 2013). Whereas optimism is thought to be most relevant within situations that allow for little personal control, hope is meant to be most relevant within situations that allow for higher levels of personal control (see Gallagher & Lopez, 2009).

Hope is a phenomenon that is experienced by people of all backgrounds. However, there are individual differences, which are still not well understood. This applies for age, but also for gender and personality variables such as optimism. Is hope more or less stable over life-span or does it change with advancing age and depending on gender? And how does the association between hope and subjective well-being vary when considering different age groups?

Subjective Well-Being and Hope Over Life-Span

Along with the demographic trend of longer life expectancy and changing values (especially individualization), the study of subjective well-being over life-span has become an increasingly prominent research topic (Ehrler et al., 2016). The topic is of high scientific and societal relevance since increasing evidence supports health protective features of subjective well-being, especially psychological well-being, in reducing risk for disease and promoting length of life (Ryff, 2014). Empirical studies provide consistent evidence that subjective well-being varies with age showing a more or less universal convex pattern over the age domain. Accordingly, well-being declines from young adulthood until age 40 and then improves gradually until age 70 (Steel, 2016; Steptoe, Deaton, & Stone, 2015; Stone, Schwartz, Broderick, & Deaton, 2010). This U-shaped course still holds when controlling for possible covariates such as gender, having children or income. Explanations for this age-typical trajectory have tried to unravel the phenomenon as a cohort effect (i.e. older generations being less demanding and more adaptive than younger ones). However, as several studies could show, cohort belonging contributes little for explaining the variance of well-being over age groups (Sutin et al., 2013). A more convincing and empirically confirmed explanation is that the level of subjective well-being changes as a function of individuals' life experiences leading to better adaption to age-specific challenges and to an improved self-regulation and emotion management (Urry & Gross, 2010). The ability of self-management and adaptive coping is strongly related to hope.

In fact and as stated above, hope has been identified as a basic and lifelong human reaction that stimulates successful coping with and adaptation to life changes and illness (Kornadt, Voss, & Rothermund, 2015; Kortte, Stevenson, Hosey, Castillo, & Wegener, 2012; Snyder, Lehman, Kluck, & Monsson, 2006; Tutton, Seers, & Langstaff, 2009). Hopeful thoughts help promote positive emotions (Gallagher & Lopez, 2009; Martínez-Marti & Ruch, 2014), which have been shown to be building blocks leading to other dimensions of well-being such as life satisfaction (Alarcon et al., 2013). Since hope has been defined as the ability to recognize the limitations of a situation while believing that opportunities exist (Parse, 1999), one could expect that hope grows with advancing age, since older age is associated with an increase of losses and limitations, but generally also with an improved self-management. However up to now, research results in this regard are very limited, since the majority of research has focused either on younger age groups, mostly on college students or on clinical samples such as individuals with cancer (e.g. Jafari et al., 2010; Sung, Turner, & Kaewchinda, 2013). In addition, the few existing results are contradictory. Some research results suggest that hope is rather stable across the life-span (Ciarrochi, Parker, Todd, Kashdan, Heaven, & Barkus, 2015; Snyder, Lopez, Shorey, Rand, & Feldman, 2003) whereas other found that older age is associated with less hope (Bailey & Snyder, 2007). A similar research gap applies for gender differences: some researchers reported higher levels of hope in women (Ciarrochi et al., 2015; Heaven & Ciarrochi, 2008; Jackson, van de Vijver, & Fouché, 2014), whereas other did not find any differences at all (Bailey & Snyder, 2007). An explanation for these inconsistencies lies in the fact, that

1. age and gender differences regarding hope were neither explored over the life-span nor in large random samples from a general population. Additionally, in most of this research, the differentiation between pathways and agency thinking was not considered.
2. possibly confounding variables such as optimism were not enough controlled for, even though hope and optimism have been shown to load on separate factors (Bryant & Cvengros, 2004).

Research Questions and Hypotheses

Considering these research gaps and taking into account findings from life-span research on well-being, our aim is to shed light on

1. age and gender differences with regard (a) to major indicators of well-being, i.e. life satisfaction (rational aspect of well-being), happiness (hedonic well-being),

meaning in life (eudemonic well-being), and (b) with regard to dispositional hope (pathways and agency);

2. the amount of hope depending on individuals' concern regarding different life domains by taking into account age and gender.
3. how dispositional hope is (a) related with the three well-being indicators (life satisfaction, hedonic and eudemonic well-being), and (b) how it predicts the variance of these well-being indicators.

We expect age differences regarding all indicators of well-being, namely highest scores in the oldest group, especially in eudemonic well-being, which is most dependent on adaptive processes and on life experience. We also predict age differences regarding dispositional hope, i.e. increasing scores with advancing age especially for pathways, since knowledge on how reaching goals might increase with advancing age and life experience. Regarding gender differences, we do not have any specific expectations. Finally, we expect highest scores of hope for more personal domains of life over all age groups, and in general higher scores with advancing age and in women regarding social concerns.

As for the predictive power of dispositional hope we hypothesize that hope is a significant predictor for more controllable indicators of well-being, namely life satisfaction and meaning in life, even after controlling for optimism age, sex and subjective health. This in contrast to the more emotional, less controllable indicator of well-being, i.e. happiness, which is expected to depend more on personality variables such as optimism than on dispositional hope.

Method

Data analysed in this chapter stem from the Hope-Barometer survey Switzerland 2015. The variables used are:

Well-Being

- *Subjective health* was measured with the single item question 'How would you rate your physical health status?', answered on a scale from 1 'I am seriously ill' to 7 'I am totally healthy'.
- *Happiness* was assessed with the Subjective Happiness Scale (Lyubomirsky & Lepper, 1999), including four items rated on a 7-point Likert scale with higher scores reflecting greater happiness (Cronbach's alpha was .83).
- *Life satisfaction* was measured with the Satisfaction with Life Scale (Diener, Emmons, Larsen, & Griffin, 1985; Schumacher, 2003). The five items are rated on a 7-point scale ranging from 1 ‚completely disagree' to 7 ‚completely agree' and loading onto one factor (Cronbach's alpha was .89).

- The presence of *meaning in life* was measured with four items of the Meaning in Life Questionnaire (Steger, Frazier, Oishi, & Kaler, 2006), rated on a scale from 1 'absolutely untrue' to 7 'absolutely true' (Cronbach's alpha was .91).
- Self-constructed items asked participants about their *domain-specific satisfaction* in private life, national politics, national economics, national social issues, and climate and environment. Satisfaction was rated from 1 'very unsatisfied' to 5 'very satisfied'.

Hope

- *Dispositional Hope* was assessed with the Adult Dispositional Trait Hope Scale (Snyder et al., 1991), comprising two subscales, one for ,agency' and one for ,pathways'. Agency is defined as the successful sense of goal-related determination, pathways stands for the belief in one's own ability to deal with goal-related obstacles. Each subscale has four items, rated on a 4-point scale from 0 ,definitely false' to 5 ,definitely true (Cronbach's alpha: .90; agency .84; pathways .84).
- *Domain-specific hope* was assessed with self-constructed items addressing:
  - *self-related hope*: harmony in life, personal health, meaningful and fulfilling task, order in my life, independence and autonomy;
  - *hope related to significant others*: happy marriage, family, partnership; good and trusting relations;
  - *hope related to others in general*: importance to help others.

All items were measured with a 4-point scale from 0 'not important' to 3 'very important'.

Sample

A total of 9103 participants answered the questionnaire in 2015 in Switzerland. For our analyses, we focus on participants 18 years and older, which were allocated to three age groups of 18–39, 40–59, and 60> years. Descriptives are presented in Table 4.1.

Statistical Analyses

In a first step, group comparisons were performed with regard to well-being and hope between the three age groups using analysis of variance with post-hoc tests. Some of the analyses were run also separately by gender. In a second step, we looked at the relationship between well-being and hope. Pearson correlation coefficients show how the different scales and subscales are associated with each other by age-group ($r > .10$ small, $>.30$ middle, $>.50$ large effect, according to Cohen, 1969). In a third step, multiple stepwise regressions were carried out to predict the three well-being indicators: happiness, life satisfaction and meaning in life. As predictors age and gender (step 1) were considered, followed by dispositional hope, i.e. agency and pathways (step 2), and optimism (step 3). All analyses were performed with the software SPSS (IBM, 2014).

Results

Well-Being and Hope in Different Age-Groups

Well-Being

Whereas subjective health decreases significantly with advancing age ($p < .01$) the opposite is true for happiness, life satisfaction and meaning in life ($p < .01$) (Fig. 4.1).

The oldest age group shows the highest scores in all three well-being indicators. Differences between age groups are smaller between young and middle aged, and most prominent from middle to older age. Whereas all well-being indicators are evenly balanced in the youngest age group, in the older age groups life satisfaction is remarkably lower than happiness and meaning. In the oldest age group meaning in life is most pronounced.

Table 4.1 Sample description by age group

	Age group		
	18–39	40–59	60>
Female	3184 (65.6%)	1488 (54.2%)	370 (39.3%)
Male	1673 (34.4%)	1256 (45.8%)	572 (60.7%)
Family status			
Living with parents	1195 (24.6%)	7 (0.3%)	1 (0.1%)
Single	941 (19.4%)	279 (10.2%)	65 (6.9%)
In relationship, not living together	532 (11%)	204 (7.4%)	38 (4.0%)
In relationship, living together	1174 (24.2%)	397 (14.5%)	103 (10.9%)
Married	920 (18.9%)	1418 (51.7%)	546 (58%)
Separated/divorced	88 (1.8%)	393 (14.3%)	130 (13.8%)
Widowed	7 (0.1%)	46 (1.7%)	59 (6.3%)
Children (yes)	915 (18.8%)	1940 (70.1%)	748 (79.4%)
Educational level			
None	39 (0.8%)	22 (0.8%)	3 (0.3%)
Primary	233 (6.9%)	144 (5.2%)	63 (6.7%)
Secondary	2705 (55.8%)	1359 (49.6%)	427 (45.3%)
Tertiary	1780 (36.7%)	1219 (44.4%)	449 (47.7%)

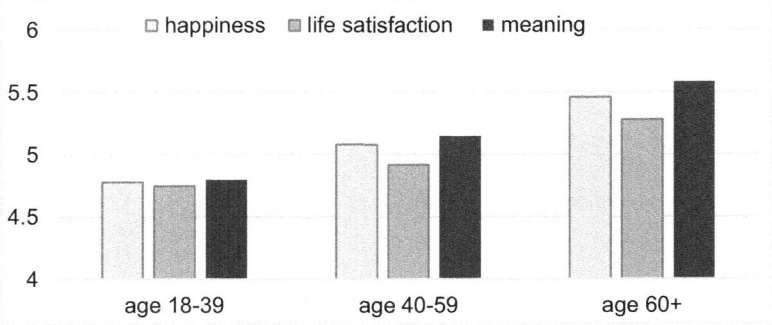

Fig. 4.1 Various well-being indicators by age (scale 1–7)

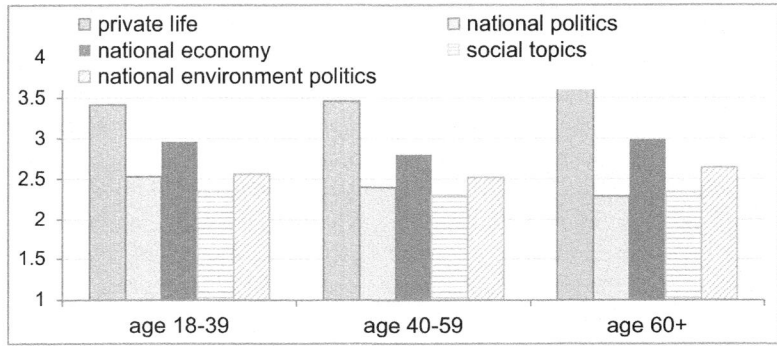

Fig. 4.2 Domain specific satisfaction by age (scale 1–5)

Gender differences were not so distinct in general, and no gender differences at all were found for meaning in life. Differences were observed mainly in the youngest age group, where women rated their health significantly lower than men ($p < .001$), but had higher scores in life satisfaction and happiness ($p < .01$). Middle aged women still have a lower subjective health ($p = .01$), but slightly higher happiness scores ($p < .01$) than men. In the oldest age group finally, the only difference was that women had a significantly lower life satisfaction than men ($p < .01$).

We get a deeper insight into individuals' life satisfaction by focusing on specific domains. Over all age groups satisfaction with one's private life is rated significantly higher than satisfaction with various public issues (Fig. 4.2). As for life satisfaction the oldest age group shows the highest ratings regarding private life, but the lowest ones for national politics. Satisfaction with national economy is lowest in the middle-aged. No age effects were observed for satisfaction for social topics and environmental politics.

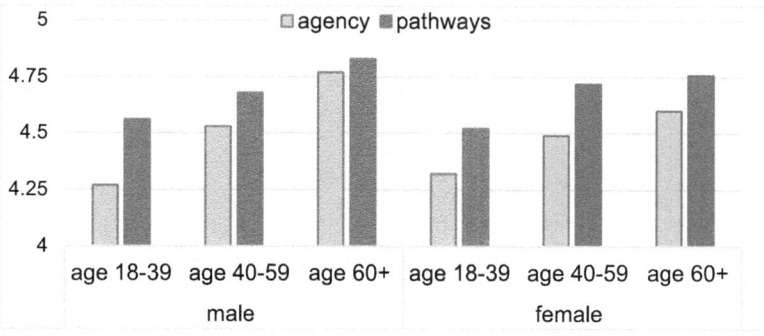

Fig. 4.3 Dispositional hope (agency and pathways) by age and gender (scale 0–5)

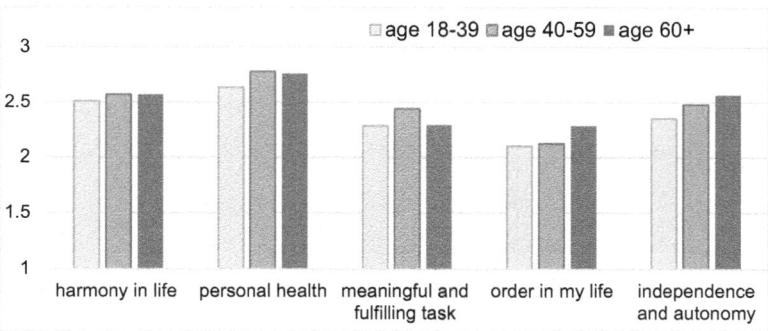

Fig. 4.4 Self-related hope by age (0 = not important – 3 = very important)

Hope

Dispositional Hope

Group comparisons show a significant age-related increase in both hope dimensions, especially in agency in men and women ($p < .01$). In all age groups pathway thinking outweighs agency, particularly in young men, and young and middle aged women (Fig. 4.3). Young women have lower scores for pathways, and older women score lower in agency compared to their male peers.

Domain-Specific Hope

With regard to *self-related hope* the highest valued concerns were personal health and harmony (middle and older age greater than younger age), and independence with a significant age-related increase (Fig. 4.4).

Hope to have a well-ordered life is expressed significantly more in the oldest age group, whereas to have a meaningful and fulfilling task is a concern of the middle aged, more than of younger and older individuals.

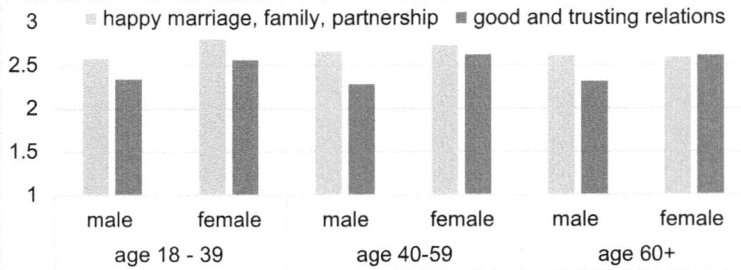

Fig. 4.5 Hope regarding partnership/family and important others by age and gender (0 = not important – 3 = very important)

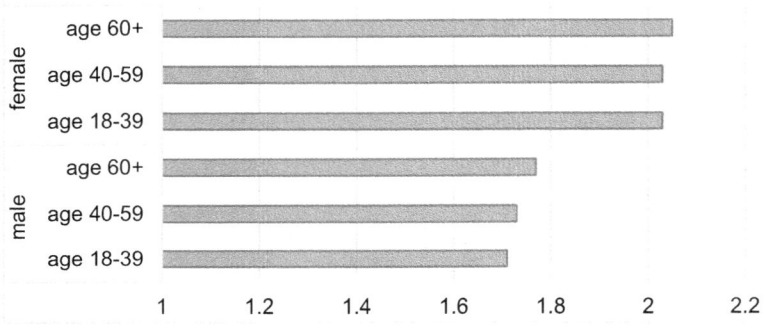

Fig. 4.6 Importance and hope for helping others by age (0 = not important – 3 = very important)

Regarding *other-oriented hope,* the hope of having a fulfilling partnership and good family relationships as well as trusting relations with friends are most expressed by the youngest age group (Fig. 4.5). However differences between men and women are more pronounced than between age groups. Women of the younger and middle-aged group outscore their male peers in both indicators, whereas in the oldest age group this is only the case for good and trusting relations with friends.

Importance to help others is – compared to personal and familial issues under-standably enough – not such a central concern, and this independently of age (Fig. 4.6). However there is a significant gender effect: Women of all age groups rate the importance and hope for helping others higher than men.

Relationship Between Hope and Well-Being

In a second step, we wanted to shed light on the relationship of hope and well-being. First, we explored the correlation between dispositional hope (agency and path-ways) and the indicators of well-being, i.e. happiness, life satisfaction and meaning.

Table 4.2 Correlations between dispositional hope and well-being

	Happiness	Life satisfaction	Meaning
Age 18–39			
Agency	.53***	.62***	.58***
Pathways	.52***	.50***	.47***
Age 40–59			
Agency	.59***	.67***	.62***
Pathways	.56***	.57***	.53***
Age 60+			
Agency	.55***	.64***	.58***
Pathways	.62***	.52***	.49***

*** = p < 0.001

Table 4.3 Dispositional hope (agency and pathways), age, gender and optimism as predictors of well-being outcomes

Outcomes	Happiness			Life satisfaction			Meaning in life		
B, SE B, β/predictors	B	SE B	β	B	SE B	β	B	SE B	β
Age	.05	.01	.06***	-.01	.01	-.01	.07	.01	.07***
Gender (F)	.16	.02	.06***	.08	.02	.03***	.10	.02	.03***
Agency	.25	.02	.17***	.55	.02	**.39***	.64	.02	**.42***
Pathways	.19	.02	.13***	.03	.02	.02	.07	.02	.05***
Optimism	.70	.01	**.48***	.56	.01	**.39***	.38	.02	.24***
Adjust. R^2	.49			.51			.42		
	1738.54***			1872.93***			1310.89***		

*** = p < 0.001

As Table 4.2 shows, all three indicators are significantly correlated to both agency and pathways in all three age groups. This is especially true for agency.

Hope as Predictor for Life Satisfaction, Happiness and Meaning in Life

Based on our empirical insights and on previous work we conducted, multiple step-wise regressions with each of the three well-being indicators (happiness, life satisfaction, meaning in life) as criteria, and dispositional hope (i.e. agency and pathways) as predictor by taking into account age and gender as well as optimism. In a first step, we entered age and gender, in a second one agency and pathways thinking, and in step 3 optimism. In Table 4.3 the final results for all well-being outcomes are presented:

Happiness For the prediction of happiness, age and gender contribute very little (R^2 = 04), agency and pathway modestly (R^2 = .35), the most variance is explained by entering the personality variable optimism (step 3) (R^2 = .48).

Life Satisfaction Here again age and gender do not explain much of the variance ($R^2 = .03$), however by entering pathways and especially agency increases the R^2 to .42. Optimism boosts the explained variance by additional 9%.

Meaning in Life For eudemonic well-being, agency is by far the strongest predictor ($\beta = .42$). Age and gender do not contribute much for predicting meaning in life ($R^2 = 0.4$), and entering optimism increases R^2 only by .04.

Overall, age and gender have a modest though significant predictive power for explaining all three well-being indicators as soon as agency and pathways are considered. Dispositional hope – especially agency – is a significant and strong predictor of life satisfaction and for meaning in life, whereas happiness is best predicted by the personality variable optimism and much less by dispositional hope.

Discussion

Despite the impressive increase of theoretical and empirical work on subjective well-being, research addressing the relationship between character strengths such as hope and various dimensions of well-being from a life-span approach is still scarce. Based on data from the Hope-Barometer 2015 Switzerland, including a large random sample covering the whole adult life-span, and focussing on the question of how well-being, hope and age are related, our results contribute to answer some open research questions. As for *subjective well-being* our results confirm existing research according to which the oldest age-group shows the highest scores in life satisfaction, happiness and especially meaning, while subjective health deteriorates (Perrig-Chiello, 2011, 2016). This so-called paradox of well-being in older age can be interpreted as a volitional effort of adaptation to age-specific challenges and an improved self-regulation and emotion management due to lessons learned from passed life events (Urry & Gross, 2010). This is mirrored – as expected – in the high scores in meaning in life compared to happiness and life satisfaction, which is known to be most dependent on adaptive processes and on life experience. However we cannot observe a U-shaped curve, but rather a J-curve, with a slight increase from the younger to the middle-aged group and a steep increase for the oldest group. A possible explanation for this can be found in the demographic characteristics of the sample, where the middle-aged group is underrepresented compared to the younger age group. Additionally, individuals of the middle-aged sample seem to be a rather positive selection in the Hope-Barometer, e.g. with regard to marital status (significantly less divorced than in the average population). Results further suggest that *domain specific satisfaction* depend primarily upon the personal concern about the issue and the control one can exert over it. This is shown by the significantly far higher scores with regard to private life for all three age groups compared to those for all other issues (economy, environment, social topics, national politics).

Since the ability of self-management and adaptive coping is strongly related to age, we expected also higher scores for *dispositional hope*. Research results so far have been rather rare and contradictory, and mostly focusing on younger age groups. Based on a large random sample from the Hope-Barometer and considering research from life-span perspective this contribution brings new and interesting insights. In fact, our results go in the predicted direction showing consistently and clearly an age-related increase independently of gender for both dimensions of hope, however especially for agency and not as expected for pathways. The steep age-related increase we found for agency suggests that the will and belief that one can reach goals is much more dependent on life experience than the knowledge about ways how to reach them effectively. This is somehow comprehensible since every phase of life has its own possibilities and limitations. Interestingly, pathways outweigh agency in all age groups particularly in women. It seems that women in our society still perceive and possibly also effectively have less possibilities of reaching their life goals than men.

With regard to *self-related hope* the scores mirror age specific demands and tasks very well: Independence and autonomy, as well as health are most valued in the older age groups, whereas having meaningful and fulfilling tasks are predominantly the concern of the middle aged. Hope related to partnership and family is a major concern across all age-groups however stronger in younger and middle-aged women than in men. This confirms empirical findings but also gender stereotypes of the more family oriented and caring women. Only in older age this gender difference does not exist any more, possibly indicating the greater dependence of older men on their spouses (Perrig-Chiello & Hutchison, 2010). The gender differences regarding social concerns become even more significant when considering the importance and hope for helping other, where women outweigh by far men across all age groups.

An innovative point of this contribution is the exploration of the power of dispositional hope in predicting the variance of the three dimensions of subjective well-being, i.e. life satisfaction, happiness and meaning in life. According to our expectation, dispositional hope, particularly agency thinking, predicted the more controllable indicators of well-being, namely life satisfaction and meaning in life, even after controlling for possible confounders such as age, gender, and optimism. In fact, agency was strongly related to meaning in life and life satisfaction ($\beta = .42$ respectively .39) and much less with happiness ($\beta = .17$). In contrast with agency, pathways thinking played a far weaker role in predicting happiness ($\beta = .13$) and meaning in life ($\beta = .05$), and was not at all correlated with life satisfaction. This finding confirms research done by Umphrey and Sherblom (2014), who found a strong and direct link between agency and life satisfaction, however not for pathways. Concerning the more emotional component of well-being, i.e. happiness, our results show that it was best predicted by optimism, while hope played a marginal role. Our data confirm the dominant role of hope – especially of agency thinking – for predicting meaning in life and life satisfaction. Nonetheless, also optimism has a non- negligible impact on well-being outcomes, essentially for happiness and to a lesser degree for life satisfaction. Compared to hope and optimism however, age and gender played only a marginal role for predicting the various well-being outcomes.

Overall, our research shows the beneficial and dominant role of having hope for the regulation of well-being across all age groups. Hereby it is not primarily the strategic knowledge about possible pathways to reach life goals decisive, but rather the will and belief that one will find solutions to overcome insecurity and obstacles. Our results also suggest that agency thinking is especially beneficial for achieving a higher sense of meaning in life and a higher life satisfaction, which in turn are both conditional upon life experiences and volitional adaptation processes. This insight is not only scientifically relevant, but has also important practical implications. Developing a deeper understanding of how people experience hope and how this is related to specific outcomes of well-being is important for designing interventions and psychological education programs for people in their middle and older age, since most intervention studies were carried out with children and college students (Feldman & Dreher, 2012; Marques, Lopez, & Pais-Ribeiro, 2011).

Although our research is innovative and opens new perspectives, it has one limitation. Our data being cross-sectional do not allow for causal interpretations and do not give a sufficient answer to the question, whether the age-effects we found are pure age effects or possibly confounded with generation- or cohort effects. However, recurring to existing longitudinal research, we can assume, that although cohort-effects could effectively play a certain role in explaining the effects, age per se is nonetheless the major predicting variable. Still, future research should try to adopt cross-sequential study designs in order to disentangle age and cohort effects and to consider multidimensional measures of subjective well-being and hope.

References

Alarcon, G. M., Bowling, N. A., & Khazon, S. (2013). Great expectations: A meta-analytic examination of optimism and hope. *Personality and Individual Differences, 54*, 821–827.

Bailey, T. C., & Snyder, C. R. (2007). Satisfaction with life and hope: A look at age and marital status. *The Psychological Record, 57*, 233–240.

Boehm, J. K., & Kubzansky, L. D. (2012). The heart's content: The association between positive psychological well-being and cardiovascular health. *Psychological Bulletin, 138*, 655–691.

Bryant, F. B., & Cvengros, J. A. (2004). Distinguishing hope and optimism: Two sides of a coin, or two separate coins? *Journal of Social and Clinical Psychology, 23*(2), 273–302.

Ciarrochi, J., Parker, P., Kashdan, T. B., Heaven, P. C. L., & Barkus, E. (2015). Hope and emotional well-being: A six-year study to distinguish antecedents, correlates, and consequences. *The Journal of Positive Psychology, 10*(6), 520–532.

Cohen, J. (1969). *Statistical power analysis for the behavioral sciences.* San Diego, CA: Academic Press.

Diener, E. D., Emmons, R. A., Larsen, R. J., & Griffin, S. (1985). The satisfaction with life scale. *Journal of Personality Assessment, 49*(1), 71–75.

Ehrler, F., Bühlmann, F., Höpflinger, F., Joye, D., Perrig-Chiello, P., & Suter, C. (2016). *Sozialbericht 2016: Wohlbefinden.* Zürich, Switzerland: Seismo.

Feldman, D. B., & Dreher, D. E. (2012). Can hope be changed in 90 minutes? Testing the efficacy of a single-session goal-pursuit intervention for college students. *Journal of Happiness Studies, 13*, 745–759.

Gallagher, M. W., & Lopez, S. J. (2009). Positive expectancies and mental health: Identifying the unique contributions of hope and optimism. *The Journal of Positive Psychology, 4*, 548–556.

Heaven, P., & Ciarrochi, J. (2008). Parental styles, gender and the development of hope and self-esteem. *European Journal of Personality, 22*(8), 707–724.

IBM Corp. Released (2014). IBM SPSS Statistics for Windows, Version 23.0. Armonk, NY: IBM Corp.

Jackson, L. T. B., van de Vijver, F. J. R., & Fouché, R. (2014). Psychological strengths and subjective well-being in South African white students. *Journal of Psychology in Africa, 24*(4), 299–307.

Jafari, E., Najafi, M., Sohrabi, F., Dehshiri, G. R., Soleymani, E., & Heshmati, R. (2010). Life satisfaction, spirituality well-being and hope in cancer patients. *Procedia – Social and Behavioral Sciences, 5*, 1362–1366.

Kornadt, A. E., Voss, P., & Rothermund, K. (2015). Hope for the best, prepare for the worst? Future self-views and preparation for age-related changes. *Psychology and Aging, 30*(4), 967–976.

Kortte, K. B., Stevenson, J. E., Hosey, M. M., Castillo, R., & Wegener, S. T. (2012). Hope predicts positive functional role outcomes in acute rehabilitation populations. *Rehabilitation Psychology, 57*, 248–255.

Luhmann, M., Hofmann, W., Eid, M., & Lucas, R. E. (2012). Subjective well-being and adaptation to life events: A meta-analysis on differences between cognitive and affective well-being. *Journal of Personality and Social Psychology, 102*(3), 592–615.

Lyubomirsky, S., & Lepper, H. S. (1999). A measure of subjective happiness: Preliminary reliability and construct validation. *Social Indicators Research, 46*(2), 137–155.

Marques, S. C., Lopez, S. H., & Pais-Ribeiro, J. L. (2011). "Building hope for the future": A program to foster strengths in middle-school students. *Journal of Happiness Studies, 12*, 139–152.

Martínez-Marti, M. L., & Ruch, W. (2014). Character strengths and well-being across the life span: Data from a representative sample of German-speaking adults living in Switzerland. *Frontiers of Psychology, 5*, 1–10.

McGrath, R. E., Rashid, T., Park, N., & Peterson, C. (2010). Is optimal functioning a distinct state? *The Humanistic Psychologist, 38*, 159–169.

Parse, R. (1999). *Hope: An international human becoming perspective*. Boston: Jones and Bartlett.

Perrig-Chiello, P. (2011). Glücklich oder bloss zufrieden? Hintergründe und Fakten zum Paradoxon des Wohlbefindens im Alter. In A. Holenstein, R. Meyer Schweizer, P. Perrig-Chiello, et al. (Eds.), *Glück. Berner Universitätsschriften* (pp. 241–255). Bern, CH: Haupt.

Perrig-Chiello, P. (2016). Glück und Zufriedenheit im Alter. *Punktum. Zeitschrift des Schweizerischen Berufsverbandes für Angewandte Psychologie, 2*, 18–20.

Perrig-Chiello, P., & Hutchison, S. (2010). Health and well-being in old age – The pertinence of a gender mainstreaming approach in research. *Gerontology, 56*(2), 208–213.

Ryff, C. (1995). The structure of psychological well-being revisited. *Journal of Personality and Social Psychology, 69*(4), 719–727.

Ryff, C. D. (2014). Psychological well-being revisited: advances in science and practice. *Psychotherapy & Psychosomatics, 83*(1), 10–28.

Schumacher, J. (2003). SWLS–satisfaction with life scale. In U. Ravens-Sieberer & M. Bullinger (Eds.), *Diagnostische Verfahren zu Lebensqualität und Wohlbefinden* (pp. 305–309). Goettingen, DE: Hogrefe.

Snyder, C. R. (2002). Hope theory: Rainbows in the mind. *Psychological Inquiry, 13*, 249–275.

Snyder, C. R., Irving, L. M., & Anderson, J. R. (1991). *Handbook of social and clinical psychology: The health perspective, Pergamon General Psychology Series, 162*. Richmond, VA: Pergamon.

Snyder, C. R., Lehman, K. A., Kluck, B., & Monsson, Y. (2006). Hope for rehabilitation and vice versa. *Rehabilitation Psychology, 51*, 89–112.

Snyder, C. R., Lopez, S. J., Shorey, H. S., Rand, K. L., & Feldman, D. B. (2003). Hope: Theory, measurements and applications to school psychology. *School Psychology Quarterly, 18*(2), 122–139.

Steel, M. (2016). *Measuring national well-being: At what age is personal well-being the highest?* UK Office of National Statistics. Retrieved August, 26, 2017, from https://www.ons.

gov.uk/peoplepopulationandcommunity/wellbeing/articles/measuringnationalwellbeing/
atwhatageispersonalwellbeingthehighest

Steger, M. F., Frazier, P., Oishi, S., & Kaler, M. (2006). The meaning in life questionnaire:
Assessing the presence of and search for meaning in life. *Journal of Counseling Psychology,*
53(1), 80–93.

Steptoe, A., Deaton, A., & Stone, A. A. (2015). Psychological wellbeing, health and ageing.
Lancet, 385(9968), 640–648.

Stone, A., Schwartz, J. E., Broderick, J. E., & Deaton, A. (2010). A snapshot of the age distribution of psychological well-being in the United States. *Proceedings of the National Academy of*
Sciences of the USA, 107(22), 9985–9990.

Sung, Y., Turner, S. L., & Kaewchinda, M. (2013). Career development skills, outcomes, and hope
among college students. *Journal of Career Development, 40*(2), 127–145.

Sutin, A. R., Terracciano, A., Milaneschi, Y., An, Y., Ferrucci, L., & Zonderman, A. B. (2013).
Cohort effects on well-being: The legacy of economic hard times. *Psychological Science,*
24(3), 379–385.

Tutton, E., Seers, K., & Langstaff, D. (2009). An exploration of hope as a concept for nursing.
Journal of Orthopaedic Nursing, 13(3), 119–127.

Umphrey, L. R., & Sherblom, J. C. (2014). The relationship of hope to self-compassion, relational social skill, communication apprehension, and life satisfaction. *International Journal of*
Wellbeing, 4(2), 1–18.

Urry, H. L., & Gross, J. J. (2010). Emotion regulation in older age. *Current Directions in*
Psychological Science, 19(6), 352–357.

Chapter 5
How Marital Status Is Related to Subjective Well-Being and Dispositional Hope

Stefanie Spahni and Pasqualina Perrig-Chiello

Intimate Partnership and Well-Being

Despite the significant decrease of marriage rate in the past decades, the majority of young adults still wishes to have a lasting intimate partnership (Perrig-Chiello, 2012). From birth on, close relationships are crucial for our survival. They are essential for our development and promote individual happiness over a lifetime (Perrig-Chiello, 2017). Having an intimate relationship is an important source of support. It is relevant for individual's psychological and social well-being but also for physical health.

Due to the increase in life expectancy, marriages entered in younger age can nowadays potentially last longer than ever before. The increasing divorce rate in long-term marriages however suggests, that this is rather perceived as a challenge than as a chance. In addition, expectations regarding the quality of the marriage have significantly risen. It has also been shown that the quality of and satisfaction with the relationship can harm or promote our health and subjective well-being (Hetherington, 2003). This is the case for ongoing relationships, but also after marital breakups and losses. It could be shown that having a supportive relationship is predictive for better well-being even after its loss (Spahni, Bennett, & Perrig-Chiello, 2016).

Considering the beneficial effect of intimate partnerships on well-being and health, spousal losses and breakups can be seen as critical life events. At the same time, such events are inevitable. Common to all is that they attack the person-environment fit causing uncertainty and emotional imbalance affecting health, well-being and everyday functioning. It has been shown that death of a spouse,

S. Spahni (✉) · P. Perrig-Chiello
Institute of Psychology, Developmental Psychology,
University of Bern, Bern, Switzerland
e-mail: stefanie.spahni@psy.unibe.ch

divorce and marital separation are rated as the most stressful life events (Holmes & Rahe, 1967). In fact, marital transitions usually entail detrimental affective, cognitive, behavioural and psychosomatic reactions (Stroebe, Schut, & Stroebe, 2007). Dependent on the type of loss differential effects on well-being can be observed. A meta-analysis by Luhmann, Hofmann, Eid, and Lucas (2012) revealed rather negative effects on affective well-being (i.e. more negative affects, lower happiness, higher depression rates) for divorce, whereas bereavement was associated with stronger and more long-lasting effects on cognitive well-being (i.e. decreased life satisfaction). Differences in well-being depending on marital status are also reported by the American Gallup-Healthways Study that considered various indicators. Accordingly, married individuals report the highest overall well-being scores, while divorced and separated individuals have the lowest ones (Brown & Jones, 2012). Furthermore Clark, Diener, Georgellis, and Lucas (2008) compared the effects of different life events on life satisfaction using 20 waves of the German Socio-Economic Panel data. They provide evidence for a negative impact on life satisfaction long before the actual event of the divorce or bereavement occurred, may it be caused by marital conflicts or spousal disease, and which was measurable up to 2 years after the event.

Taken together we can say that there seems to be a differential impact of marital breakup and marital bereavement on well-being outcomes. However, the determinants of this finding is still unclear.

The Role of Personal Resources

Although the consequences of marital break-up and loss on psychological, social, and physical well-being are in general negative, there is a great variability in the extent and the adaptation process. These individual differences depend on personal and social resources (Spahni, Morselli, Perrig-Chiello, & Bennett, 2015; Halford & Sweeper, 2013; Knoepfli, Morselli, & Perrig-Chiello, 2016; Lucas, Clark, Georgellis, & Diener, 2003; Pudrovska & Carr, 2008; Wang & Amato, 2000). The majority of empirical results can be explained by the prominent well-established paradigm, the vulnerability-stress model (Wittchen & Hoyer, 2006). According to this model, biological, psychological and social/contextual factors explain the reaction to stressful life experience. Depending on the available protective factors and the experienced stress, a person is more or less vulnerable. While good personal resources can protect against adverse consequences, poor or missing resources increase vulnerability and therefore the risk of enduring psychological impairment (Ingram & Luxton, 2005). In the same vein, Amato proposed a divorce-stress-adjustment model, according to which the impact of marital breakup on people's psychological health depends largely on protective factors, especially on individual resources (personality variables such as emotional stability) and social (having a supportive social network) ones (Amato, 2000).

As for bereavement Stroebe et al. (2007) give a review on potential risk and protective factors. Similar to the above mentioned theoretical models, the authors differentiate between personal (intrapersonal, interpersonal) and non-personal resources, and circumstances of death as relevant determinants of recovery from loss experience.

Although the particular importance of personal resources for coping with negative life events has been emphasized in literature, little is known about the interdependence of personality variables such as optimism, dispositional hope, psychological well-being and life satisfaction after divorce or bereavement. Dispositional hope as well as optimism were found to be associated with better positive well-being outcomes when facing adverse life events (Goodman, Disabato, Kashdan, & Machell 2017; Michael & Snyder, 2005). Both concepts refer to positive expectations about one's future, however they are not interchangeable (Bryant & Cvengros, 2004; Gallagher & Lopez, 2009). Optimism refers to the expectation that one's own outcomes will generally be positive, it incorporates a belief that a stressful present can change to become better in the future (Carver & Scheier, 2014). A large majority of evidence has shown the beneficial effect of optimism in many life domains. However there are significant gaps in knowledge concerning its role in moderating negative life events such as marital breakup or loss. In contrast to optimism, which is thought to be relevant in situations allowing for little personal control, dispositional hope plays a crucial role within situations allowing for higher levels of control. Dispositional hope is defined as a cognitive set that includes agency and pathways (Snyder et al., 1991). Pathways thinking refers to developing different ways to handle issues, whereas agency is about motivation to pursue the different options for addressing problems. Similar to optimism the role of dispositional hope for adjusting to these negative life events is understudied. In fact most research on hope has been carried out with children, youth or college students.

Another important resource for adapting to spousal loss or breakup is social support, since both events are usually associated with a decline in emotional (and maybe also instrumental) support. The ability to form new supportive relationships or to intensify available networks, is relevant for compensation. However, the ability to get new positive relations and to accept support is very individual, and also related to one's personality. Although the beneficial effect of social support has been widely acknowledged in research, little is known about its differential effect on marital loss and breakup.

In this contribution, we want to address some of the research gaps mentioned above. In order to have a more comprehensive view of well-being we will consider various indicators: emotional dimension (depression), cognitive dimension (life satisfaction), social dimension (loneliness), and physical dimension (subjective health). As for the personal and social resources, we focus on three variables: positive relations, dispositional hope, and optimism.

Aims

Considering the current state of research and based on data from the Swiss Hope-Barometer, this contribution aims at:

- analyzing how several indicators of subjective well-being – i.e. cognitive (life satisfaction), social (loneliness), affective (depression), and physical (subjective health) – differ by marital status.
- exploring to what extent marital status groups, namely being married, divorced or widowed, differ with regard to intrapersonal resources, i.e. dispositional hope and optimism, as well as social resources (positive relations).
- examining the predictive effect of these resources for well-being.

Method

Procedure and Sample

Data stem from the Hope-Barometer 2015 collected in the German and French speaking part of Switzerland. A total of 9103 participants fully answered the questionnaire. We focus on the 3607 participants aged 18 or older, who indicated their marital status as married (80%, n = 2884), separated/divorced (16.9%, n = 611) or widowed (3.1%, n = 112). The married ones are used as controls to contextualize the well-being outcomes of the two loss groups. The sample description is reported in Table 5.1.

Table 5.1 Demographic characteristics of the sample

	Total n (%)	Married n (%)	Break-up[a] n (%)	Widowed n (%)	Group comparison[b]
Gender					***
Male	1611 (44.7)	1377 (47.7)	203 (33.2)	31 (27.2)	
Female	1996 (55.3)	1507 (52.3)	408 (66.8)	81 (72.8)	
Age group					***
18–39	1015 (28.1)	920 (31.9)	88 (14.4)	7 (6.3)	
40–59	1857 (51.5)	1418 (49.2)	393 (64.3)	46 (41.1)	
60 >	735 (20.4)	546 (18.9)	130 (21.3)	59 (52.7)	
Educational level					**
Primary	413 (11.4)	316 (11.0)	80 (13.1)	17 (15.2)	
Secondary	1593 (44.2)	1244 (43.1)	299 (48.9)	50 (44.6)	
Tertiary	1578 (43.7)	1308 (45.4)	225 (36.8)	45 (40.2)	
Having children	2865 (79.4)	2278 (79.0)	500 (81.8)	87 (77.7)	*ns*

[***]$p < 0.001$, [**]$p < 0.01$, ns = non significant

[a]Break-up = separated or divorced

[b]Group comparisons were made using Pearson Chi-Square Tests

Group comparisons in Table 5.1 show that the proportion of women is significantly higher in the two loss groups than in the married. While married ones are more likely to be in the younger age group, separated/divorced individuals show a higher proportion in the middle, and widowed individuals in the old age group. Education is not equally distributed, separated/divorced are more likely to report education on secondary level. The proportion of individuals having children does not differ by marital status.

Measures

Well-Being

- Life satisfaction was assessed with the Satisfaction With Life Scale (Diener, Emmons, Larsen, & Griffin, 1985; Schumacher, 2003), with 5 items rated on a 7-point scale from 1 'completely disagree' to 7 'completely agree' (Cronbach's alpha .90).
- Loneliness was measured with the Three-Item Loneliness Scale (Hughes, Waite, Hawkley, & Cacioppo, 2004), containing questions answered on a 5-point scale as 1 'never', 2 'hardly ever', 3 'some of the time', 4 'often', 5 'all of the time' (Cronbach's alpha .88).
- Depression was assessed with the Patient Health Questionnaire for Depression and Anxiety (PHQ-4) (Kroenke, Spitzer, Williams, & Löwe, 2009), containing 4 items rated on a 4-point scale from 0 'not at all' to 3 'nearly every day' (Cronbach's alpha .87).
- Subjective health was measured with a single item 'How would you rate your physical health status?', indicated on a 6-point likert scale from 1 'I am seriously ill' to 6 'I am totally healthy'.

Resources

- Dispositional hope was assessed with the Adult Dispositional Hope Scale (Snyder et al., 1991), containing two subscales for 'agency' and 'pathways', each measured with 4 items rated on a 6-point scale from 0 'definitely false' to 5 'definitely true'. The total score of both subscales was used as hope scale (Cronbach's alpha .91).
- Optimism was measured with the Life Orientation Test (LOT-R, without the four filler items) (Scheier, Carver, & Bridges, 1994) with 3 items for optimism and 3 for pessimism rated on a 6-point scale from 1 'strongly disagree' to 6 'strongly agree' (Cronbach's alpha .76).
- Positive relations is a subscale from the Ryff's Scales of Psychological Well-Being (Ryff & Keyes, 1995; Springer & Hauser, 2006). Four positive and 5 negative items were indicated on a 6-point Likert scale from 1 'strongly disagree' to 6 'strongly agree' (Cronbach's alpha .81).

Data Analysis

Firstly, we compared the separated/divorced and widowed group with the married one with regard to the well-being indicators, and personal and social resources. Second, the predictive role of the resources for well-being was assessed.

The two loss groups were compared with married individuals regarding well-being (life satisfaction, loneliness, depression, physical health), and resources (dispositional hope, optimism, positive relations) using Analysis Of Variance (ANOVA), followed by post-hoc tests with Games-Howell correction, because data did not meet the homogeneity of variances assumption, very likely caused by the very unequal group sizes. Multiple stepwise regression analyses were used to examine how far the selected resources predict the various indicators of subjective well-being. Predictors were entered in two steps with (1) marital status and demographics: age group, gender, educational level and (2) resources: dispositional hope, optimism, and positive relations. Effect size f from Cohen (1992) is calculated, with $f \geq 0.10$ for small, $f \geq 0.25$ medium, and $f \geq 0.40$ large effects. Analyses were made using IBM SPSS Advanced Statistics 23.

Results

Well-Being by Marital Status

The main effects of the group membership are significant for all four well-being indicators (all $p < .001$) with medium to small effect sizes (life satisfaction $f = 0.27$, loneliness $f = 0.14$, depression $f = 0.12$, physical health $f = 0.10$). Life satisfaction significantly differs between all three groups: Married individuals report higher satisfaction than the widowed group ($p < .05$) which both in turn show higher values than the breakup group (both $p < .001$). Regarding loneliness and depression, there are significant differences only between the married and the separated/divorced group, with higher values in the latter one (both $p < .001$). The widowed group shows values in loneliness and depression in between the married and separated/divorced group, and none of the differences is significant. Nevertheless, the widowed show lower physical health than the married ones ($p < .001$), while they do not differ significantly from the separated/divorced. Because widowed individuals are more often in older age, which in turn is assumed to be associated with more physical complaints, further analysis considering age were conducted. Two-way analysis of variance shows a significant main effect of marital status ($F(2, 3587) = 3.76$, $p < .05$), but a non-significant effect of age ($F(6, 3587) = 1.86$, $p = 0.08$) on subjective physical health. Means and standard deviations of all well-being indicators by marital status are presented in Fig. 5.1.

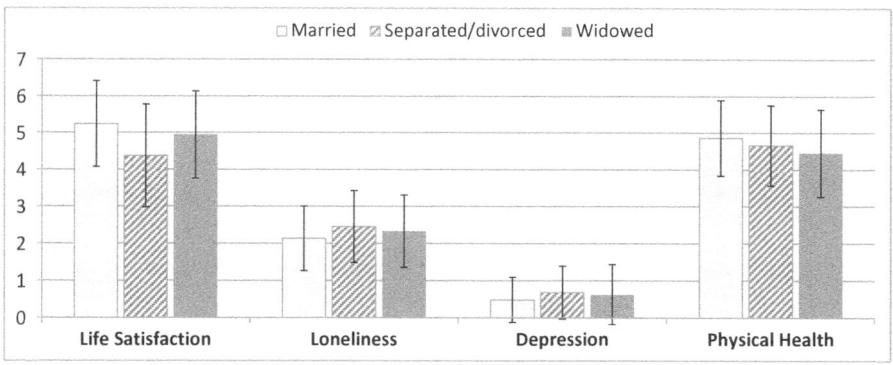

Fig. 5.1 Well-being indicators compared by marital status. Range: Life Satisfaction 1–7, Loneliness 1–5, Depression 0–3, Physical health 1–6

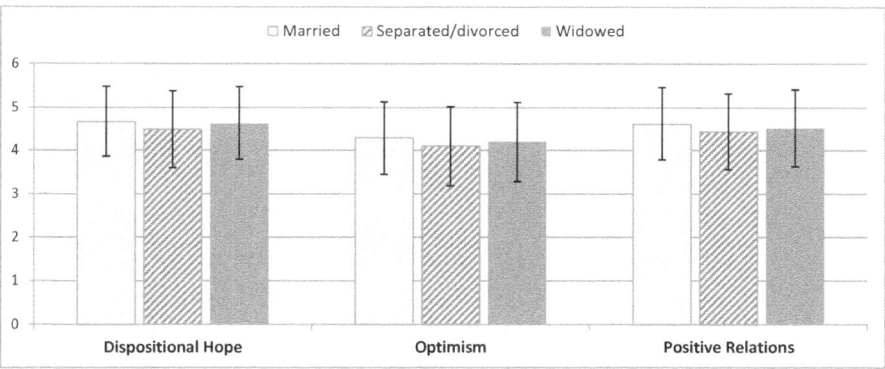

Fig. 5.2 Resources compared by marital status. Range: Dispositonal Hope 0–5, Optimism 1–6, Positive Relations 1–6

Resources by Marital Status

Marital status shows also highly significant main effects regarding the available resources (all $p < .001$), but only with very small effect sizes (all $f = 0.08$). The post hoc tests show that the breakup group report lower dispositional hope, optimism, and positive relations than the married group ($p < .001$). The mean values of the widowed group do not differ either from the separated/divorced or from the married ones significantly (Fig. 5.2).

Table 5.2 Predictors of various indicators of well-being

	Life satisfaction		Loneliness		Depression		Physical Health	
	Model 1	Model 2	Model 1	Model 2	Model 1	Model 2	Model 1	Model 2
Step 1								
Marital status								
Married[a]								
Separated/divorced	-0.26^{***}	-0.20^{***}	0.13^{***}	0.06^{***}	0.12^{***}	0.07^{***}	-0.05^{**}	-0.02
Widowed	-0.06^{***}	-0.04^{***}	0.05^{**}	0.03^{*}	0.07^{***}	0.05^{***}	-0.05^{**}	-0.04^{*}
Age group								
18–39[b]								
40–59	0.02	-0.02	-0.05^{**}	-0.01	-0.08^{***}	-0.04^{**}	-0.13^{***}	-0.15^{***}
60+	0.13^{***}	0.07^{***}	-0.11^{***}	-0.08^{***}	-0.22^{***}	-0.17^{***}	-0.16^{***}	-0.19^{***}
Gender (female)	0.05^{**}	0.03^{**}	0.05^{**}	0.13^{***}	0.01	0.02	0.00	-0.01
Educational level								
Primary[c]								
Secondary	0.07^{**}	0.04^{*}	-0.07^{*}	-0.01	-0.05^{*}	-0.03	0.04	0.03
Tertiary	0.23^{***}	0.08^{***}	-0.16^{***}	-0.00	-0.16^{***}	-0.02	0.13^{***}	0.07^{*}
Step 2								
Dispositional hope		0.34^{***}		-0.07^{***}		-0.22^{***}		0.09^{***}
Optimism		0.30^{***}		-0.16^{***}		-0.32^{***}		0.19^{***}
Positive relations		0.13^{***}		-0.57^{***}		-0.13^{***}		0.05^{*}
R^2	0.12	0.52	0.05	0.52	0.07	0.37	0.04	0.12
Change in R^2	0.12	0.40	0.05	0.47	0.07	0.30	0.04	0.08
F (change)	66.87	989.06	26.70	1178.98	36.91	569.76	20.12	106.11
df	7	3	7	3	7	3	7	3
p	$.000$	$.000$	$.000$	$.000$	$.000$	$.000$	$.000$	$.000$

Standardized coefficients (β) are reported
[a, b, c]Reference category
$^{***}p < .001,\ ^{**}p < .01,\ ^{*}p < .05$

The Predictive Effects of Resources for Well-Being

To examine how far the resources dispositional hope, optimism, and positive relations account for well-being, we calculated multiple stepwise regression analyses with the resources as predictors and the four well-being indicators life satisfaction, loneliness, depression and physical health as criteria. Predictors were entered in the model stepwise, first marital status and other demographics (age group, gender, educational level) (Step 1), followed by the three resources in Step 2. The results are presented in Table 5.2.

The resources explain more variance in all the well-being indicators than the demographics can and the total explained variance by all factors together is quite high, especially for life satisfaction (52%, $f = 1.04$) and loneliness (52%, $f = 1.04$) (depression 37%, $f = 0.77$; physical health 11%, $f = 0.35$). Moreover, when entering individual resources in Step 2, marital status remains a significant predictor. Compared to the comparison group of married ones, being separated/divorced is associated with higher negative effects on well-being than being widowed. The strongest predictors of life satisfaction are dispositional hope, optimism, and being separated/divorced (negatively). Loneliness is highly associated with lower positive relations, but also with lower optimism and being female. Depression is strongly predicted negatively by optimism, dispositional hope, and positive relations. In contrast to many other studies, there was no effect of gender for depression. The strongest predictors of physical health are optimism and being in middle or older age (negatively).

Discussion

In our analyses we examined how subjective well-being and health are affected by marital status and to what extent resources such a dispositional hope, optimism and social resources can explain these outcomes. Using various indicators of well-being we could show that: Being separated or divorced is associated with lower life satisfaction, higher loneliness, more depressive symptoms and lower physical health compared to married controls. Widowed individuals report in average lower life satisfaction than married ones, but higher values than the separated/divorced group. They do not differ significantly in loneliness and depression either from married or separated/divorced group, but they also report lower physical health compared to the married ones. This could be due to their higher proportion of individuals aged 60+, because physical complaints increase with age and are reflected in perceived subjective health.

We could further show that resources vary with marital status, however the effects are small: Separated and divorced individuals show significantly lower scores of dispositional hope, optimism, and positive relations compared to married ones. The widowed group again ranks between the married and the separated/ divorced group showing average values with no significant differences. After controlling for marital status, age, gender, and education, results from regression analyses show strong predictive effects of the three selected resources for the various well-being indicators. Dispositional hope and optimism are strongly associated with higher life satisfaction and lower depressive symptoms. Positive relations, on the other hand, are strongly related with lower feelings of loneliness. Furthermore, optimism is positively associated with subjective health.

Our results from the Hope-Barometer show, that the negative effect of separation and divorce on well-being is stronger and concerns more dimensions than widowhood. This is in line with the results of the American Gallup study (Brown & Jones, 2012).

Our study further shows, that widowed individuals report lower life satisfaction than the married ones, but do not differ in depression or loneliness. The meta-analysis of Luhmann et al. (2012) as well as the review of Diener, Suh, Lucas, and Smith (1999) both showed an impact of spousal bereavement on cognitive well-being initially worse and more persistent than on affective well-being. Cognitive and affective well-being are not equally responsive to life events and thus there are different interventions needed to influence these two components (Larsen & Prizmic, 2008). Efforts in policy addressing changes in people's life circumstances are assumed to be more relevant for cognitive well-being, while interventions that focus on individual activities are assumed to be more relevant for affective well-being (Luhmann et al., 2012). Both dimensions are essential for subjective well-being.

Differences between separated/divorced and widowed individuals can be based on the different causes these events have. While spousal death is mostly natural and unintentional, the reasons for marital break-up are mostly caused by personal deficits and lack of love. This is often more challenging for the individual to overcome. As Wilson and Gilbert (2008) propose, people adapt better as soon as they find an explanation for the event. Therefore especially separated and divorced individuals, but also bereaved ones with an unexpected loss, should be supported in finding new meaning in life with the help of their social network or by professional support in counseling practice and psychotherapy.

Even if on average the effect of marital breakup and loss on well-being is negative, there are large individual differences. Research shows different patterns of adaptation to divorce and bereavement. The majority succeeds in adapting to the new living situation over time, but there are also individuals with high risk factors and vulnerability for constant poor physical and psychological health (Spahni, Morselli, Perrig-Chiello, & Bennett, 2015; Bonanno, 2008; Knoepfli, Morselli, & Perrig-Chiello, 2016). Personal and social resources are essential for adaptation and maintenance of well-being, and trajectories depend on the available resources and the context of loss. Our results confirm that dispositional hope and optimism are crucial personal characteristics associated with better well-being after facing separation, divorce or death. Optimism as the tendency to look on the favorable side of an event and to expect the most favorable outcome can support individuals in finding meaning in their loss experience. Dispositional hope on the other hand, can enable individuals to evolve different strategies to handle the new life circumstances and strengthen the motivation to reach their goals. Social relations are a further important resource. Marital breakup or loss means losing and intimate relationship and the emotional support associated with it. Having other close relationships with friends or relatives can help compensate, reduce loneliness, and give support in handling daily life and stressors.

Although these findings help closing important research gaps, some limitations have to be considered. The Hope-Barometer 2015 is a cross-sectional study and does not allow for any causal conclusion. In the current work we considered only marital status and did not control, whether marriages are satisfying and if separated/divorced and widowed individuals are in a new relationship. We also could not controll for the time since and the context of loss (e.g. initiator status or expectedness of loss).

Conclusions

The protective effect of marriage is explained with the common life goals and the (emotional, social, instrumental) support received from the partner. The loss of a partner by separation/divorce or death therefore means a loss of support and challenges the individual in its self-view and view of life. Dispositional hope is confirmed as strong predictor of subjective well-being and assumed to be a crucial resource for promoting adaptation. It enables individuals reorientation, to find a way to new daily routine and desirable goals after a critical life event like marital breakup or loss and sould therefore be promoted.

References

Amato, P. R. (2000). The consequences of divorce for adults and children. *Journal of Marriage and the Family, 62*, 1269–1287. https://doi.org/10.1111/j.1741-3737.2000.01269.x

Bonanno, G. A. (2008). Loss, trauma, and human resilience: Have we underestimated the human capacity to thrive after extremely aversive events? *Psychological Trauma: Theory, Research, Practice, & Policy, S*(1), 101–113. https://doi.org/10.1037/0003-066X.59.1.20

Brown, S. L., & Jones, J. M. (2012). *Separation, divorce linked to sharply lower well- being.* http://www.gallup.com/poll/154001/Separation-Divorce-Linked-Sharply-Lower-Wellbeing.aspx?g_source=marital+status&g_medium=search&g_campaign=tiles

Bryant, F. B., & Cvengros, J. A. (2004). Distinguishing hope and optimism: Two sides of a coin, or two separate coins? *Journal of Social and Clinical Psychology, 23*, 273–302. https://doi.org/10.1521/jscp.23.2.273.31018

Carver, C. S., & Scheier, M. F. (2014). Dispositional optimism. *Trends in Cognitive Sciences, 18*(6), 293–299. https://doi.org/10.1016/j.tics.2014.02.003

Clark, A. E., Diener, E., Georgellis, Y., & Lucas, R. E. (2008). Lags and leads in life satisfaction: A test of the baseline hypothesis. *Economic Journal, 118*(529), 222–243. https://doi.org/10.1111/j.1468-0297.2008.02150.x

Cohen, J. (1992). A power primer. *Psychological Bulletin, 122*(1), 155–159.

Diener, E., Emmons, R. A., Larsen, R. J., & Griffin, S. (1985). The satisfaction with life scale. *Journal of Personality Assessment, 49*(1), 71–75.

Diener, E., Suh, E. M., Lucas, R. E., & Smith, H. L. (1999). Subjective well-being: Three decades of progress. *Psychological Bulletin, 125*(2), 276–302. https://doi.org/10.1037/0033-2909.125.2.276

Gallagher, M. W., & Lopez, S. J. (2009). Positive expectancies and mental health: Identifying the unique contributions of hope and optimism. *The Journal of Positive Psychology, 4*, 548–556. https://doi.org/10.1080/17439760903157166

Goodman, F. R., Disabato, D. J., Kashdan, T. B., & Machell, K. A. (2017). Personality strengths as resilience: A one-year multiwave study. *Journal of Personality, 85*(3), 423–434. https://doi.org/10.1111/jopy.12250

Halford, K. W., & Sweeper, S. (2013). Trajectories of adjustment to couple relationship separation. *Family Process, 52*(2), 228–243. https://doi.org/10.1111/famp.12006

Hetherington, E. M. (2003). Intimate pathways: Changing patterns in close personal rela- tionships across time. *Family Relations, 52*, 318–331.

Holmes, T. H., & Rahe, R. H. (1967). Social readjustment rating scale. *Journal of Psychosomatic Research, 11*(2), 213–218. https://doi.org/10.1016/0022-3999(67)90010-4

Hughes, M. E., Waite, L. J., Hawkley, L. C., & Cacioppo, J. T. (2004). A short scale for measuring loneliness in large surveys: Results from two population-based studies. *Research on Aging, 26*(6), 655–672. https://doi.org/10.1177/0164027504268574

Ingram, R. E., & Luxton, D. D. (2005). Vulnerability-stress models. In B. L. Hankin & J. R. Z. Abela (Eds.), *Development of psychopathology: A vulnerability stress perspective* (pp. 32–46). Thousand Oaks, CA: Sage publications Inc.

Knoepfli, B., Morselli, D., & Perrig-Chiello, P. (2016). Trajectories of psychological adaptation to marital breakup after long-term marriage. *Gerontology, 62*, 541–552. https://doi.org/10.1159/000445056

Kroenke, K., Spitzer, R. L., Williams, J., & Löwe, B. (2009). An ultra-brief screening scale for anxiety and depression: The PHQ-4. *Psychosomatics, 50*, 613. https://doi.org/10.1176/appi.psy.50.6.613

Larsen, R. J., & Prizmic, Z. (2008). Regulation of emotional well-being: Overcoming the hedonic treadmill. In M. Eid & R. J. Larsen (Eds.), *The science of subjective well-being* (pp. 258–289). New York: Guilford Press.

Lucas, R. E., Clark, A. E., Georgellis, Y., & Diener, E. (2003). Reexamining adaptation and the set point model of happiness: Reactions to changes in marital status. *Journal of Personality and Social Psychology, 84*(3), 527–539. https://doi.org/10.1037/0022-3514.84.3.527

Luhmann, M., Hofmann, W., Eid, M., & Lucas, R. E. (2012). Subjective well-being and adaptation to life events: A meta-analysis. *Journal of Personality and Social Psychology, 102*(3), 592–615. https://doi.org/10.1037/a0025948

Michael, S. T., & Snyder, C. R. (2005). Getting unstuck: The roles of hope, finding meaning, and rumination in the adjustment to bereavement among college students. *Death Studies, 29*(5), 435–458. https://doi.org/10.1080/07481180590932544

Perrig-Chiello, P. (2012). Familienglück – eine zwingende Option? Junge Erwachsene vor der grossen und entscheidenden Frage. In P. Perrig-Chiello, F. Hoepflinger, A. Spillmann, & C. Kuebler (Eds.), *Familienglück – Was ist das?* (pp. 117–125). Zurich, Switzerland: NZZ Libero.

Perrig-Chiello, P. (2017). *Wenn die Liebe nicht mehr jung ist – Warum viele langjährige Partnerschaften zerbrechen und andere nicht.* Bern, Switzerland: Hogrefe.

Pudrovska, T., & Carr, D. (2008). Psychological adjustment to divorce and widowhood in mid- and later life: Do coping strategies and personality protect against psychological distress? *Advances in Life Course Research, 13*, 283–317. https://doi.org/10.1016/S1040-2608(08)00011-7

Ryff, C. D., & Keyes, C. L. M. (1995). The structure of psychological well-being revisited. *Journal of Personality and Social Psychology, 69*(4), 719–727. https://doi.org/10.1037/0022-3514.69.4.719

Scheier, M. F., Carver, C. S., & Bridges, M. W. (1994). Distinguishing optimism from neuroticism (and trait anxiety, self-mastery, and selfesteem) – A revaluation of the life orientation test. *Journal of Personality and Social Psychology, 67*, 1063–1078. https://doi.org/10.1037/0022-3514.67.6.1063

Schumacher, J. (2003). SWLS - satisfaction with life scale. In J. Schumacher, A. Klaiberg, & E. Brähler (Eds.), *Diagnostische Verfahren zu Lebensqualität und Wohlbefinden (Diagnostik für Klinik und Praxis, Band 2)* (pp. 305–309). Göttingen, Germany: Hogrefe.

Snyder, C. R., Harris, C., Anderson, J. R., Holleran, S. A., Irving, L. M., Sigmon, S. T., et al. (1991). The will and the ways – Development and validation of an individual-differences measure of hope. *Journal of Personality and Social Psychology, 60*(4), 570–585. https://doi.org/10.1037/0022-3514.60.4.570

Spahni, S., Bennett, K. M., & Perrig-Chiello, P. (2016). Psychological adaptation to spousal bereavement in old age. The role of trait resilience, marital history, and context of death. *Death Studies., 40*, 182. https://doi.org/10.1080/07481187.2015.1109566

Spahni, S., Morselli, D., Perrig-Chiello, P., & Bennett, K. M. (2015). Patterns of psychological adaptation to spousal bereavement in old age. Gerontology, 61, 456–468. https://doi.org/10.1159/000371444

Springer, K. W., & Hauser, R. M. (2006). An assessment of the construct validity of Ryff's scales of psychological well-being: Method, mode, and measurement effects. *Social Science Research, 35*(4), 1080–1102. https://doi.org/10.1016/j.ssresearch.2005.07.004

Stroebe, M. S., Schut, H., & Stroebe, W. (2007). Health outcomes of bereavement. The Lancet, 370(9603), 1960–1973. https://doi.org/10.1016/S0140-6736(07)61816-9

Wang, H. Y., & Amato, P. R. (2000). Predictors of divorce adjustment: Stressors, resources, and definitions. *Journal of Marriage and the Family, 62*(3), 655–668. https://doi.org/10.1111/j.1741-3737.2000.00655.x

Wilson, T. D., & Gilbert, D. T. (2008). Explaining away: A model of affective adaptation. *Perspectives on Psychological Science, 3*, 370–386. https://doi.org/10.1111/j.1745-6924.2008.00085.x

Wittchen, H.-U., & Hoyer, J. (2006). Was ist Klinische Psychologie? Definitionen, Konzepte und Modelle. In H.-U. Wittchen & J. Hoyer (Eds.), *Klinische Psychologie & Psychotherapie* (2nd ed., pp. 3–25). Heidelberg: Springer.

Chapter 6
The Association Between Spirituality/Religiosity and Well-Being in Young, Middle and Old Age in Switzerland

Katja Margelisch

Introduction

It is widely assumed that religiosity and spirituality play a positive role in providing a sense of identity and hope, a network of social support, and a coherent framework for responding to existential questions (Elliott & Hayward, 2007). This framework can help people to cope with critical life events or illness (Ivtzan, Chan, Gardner, & Prashar, 2013), and lead to a sense of shared understanding of a loss (Ellens, 2007). Yet, individuals who take their religions seriously can also exhibit poorer mental health (Greenway, Phelan, Turnbull, & Milne, 2007), because it can be judgemental and exclusive (Williams & Sternthal, 2007). As a consequence, it can lead to stress or guilt.

There have been different reviews on the various mechanisms through which religion is beneficial as well as detrimental, on specific aspects of psychological health (e.g. Bonelli & Koenig, 2013; Koenig, 2009, 2015). Recent research that has more finely delineated the constructs of religion and spirituality points to a largely positive association with psychological well-being (Hill & Pargament, 2008). However, most of the studies were conducted in the United States, whereas research about the connection of religiosity and spirituality to well-being hardly exists in Switzerland. This chapter deals with the question of how important religiosity and spirituality are for persons in Switzerland from young adulthood to old age and how they are related to subjective well-being and health.

The chapter is structured as follows: First, the concepts of religiosity and spirituality were defined, followed by theoretical considerations concerning the association of religiosity/spirituality and well-being and the role of age and gender in this association. Second, in the empirical part, data of the "Swiss Hope-Barometer 2015" (on the topics religiosity/spirituality and well-being in young, middle and old age) were analysed and discussed. The chapter closes with important conclusions for research and practice.

K. Margelisch (✉)
Institute of Psychology, Developmental Psychology, University of Bern, Bern, Switzerland
e-mail: katja.margelisch@psy.unibe.ch

© Springer International Publishing AG, part of Springer Nature 2018   109
A. M. Krafft et al. (eds.), *Hope for a Good Life*, Social Indicators Research
Series 72, https://doi.org/10.1007/978-3-319-78470-0_6

Theoretical Background

Conceptualisation of Religiosity and Spirituality

In the last century, a variety of classifications of the two terms, religion and spirituality, were witnessed, but there was no explicit distinction between the two (Ivtzan et al., 2013). This lack of consensus has presented a critical challenge in the field. A degree of agreement is necessary to produce consistent findings to allow for progress (Zinnbauer & Pargament, 2005). Through the rise of secularism in the middle of the last century, spirituality became separated from religion and began to acquire distinct connotations. Due to its association with the individual experiences of the transcendent, spirituality began to be regarded in a more positive light, while religion, with its formal structure and prescribed rituals restricted such experiences (e.g. Miller & Thoresen, 2003; Zinnbauer & Pargament, 2005).

According to Ellens (2008), spirituality describes an inner, personal experience that provides a strong interest in understanding the meaning of things in life. This makes spirituality the longing or internal motivation to seek out anything beyond the merely empirical, be that religious or otherwise (Ellens, 2008). Religion involves practices engaged in by members of a social organisation (Miller & Thoresen, 2003), which refers to the outward worship, creeds, and theology, which reflect an understanding of the devine and the world (Ellens, 2008).

However, often religion and spirituality go hand in hand (Sheldrake, 2007). The two words are overlapping constructs that share some characteristics (Miller & Thoresen, 2003) and personality factors (Paloutzian & Park, 2005). Thus, the polarisation of religion and spirituality has been criticised by researchers. Hill et al. (2000) stated that both spirituality and religion are multidimensional and complex phenomena, and any single definition is likely to reflect a limited perspective. The authors argued that past attempts at defining the constructs have often either been too narrow, resulting in operational definitions that have produced empirical research with limited value, or too broad, resulting in a loss of a clear distinction between the two (Hill et al., 2000). Hill et al. (2000) have emphasised that the search for the sacred, which can be a divine being, a divine object, the ultimate reality or the ultimate truth, is central for spirituality as well as for religion. The search involves a number of processes, including the attempt to identify what is sacred, to maintain the sacred within the individual religious or spiritual experience, and finally to transform the sacred or modify it through a process of searching. Religion involves organised means and methods for the search for the sacred that are validated and supported by a community, whereas spirituality only necessitates the search for the sacred. Such a framework suggests that spirituality is an essential component of religion that often occurs within the context of religion. According to Ivtzan et al. (2013), religion must be said to be composed of (1) a spiritual core and (2) participation in religious activity, or religious involvement.

Theoretical Models Concerning the Association Between Religiosity/Spirituality and Well-Being

Previous research investigated the associations of religiosity/spirituality (R/S) and well-being (e.g., subjective well-being, self-rated health) in different cultures and ages. Subjective well-being can be defined as positive evaluation of one's life associated with good feelings (Pinquart & Sörensen, 2000). It is determined by emotional and cognitive components such as frequent positive affect, infrequent negative affect, and high life satisfaction (Diener, Suh, & Smith, 1999; Diener, Lucas, & Oishi, 2005). Much research has been devoted to investigating the impact of religiosity and spirituality on well-being within a *stress and coping framework*, which concerns the use of coping resources (e.g., belief in a higher power or social support network) in order to maintain the capacity to function in the face of a stressor (e.g., experiencing an illness or losing a spouse; see Pargament [1997] for a discussion). In this context, the R/S resource provides a buffer against the negative impact of a stressor on well-being (Ellison, 1991).

Another view concerning the impact of religiosity and spirituality on well-being is the *resiliency framework*, which goes beyond the specific context of coping with a stressor and emphasizes the building of adaptive resources that are available in times of need (Masten, 2001). Resiliency theory concerns the presence of risk factors (e.g., trauma, chronic stress) and resilience resources (e.g., social support, a hardy personality, a strong faith), and how the negative outcomes generally associated with vulnerabilities can be ameliorated or even eliminated by the presence of these protective factors (Masten, 2001). Although R/S can be conceptualized as either resiliency or coping resources, they are considered to be resiliency resources in the present context, because the association of these factors with well-being on a global level are of interest, not only within the context of stress.

So far, the evidence suggests that religion offers a moderate, protective effect on mental and physical health, as well as subjective well-being (Koenig, McCullough, & Larson, 2001). Research from the US and Western Europe shows a small, inverse association between religious engagement and negative psychological outcomes. For an example, a meta-analysis of 147 studies revealed a small, but statistically significant relationship ($r = 0.10$, $p < 0.001$) between religiosity and depressive symptoms (Smith, McCullough, & Poll, 2003). A second meta-analysis of studies on religiosity and psychological adjustment (including psychological distress) found that the overall association between a number of types of religiosity and psychological adjustment was $r = 0.10$, $p < 0.001$ (Hackney & Sanders, 2003). While the overall associations are positive, numerous studies have found no association between R/S and well-being (e.g., Maselko & Kubzansky, 2006).

In positive psychology, R/S is defined and measured as a *character strength*. Character strengths have become important topics of research in positive psychology (Dahlsgaard, Peterson, & Seligman, 2005), and are defined as positively valued trait-like individual differences with demonstrable generality across different situations and stability across time (Peterson & Seligman, 2004). As individual differences, strengths are not either present or absent, but exist in degrees (Park & Peterson, 2009). Character strengths manifest in the range of individual thoughts, feelings, and behaviours. They are recognised and desired across cultures (Peterson & Seligman, 2004). Peterson and Seligman derived their classification from an extensive review of literature in different areas (e.g., philosophy, psychology, popular culture, and religion).

The Association Between R/S and Well-Being in Older Age

Interestingly, in younger adults, the character strength of R/S seems to be related neither to the cognitive component of subjective well-being and life satisfaction (cf., Ruch, Proyer, & Weber, 2010), nor to the affective component of positive affect (Azañedo, Fernández-Abascal, & Barraca 2014), However, in older life questions concerning the meaning of life can step forward (cf. Ardelt, Landes, Gerlach, & Fox, 2013). Spirituality often provides a positive perspective for older adults (Ai, Wink, & Ardelt, 2010). Therefore, different empirical results confirm the correlation between spirituality and life satisfaction in later age (e.g., Tomer, Eliason, & Wong, 2008; Van Ranst & Marcoen, 2000). One theoretical explanation for the age differences of the associations between R/S and well-being could *be Erikson's theory of psychosocial development* (Erikson, 1982). Based on his account of the eight stages of psychosocial development it can be proposed that character strengths may help individuals adapt successfully to the different stages of life, and their relative importance might be reflected in their relationship with well-being (Martínez-Marti & Ruch, 2014).

According to Erikson, the goal of old age is to acknowledge the inalterability of the past (Erikson, Erikson, & Kivnick, 1986) and to accept the totality of one's life. People achieve integrity if they embrace the lives they have lived, including their own accomplishments and shortcomings. Elders who have discovered meaning and purpose in their lives tend to be less afraid of death and more willing to let go (Ardelt & Koenig, 2007). R/S can be used to generate existential meaning and forge connections to the larger universe while confronting senescence and death, helping aging adults to achieve a sense of both meaning and completion in relationship to themselves, others, and the transcendent realm (Staton, Shuy, & Byock, 2001).

Ageing is often considered a time of loss and decline (Cohen & Koenig, 2003), with a focus on decrease in physical function, mental capabilities, and the loss of friends and family members (MacKinlay, 2001). This focus tends to neglect exploration of ageing as a time of growth and vitality. Ageing can also be a period when an individual develops and grows, emotionally and spirituality (Shaw, Gullifer, & Wood, 2016). The *socioemotional selectivity theory* (Carstensen & Charles, 1998) proposes that as people age they invest more time in relationships that have meaning for them rather than in those that do not. Therefore, older people may have fewer relationships, but the ones they have will be strong and supportive (Cohen & Koenig, 2003). According to the theory, as people age they shift their focus from external goals such as career development, to internal goals such as spiritual development (Dalby, 2006).

In line with *Erikson's theory of psychosocial development* (Erikson, 1982) and the *socioemotional selectivity theory* (Carstensen & Charles, 1998), empirical research shows that older persons tend to be more religious than younger ones (e.g., Van Cappellen, Toth-Gauthier, Saroglou, & Fredrickson, 2016; Zimmer et al., 2016 for a review). However, on the one hand, this could be a function of cohort differences, with the current older generation coming from a background and a time where religion was valued to a greater degree and thus they carry those values into old age (Wilhelm, Rooney, & Tempel, 2007). On the other hand, there is evidence to suggest that people become more involved with religion and their sense of spirituality increases with age (Moberg, 2005; Wink & Dillon, 2001).

Religion and spirituality affect the physical and mental well-being of older adults, including satisfaction with the relationship they have with their family, friends and their chosen god (Cohen & Koenig, 2003). Older people tend to find a sense of control through their religion (Emery & Pargament, 2004), which may help bring meaning to their lives. This meaning may help them adjust to the changes that accompany ageing (Sadler & Biggs, 2006). Religion and spirituality can enhance one's relationship with one's god and can bring comfort and satisfaction in relationships that are developed within the church community (Yoon & Lee, 2004). The use of religion and spirituality to manage problems is not uncommon among older adults (Shaw et al., 2016). Some find comfort through prayer and support through their connections with other older adults who use similar coping mechanisms (Cohen & Koenig, 2003).

Religion has also been found to have a positive impact on disability and depression in older adults (Lavretsky, 2010). Correlation between R/S and health has been found to apply for example to cardiovascular conditions, chronic pain, cancer and self-rated overall health (e.g., Hank & Schaan, 2008; Hidajat, Zimmer, Saito, & Lin, 2013; Koenig, King, & Carson, 2012).

The Role of Gender in the Association Between R/S and Well-Being

Women are generally more religious than men (Maselko & Kubzansky, 2006) and there is some evidence from US studies that the association between R/S and well-being is not the same across genders (e.g., McCullough, Hoyt, Larson, Koenig, & Thoresen, 2000). The direction or magnitude of this difference is not clear and very few studies have examined gender in this context explicitly. Gender is most commonly treated as a potential confounder and statistically controlled for in analyses

(Thoresen & Harris, 2002). In the study by McCullough and Laurenceau (2005) on religion and self-rated health, no significant relationship was found between the one and the other among men. Several other studies on physical outcomes (notably mortality) have also found a stronger association between R/S and health among women than men (Koenig, 1999; McCullough et al., 2000). However, in the study by Maselko and Kubzansy (2006), public religious activity was associated with self-rated health, happiness, and lower psychological distress more among men than among women, whereas private religious activities were not significantly associated with any well-being outcomes for either gender. Spiritual experiences were associated with happiness in women, but not in men. Gender effects could not be explained through group differences in education income or other demographic factors (Maselko & Kubzansky, 2006). Although the role of gender in the association between R/S and well-being seems not to be clear at this time, it seems that different aspects of R/S could have a different influence on psychological and physical well-being in women and men.

Research Questions

1. What role does R/S play in the life of people in young adulthood, middle age and old age in Switzerland?
2. How is R/S associated with gender?
3. How is R/S associated with well-being and health at different ages?
4. Is there a gender difference in the association between R/S and well-being?

We Expect:

1. In accordance with empirical work (e.g., Van Cappellen et al., 2016; Zimmer et al., 2016), and according to Erikson's theory of psychosocial development (Erikson, 1982), as well as the theory of socioemotional selectivity (Carstensen & Charles, 1998), we assume R/S to be more pronounced in older age than in middle age and younger adulthood.
2. According to empirical results (e.g., Maselko & Kubzansky, 2006), R/S is more pronounced in women than in men.
3. Based on the theories of hypothesis 1 and empirical results (e.g., Ardelt et al., 2013; Ruch et al., 2010), we expect the correlation between R/S and well-being to be more pronounced in persons of older age, than in persons of middle age and younger adults.
4. In accordance with empirical research (e.g., Maselko & Kubzansky, 2006; McCullough & Laurenceau, 2005), we assume the correlation between R/S and well-being to be different for women and men.

Methods

Sample of the Hope-Barometer (2015)

The Hope-Barometer was launched in 2009. The internet survey is conducted annually. The 2015 Hope-Barometer survey questioned 9'103 people about their expectations of the coming year. Not included in the calculations for this book chapter were 560 persons less than 18 years old. The remaining sample consists of 8543 persons (3501 men and 5042 women). Most participants were Swiss ($n = 7572$, 89%), 971 had other nationalities other than Swiss. Most participants were married or in a relationship (n = 5332; 62%), 2488 were single (29%), 611 were separated or divorced (7%) and 112 were widowed. 4940 persons (58%) stated that they had no children, whereas 3603 said they had one or more children. Regarding the educational level, 1709 participants (20%) had completed tertiary education (e.g., university), 6320 (74%) had finished secondary education (e.g., vocational training or middle school), 540 (6%) had finished primary education and 64 had not yet completed their education.

Concerning religion, 2063 persons (24%) belonged to the Protestant church/ Evangelical reformed, 2498 (29%) to the Roman Catholic church, 406 (5%) to other Christian communities, 219 (2%) to Islamic communities, 65 (1%) to other churches and religious communities, 2616 (31%) had no religious affiliation, and 530 (6%) claimed to be spiritual, but outside the traditional world religions. Three age subgroups (according to Erikson's stages of psychosocial development) were created: The first group ($n = 4857$) comprised participants with ages ranging from 18 to 39 years (young adults), the second group ($n = 4857$) consisted of participants with ages ranging from 40 to 59 years ($n = 2744$, middle-aged group) and the third group ($n = 942$, older age) comprised participants with ages from 60 and older. The age distribution is shown in Table 6.1.

Instruments

Dependent Variable/Well-Being Measures

Cognitive aspect of subjective well-being: Life satisfaction was measured with the German version of the *Satisfaction with Life Scale* (SWLS; Diener, Emmons, Larsen, & Griffin 1985). The SWLS is a 5-item questionnaire for the subjective

Table 6.1 Age group distribution Hope-Barometer 2015

Age group	Female	Male	Total
18–39 years (young adulthood)	3184 (63.1%)	1673 (47.8%)	4857 (56.9%)
40–59 years (middle age)	1488 (35.9%)	1256 (35.9%)	2744 (32.1%)
60+ years (older age)	370 (7.3%)	572 (16.3%)	942 (11.0%)
	5042 (100%)	3501 (100%)	8543 (100%)

assessment of overall life satisfaction (e.g., "I am satisfied with my life"), utilising a 7-point answer format (from 1 = strongly disagree to 7 = strongly agree.). Cronbach's alpha in the present study was 0.89.

Affective aspect of subjective well-being: Happiness was measured with *The Subjective Happiness Scale* (SHS, Lyubomirsky & Lepper, 1999), using a 7-point answer format (from 1 = strongly disagree to 7 = strongly agree). Cronbach's alpha was 0.83. As a negative aspect of emotional well-being, depression/anxiety was measured by the *ultra-brief Depression/Anxiety Screening Scale* (PHQ-4; Kroenke, Spitzer, Williams, & Loewe, 2009), using a 4-point answer format (0 = not at all, 1 = several days, 2 = more than half the days, 3 = nearly every day).

Self-rated health is a measure that is regularly used and has been found predictive of future health events including mortality (e.g., Perruccio, Katz, & Losina 2012). In the present study, health status is measured through self-reported assessments of physical and psychological health. Respondents were asked to rate their actual physical and psychological health status on a Likert scale (1= "I am seriously ill", to 7 = "I am completely well"). A composite score of physical and psychological health items was computed.

Independent Variables: Measures of Religiosity/Spirituality

Spirituality was measured with the subscale Importance of Spiritual Beliefs in Life of the The Spirituality Questionnaire, (SQ; Parsian & Dunning, 2009), using a Likert scale from 1 = strongly disagree to 4 = strongly agree. Cronbach's alpha was 0.97. Religiosity was measured by five items of the ten-item scale of The Santa Clara Strength of Religious Faith Questionnaire (Plante & Boccaccini, 1997) on a Likert scale from 1 = strongly disagree to 4 = strongly agree. Principal component analysis showed an explained variation of 76.11%, and Cronbach's alpha was 0.92. Additionally, three different R/S activities (praying, going to church, trusting in a god) were investigated (scaled from 0 = not at all to 3 = very often). A composite score of the three measures was calculated; Cronbach's alpha for R/S activities was 0.85.

Results

Descriptive Analyses

The age distribution of the affiliation with religious groups is shown in Fig. 6.1. In the younger adult group (18–39 years) the Islamic religion is more represented than in the older age groups. Spirituality outside a world religion is more represented in the younger and middle adult group than in the older adult group (60+ years).

In Table 6.2, the means and standard deviations of the whole sample and the three age groups were shown. We carried out a series of one-way analyses of variance to explore differences in well-being between different age groups. Age groups

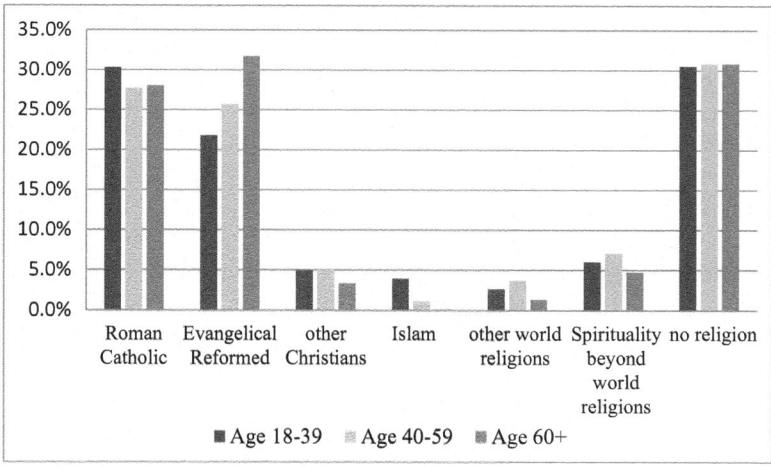

Fig. 6.1 Distribution of the affiliation with religious groups by age group

Table 6.2 Means and standard deviations of R/S and well-being indicators in the total sample, and across age groups

	Total		Age 18–39		Age 40–59		Age 60+	
	M	SD	M	SD	M	SD	M	SD
Well-being								
Life satisfaction (1–7)	4.86	1.31	4.75	1.33	4.92	1.32	5.28	1.12
Happiness (1–7)	4.93	1.34	4.77	1.36	5.08	1.32	5.46	1.12
Depression (0–3)	0.64	0.68	0.75	0.69	0.56	0.67	0.32	0.50
Health (1–7)	4.92	0.88	4.95	0.85	4.88	0.94	4.87	0.89
Religiosity/Spirituality								
R/S activities (0–3)	0.90	0.89	0.78	0.84	1.03	0.92	1.15	0.95
Religiosity (1–4)	1.73	0.86	1.64	0.82	1.82	0.89	1.94	0.92
Spirituality (1–4)	1.91	0.99	1.80	0.95	2.04	1.04	2.11	1.01

significantly differed in life satisfaction ($F(2,8540) = 68.98$, $p < 0.001$), happiness ($F(2,8540) = 124.17$, $p < 0.001$), depression ($F(2,8540) = 200.21$, $p < 0.001$), and health ($F(2,8540) = 7.32$, $p < 0.01$). Post hoc comparisons with Bonferroni correction showed that the 18–39 years group scored significantly lower in life satisfaction than the 40–59 years group ($d = 0.13$) and the 60+ years group ($d = 0.41$); and the 40–59 years group scored significantly lower in life satisfaction than the 60+ years group ($d = 0.28$), all p's < 0.001. The 18–39 years group also scored lower in happiness than the 40–59 years group ($d = 0.24$) and the 60+ years group ($d = 0.52$), as well as the 40–59 years group scored lower in happiness than the 60+ years group ($d = 0.30$), all p's < 0.001. The scores for depression/anxiety showed the reverse pattern: The 18–39 years group scored significantly higher in depression/anxiety than the 40–59 years group ($d = -0.28$), and the 60+ years group ($d = -0.65$), and the 40–59 years group scored significantly higher than the 60+ years group

($d = -0.38$), all p's < 0.001. In sum, older persons have higher levels of subjective well-being than younger persons. However, the 18–39 years group scored higher in subjective health than the 40–59 years group ($p < 0.01$, $d = -0.08$), and the 60+ group ($p < 0.05$, $d = -0.09$). No significant differences in subjective health were found between the 40–59 years and the 60+ years group.

Concerning gender differences across age groups, men scored significantly lower in depression than women ($t(8541) = -8.74$, $p < 0.001$, $d = 0.43$), and men scored higher in self-rated health than women $t(8541) = 3.49$, $p < 0.001$, $d = 0.08$). No gender differences were found in life satisfaction and happiness.

To investigate age differences in religiosity and spirituality, another series of one-way analyses of variances were calculated to explore differences between age groups. Age groups differed significantly in R/S activities ($F(2,8540) = 117.75$, $p < 0.001$), religiosity ($F(2,8540) = 73.05$, $p < 0.001$), and spirituality ($F(2,8540) = 73.02$, $p < 0.001$). Post hoc comparisons with the Bonferroni correction showed that the 18–39 years group scored significantly lower in R/S activities than the 40–59 years group ($p < 0.001$, $d = 0.29$), and the 60+ years group ($p < 0.001$, $d = 0.43$), whereas the 40–59 years group scored significantly lower than the 60+ years group ($p < 0.01$, $d = 0.31$). The 18–39 years group scored significantly lower in religiosity than the 40–59 years group ($p < 0.001$, $d = 0.29$), and the 60+ years group ($p < 0.001$, $d = 0.36$), whereas the 60+ group scored significantly higher in religiosity than the 40–59 years group ($p < 0.011$, $d = 0.13$). Finally, the 18–39 years group scored significantly lower in spirituality than the 40–59 years group ($p < 0.001$, $d = 0.24$), and the 60+ years group (($p < 0.001$, $d = 0.32$), whereas no significant differences between the 40–59 years and the 60+ years group were found.

Hypothesis 1 that R/S is more pronounced in older age than in middle age and younger adulthood can therefore be confirmed for R/S activities as well as for religiosity. However, age differences for spirituality were found only between young adults and middle-aged/older adults, but not between middle-aged and older adults.

In a next step, a series of *t*-tests were carried out to explore gender differences in R/S activities, religiosity and spirituality. In order to control for the number of comparisons performed, all significance levels were adjusted by the Bonferroni-Holm correction. The means and standard deviations for R/S activities, religiosity and spirituality for women and men in the whole sample and in the different age groups were shown in Table 6.3. In the whole sample, significant gender differences in R/S activities ($t(8541) = -4.95$, $p < 0.001$, $d = 0.11$) and in spirituality ($t(8541) = -2.43$, $p < 0.05$, $d = 0.05$) in favor of women were found, whereas the gender difference in religiosity did not reach significance level.

Concerning gender differences in the 18–39 years group, women scored significantly higher in R/S activities than men ($t(4855) = -3.28$, $p < 0.001$, $d = 0.10$), whereas no significant gender differences were found in religiosity and spirituality. In the 40–59 years group, women scored significantly higher than men in R/S activities ($t(2742) = -7.03$, $p = 0.003$, $d = 0.27$), in religiosity ($t(2742) = -4.51$, $p = 0.003$, $d = 0.17$), and spirituality ($t(2742) = -5.31$, $p = 0.003$, $d = 0.20$). In the

Table 6.3 Gender-related means and standard deviations of religiosity and spirituality in the total sample, and across the age groups

	R/S activities		Religiosity		Spirituality	
	Men	Women	Men	Women	Men	Women
	M (SD)	M (SD)	M (SD)	M (SD)	M (SD)	M (SD)
Whole sample	0.89 (0.90)	0.93 (0.88)	1.72 (0.87)	1.74 (0.85)	1.88 (0.99)	1.93 (1.00)
Age 18–39	0.72 (0.86)	0.80 (0.83)	1.63 (0.84)	1.64 (0.81)	1.78 (0.96)	1.81 (0.94)
Age 40–59	0.90 (0.91)	1.15 (0.92)	1.74 (0.88)	1.89 (0.90)	1.92 (1.02)	2.13 (1.06)
Age 60+	1.07 (0.95)	1.27 (0.94)	1.92 (0.93)	1.96 (0.89)	2.07 (1.00)	2.18 (1.02)

60+ years group, women scored significantly higher in R/S activities than men ($t(940) = -3.17$, $p = 0.006$, $d = 0.21$), whereas no significant gender differences were found in religiosity and spirituality.

Hypothesis 2 that R/S is more pronounced in women than in men, is confirmed for the 40–59 years group, whereas in the other age groups, gender differences in favor of women were only found for R/S activities, but not for religiosity and spirituality.

Correlations Between R/S and Well-Being

Correlations between R/S activities, religiosity and spirituality and the different well-being indicators (life satisfaction, happiness, depression/anxiety and self-rated health) on the total sample, separated for gender and the different age groups are presented in Table 6.2. R/S activities, religiosity and spirituality were significantly associated with life satisfaction and happiness across all age groups and both gender. A negative correlation of R/S activities, as well as religiosity and spirituality with depression/anxiety was found in the 18–39 years group, but not in the other age groups. No correlation was found between the indicators of R/S and health. (Table 6.4)

In order to test whether the size of correlations between R/S indicators and well-being were statistically different among the three age groups, a series of Z tests were conducted. In order to control for the number of comparisons performed, here only the comparisons were reported that were significantly different at $p < 0.01$. The remaining Z-tests are available in Table 6.5. The correlation of religiosity and life satisfaction was significantly higher for men than for women. All other correlations among age groups or gender were not significantly different.

Hypothesis 3 that the correlation between R/S and well-being is more pronounced in persons of older age, compared with persons of middle age and younger adults, can be rejected. Z-tests revealed no significant correlation differences between the different age groups.

Table 6.4 Correlations between R/S and different indicators of well-being

	Life satisfaction	Happiness	Depression Anxiety	Health
Whole sample				
R/S activities	0.10***	0.12***	−0.04**	−0.00
Religiosity	0.09***	0.11***	−0.03*	−0.01
Spirituality	0.09***	0.13***	−0.04***	0.01
Age 18–39	(n = 4857)			
R/S activities	0.08***	0.11***	−0.01	0.02
Religiosity	0.07***	0.10***	−0.01	0.01
Spirituality	0.07***	0.13***	−0.02	0.02
Age 40–59	(n = 2744)			
R/S activities	0.09***	0.08***	0.01	−0.02
Religiosity	0.07***	0.08***	0.01	−0.03
Spirituality	0.08***	0.11**	−0.01	0.01
Age 60+	(n = 942)			
R/S activities	0.10***	0.08***	0.02	−0.01
Religiosity	0.09***	0.07*	0.01	−0.02
Spirituality	0.09***	0.09***	−0.00	−0.01
Men only	(n = 3501)			
R/S activities	0.13***	0.13***	−0.05**	0.00
Religiosity	0.12***	0.12***	−0.04*	0.00
Spirituality	0.10***	0.13**	−0.03	−0.01
Women only	(n = 5042)			
R/S activities	0.08***	0.11***	−0.04*	−0.01
Religiosity	0.06***	0.10***	−0.02	−0.02
Spirituality	0.08***	0.13***	−0.05**	0.02

Note: *** = $p < 0.001$, ** = $p < 0.01$, * = $p < 0.05$

Hypothesis 4 that the correlation between R/S and well-being is different for women and men can be confirmed only for religiosity and life satisfaction. No other gender differences in the correlation between R/S activities or spirituality and well-being indicators were found.

Discussion

The purpose of the study was to investigate both the importance of R/S in young, middle-aged and older aged persons in Switzerland, and the association between R/S indicators and well-being. A comparatively large sample of a population was questioned that was not exclusively religious or spiritual. Given that most of the previous research on R/S has been carried out in America, where about 81% of adults report an affiliation with some form of religious/spiritual group (Jackson & Bergeman, 2011), this was an opportunity to investigate the importance of R/S in a

Table 6.5 Z-tests and associated *p* values for comparing the correlations between R/S indicators and well-being indicators across age groups

	1 vs. 2		1 vs. 3		2 vs. 3		Men vs. women	
	Z	*p*	Z	*p*	Z	*p*	Z	*p*
	Life satisfaction							
R/S activities	−0.34	0.37	−0.62	0.27	−0.37	0.35	2.07	0.02
Religiosity	0.25	0.40	−0.59	0.28	−0.72	0.24	2.34	0.01
Spirituality	−0.55	0.31	−0.51	0.31	−0.13	0.45	0.69	0.25
	Happiness							
R/S activities	1.35	0.09	1.02	0.15	0.11	0.46	0.78	0.22
Religiosity	1.18	0.12	1.05	0.15	0.24	0.41	1.20	0.12
Spirituality	0.85	0.20	1.02	0.15	0.43	0.34	−0.05	0.48
	Depression/anxiety							
R/S activities	−0.67	0.25	−0.79	0.22	−0.32	0.38	−0.55	0.29
Religiosity	−1.01	0.16	−0.59	0.28	0.08	0.47	−0.91	0.18
Spirituality	−0.59	0.28	−0.51	0.31	−0.11	0.46	0.68	0.25
	Self-rated health							
R/S activities	1.76	0.04	1.01	0.16	−0.16	0.44	0.45	0.33
Religiosity	1.63	0.05	0.98	0.16	−0.11	0.46	0.77	0.22
Spirituality	0.34	0.37	0.67	0.25	0.42	0.34	−1.05	0.15

Note: 1 vs. 2, difference between the 18–39 years group and the 40–59 years group, 1 vs. 3, difference between the 18–39 years group and the 60+ group, 2 vs. 3, difference between the 40–59 years group and the 60+ years group.

Swiss sample, where only 69% reported an affiliation with a religious/spiritual group. Results revealed that R/S activities and religiosity in this group are valued more highly with advancing age, and that R/S activities are more frequent among women than among men. Additionally, R/S activities, religiosity and spirituality were significantly associated with cognitive and affective aspects of subjective well-being, but not with self-rated health.

R/S activities and religiosity are more pronounced in older age than in middle age and younger adulthood, confirming *Hypothesis 1*. These results are in line with empirical research (e.g., Van Cappellen et al., 2016; Zimmer et al., 2016). Additionally, the results can be explained by Erikson's theory of psychosocial development. Some researchers have suggested that psychological resources such as religiosity increase in salience with age because they are less affected by the physical declines associated with aging than are resources more contingent on physical health and activity (Hood, Hill, & Spilka, 2009).

Interestingly, no differences in spirituality were found between the middle-aged and the older aged group, whereas spirituality is less pronounced in younger age. Jackson and Bergeman (2011) argued that life's triumphs and challenges typically change in middle age. In younger adulthood, people have primary identifications as parents, are generally physically healthy and work on their career, whereas in middle age, people begin experiencing the challenges of failing health, the "empty nest," and approaching retirement (Lachmann, 2004). Young adults use their professional skills and their physical prowess, when they are seeking control in their life, whereas in middle adulthood, spirituality can be an important source of control in the consciousness of the transitoriness of things and the personal confrontation with one's own finiteness. In sum, when people get older, certain worldly interest can take a back seat, where some transcendent values can become more important.

The examination of *hypothesis 2*, that R/S is more pronounced in women than men, showed various results for different age groups. In all age groups, R/S activities were more pronounced in women. These results are in line with other studies (e.g., Maselko & Kubzansky, 2006) and seem to be a cross-cultural phenomenon (Trzebiatowska & Bruce, 2012). However, our results revealed that women were more religious and more spiritual than men only in the 40–59 years group, whereas in the other age groups no gender differences were found. There is a lack of research concerning gender differences at different age stages. However, a few studies have shown that R/S could have different functions for women and men because of their different roles in society (e.g., Maselko & Kubzansky, 2006). Women in middle age often have a greater role to play in managing job and family, and they are frequently burdened with heavy responsibilities with regard to their aging parents (cf., Perrig-Chiello & Höpflinger, 2012) and their own children. At the same time, women in middle age have to adapt to physical changes (menopause). In sum, middle age can be a very stressful time for women. In accordance with the stress and coping framework (Pargament, 1997), R/S appears to be a central coping resource, especially in times of distress (Perrig-Chiello & Margelisch, 2017).

R/S can present important resiliency resources, not only within the context of stress, as conceptualized in the resiliency framework (Masten, 2001). Every age has his own challenges and R/S can boost the overall resiliency as well as provide strategies for coping with specific life stressors. Such resources can include a broad social support network, a sense of meaning and purpose (Park, 2007), and enhanced perceptions of control (Fiori, Antonucci, & Cortina 2006). The current study revealed that R/S activities, religiosity and spirituality were positively associated with happiness and life satisfaction in all age groups, and no differences in the strength of the correlation across age groups were found. Therefore, *Hypothesis 3*, that the association between R/S and well-being is more pronounced in older age than in middle and younger age, can be rejected.

These results contradict the research results of Ruch et al. (2010) and Azañedo et al. (2014), who investigated the association of the character strengths R/S and well-being in adult samples. However, the link between R/S and well-being is still far from understood. Note that different measurement methods are used to determine R/S in scholarly research. This makes it difficult to compare research results on the association between R/S and well-being. At the same time, religion and spirituality are not clearly defined, and therefore, the scientific research of their relationship is not clear or without fault (Ivtzan et al., 2013). In the current study, no differentiation between various aspects of spirituality were made, only the role of the construct spirituality in different life aspects (i.e., regarding decision making, aim definition, access to the life and to oneself) was asked. In future research, behavioural, emotional, and cognitive aspects of religion and spirituality should be considered to explain the functions of R/S in different life stages.

It is possible that the various aspects of R/S have different functions in younger and older life, related to different roles that people have to fulfil at certain life stages. In younger and middle age, R/S could provide an important buffer against stressors of daily life, as part of a stress and coping framework (Pargament, 1997). In older life, the sense of meaning and purpose in life could play a most prominent role (Ai et al., 2010; Ardelt et al., 2013), in accordance with Erikson's theory of psychosocial development (Erikson, 1982). Additionally, the social aspect of R/S could be of greater importance for older people, who are likely to have lost partners, friends and significant others (e.g., Liam & Putnam, 2010).

However, in all ages, R/S activities, religiosity and spirituality can provide social and cognitive resources that help believers to experience greater well-being (Van Cappellen et al., 2016). Religiosity and spirituality are a fertile ground for the experience of positive emotions such as happiness (Van Cappellen & Rimé, 2014). Through involvement in R/S practices, believers may experience positive emotions on a weekly or even daily basis, and over time the positive effect accumulates and builds important personal and social resources (Fredrickson, 2013).

Nevertheless, it has to be mentioned that correlations between R/S and well-being were small (Cohen, 1988). These findings are in line with other studies (e.g. Koenig et al., 2012; Van Cappellen et al., 2016). A meta-analysis of Hackney and Sanders (2003) estimated an average effect of $r = 0.10$ between R/S and psychological well-being. Although small, the effects are consistent across a large number of studies using a variety of design and methodologies, and are therefore not negligible (Van Cappellen et al., 2016).

Concerning gender differences in the correlations between R/S and well-being (*Hypothesis 4*), no differences were found for R/S activities and spirituality, whereas a stronger relationship between religiosity and life satisfaction was found for women than for men. Therefore, Hypothesis 4 was only partially confirmed. Considering the fact that women were more involved in R/S activities than men, it is possible that women find social support in religious activities (Krause, Ellison, & Marcum, 2002), which thus enhance their life satisfaction. A place of worship is often a location where social interaction happens, friends meet, families gather, and supportive activities take place.

In sum, this study adds to a large body of evidence that shows that there is a positive correlation between R/S and well-being. It emphasizes the fact that the association between R/S and well-being is also important to consider in secularized countries and in different age groups. However, the link between spiritual/religious engagement, subjective well-being and health is still far from understood. For example, it is still not well understood how different aspects of spirituality/religiousness, whether independently or in concert, affect well-being (Maselko & Kubzansky, 2006). Little data is available concerning the effects of prayer, beliefs, and faith in well-being. Future research should continue to investigate the psychological aspects of R/S that are beneficial for people's well-being.

The current findings must be interpreted in light of limitations to the study. One of the limits of the present work is that it is cross-sectional. Causality cannot be determined with data collected at a single moment. Nevertheless, different longitudinal studies have shown that R/S has led to greater well-being (e.g., Kashdan & Nezlek, 2012; Park & Slattery, 2012). Causal influence need not be unidirectional: positive experiences (i.e., life satisfaction, happiness) have been shown to operate as a positive self-reinforcing process (Garland, Gaylord, & Fredrickson, 2011; Kok & Fredrickson, 2010). Feeling good about one's life and future can lead to increased religious and spiritual beliefs (Van Cappellen et al., 2016). Future longitudinal studies are necessary to pinpoint causal direction(s). Second, the cross-sectional nature of the data makes it impossible to differentiate age from cohort effects. Third, as described by Hill and Pargament (2008), religiosity and spirituality are complex constructs involving cognitive, emotional, behavioural and interpersonal dimensions, and the current study considered only a partial and incomplete selection of these components. Finally, the s online sample was not randomized and the number of participants was somewhat different across groups.

Nevertheless, the current study has contributed to the understanding of the associations between R/S activities, religiosity and spirituality among different age groups in Switzerland. Future research should continue to investigate the psychological aspects of spirituality and religiosity that benefit people's well-being. Understanding the relationship between R/S and well-being will require consideration of the conditions under which particular dimensions of R/S may be related to specific well-being outcomes. For example, not all effects of religious attendance may be inherently spiritual or cultural. Future research needs to distinguish aspects of R/S that may be more social and cultural than primarily religious or spiritual. The study also offers implications for professional counselling and intervention. Interventions that adapt cognitive-behavioural methods to work with religious and spiritual issues are available and may be useful adjuncts to other treatment (Cowlishaw, Niele, Teshuva, Browning, & Kendig, 2013). However, previous studies indicate that health practitioners may under-use spiritual and religious beliefs as a resource with which to maintain well-being for patients and their families (Silvestri, Knittig, Zoller, & Nietert, 2003). This could be especially important for older patients, in their quest to find meaning in life and to maintain well-being in the face of physical deterioration. In general, researchers and clinicians could profitably pay more attention to R/S, neglected but important aspects of life that may have significant importance for lifelong development and well-being.

References

Ai, A. L., Wink, P., & Ardelt, M. (2010). Spirituality and aging: A journey from meaning through deep interconnection in humanity. In. J. C. Cavanaugh & C. K. Cavanaugh (Eds.), *Aging in America* (Vol. 3 Societal Issues, pp. 222–246). Santa Barbara, CA: Praeger.

Ardelt, M., & Koenig, C. S. (2007). The importance of religious orientation in dying well: Evidence from three case studies. *Journal of Religion, Spirituality & Aging, 19*(4), 61–79.

Ardelt, M., Landes, S. D., Gerlach, K. R., & Fox, L. P. (2013). Rediscovering internal strengths of the aged: The beneficial impact of wisdom, mastery, purpose in life, and spirituality on aging well. In J. D. Sinnott (Ed.), *Positive psychology* (pp. 97–119). New York: Springer.

Azañedo, C. M., Fernández-Abascal, E. G., & Barraca, J. (2014). Character strengths in Spain: Validation of the Values in Action Inventory of Strengths (VIA-IS) in a Spanish sample. *Clínica y Salud, 25*(2), 123–130.

Bonelli, R. M., & Koenig, H. G. (2013). Mental disorders, religion and spirituality 1990 to 2010: A systematic evidence-based review. *Journal of Religion and Health, 52*(2), 657–673.

Carstensen, L. L., & Charles, S. T. (1998). Emotion in the second half of life. *Current Directions in Psychological Science, 7*(5), 144–149.

Cohen, A. B., & Koenig, H. G. (2003). Religion, religiosity and spirituality in the biopsychosocial model of health and ageing. *Ageing International, 28*(3), 215–241.

Cohen, J. (1988). *Statistical power analysis for the behavioral sciences*. Hillsdale, NJ: Lawrence Erlbaum Associates.

Cowlishaw, S., Niele, S., Teshuva, K., Browning, C., & Kendig, H. (2013). Older adults' spirituality and life satisfaction: A longitudinal test of social support and sense of coherence as mediating mechanisms. *Ageing & Society, 33*(7), 1243–1262.

Dahlsgaard, K., Peterson, C., & Seligman, M. E. P. (2005). Shared virtue: The convergence of valued human strengths across culture and history. *Review of General Psychology, 9*, 203–213.

Dalby, P. (2006). Is there a process of spiritual change or development associated with ageing? A critical review of research. *Ageing & Mental Health, 10*(1), 4–12.

Diener, E. D., Emmons, R. A., Larsen, R. J., & Griffin, S. (1985). The satisfaction with life scale. *Journal of Personality Assessment, 49*(1), 71–75.

Diener, E. F., Lucas, R. E., & Oishi, S. (2005). Subjective well-being: The science of happiness and life satisfaction. In C. R. Snyder & S. J. Lopez (Eds.), *Handbook of positive psychology* (pp. 63–73). New York: Oxford University Press.

Diener, E. F., Suh, E. M., & Smith, R. L. H. (1999). Subjective well-being: Three decades of progress. *Psychological Bulletin, 125*(2), 276–302.

Ellens, J. H. (2007). *Radical grace: How belief in a benevolent God benefits your health*. Westport, CT: Praeger.

Ellens, J. H. (2008). *Understanding religious experiences: What the Bible says about spirituality*. Westport, CT: Praeger.

Elliott, M., & Hayward, R. D. (2007). Religion and the search for meaning in life. *Journal of Counselling Psychology, 53*(1), 80–93.

Ellison, C. G. (1991). Religious involvement and subjective well-being. *Journal of Health and Social Behavior, 32*(1), 80–99.

Emery, E. E., & Pargament, K. I. (2004). The many faces of religious coping in late life: Conceptualization, measurement, and links to well-being. *Ageing International, 29*(1), 3–27.

Erikson, E. H. (1982). *The life cycle completed*. New York: Norton & Company.

Erikson, E. H., Erikson, J. M., & Kivnick, H. Q. (1986). *Vital involvement in old age: The experience of old age in our time*. New York: Norton.

Fiori, K. L., Antonucci, T. C., & Cortina, K. S. (2006). Social network typologies and mental health among older adults. *The Journals of Gerontology Series B: Psychological Sciences and Social Sciences, 61*(1), P25–P32.

Fredrickson, B. L. (2013). Positive emotions broaden and build. In P. Devine & A. Plant (Eds.), *Advances in experimental social psychology* (Vol. 47, pp. 1–53). Burlington, VT: Academic Press.

Garland, E. L., Gaylord, S. A., & Fredrickson, B. L. (2011). Positive reappraisal mediates the stress-reductive effects of mindfulness: An upward spiral process. *Mindfulness, 2*(1), 59–67.

Greenway, A. P., Phelan, M., Turnbull, S., & Milne, L. C. (2007). Religious coping strategies and spiritual transcendence. *Mental Health, Religion and Culture, 10*(4), 325–333.

Hackney, C. H., & Sanders, G. S. (2003). Religiosity and mental health: A meta-analysis of recent studies. *Journal for the Scientific Study of Religion, 42*(1), 43–55.

Hank, K., & Shaan, B. (2008). Cross-national variations in the correlations between frequency of prayer and health among older Europeans. *Research on Aging, 30*, 36–54.

Hidajat, M., Zimmer, Z., Saito, Y., & Lin, H.-S. (2013). Religious activity, life expectancy, and disability-free life expectancy in Taiwan. *European Journal of Ageing, 10*, 1–8.

Hill, P. C., & Pargament, K. I. (2008). Advances in the conceptualization and measurement of religion and spirituality: Implications for physical and mental health research. *Psychology of Religion and Spirituality, S*(1), 3–17.

Hill, P. C., Pargament, K. I., Hood, R. W., McCullough, M. E., Jr., Swyers, J. P., Larson, D. B., & Zinnbauer, B. J. (2000). Conceptualizing religion and spirituality: Points of commonality, points of departure. *Journal for the Theory of Social Behaviour, 30*(1), 51–77.

Hood, R. W., Hill, P. C., & Spilka, B. (2009). *The psychology of religion: An empirical approach* (4th ed.). New York: Guilford Press.

Ivtzan, I., Chan, C. P. L., Gardner, H. E., & Prashar, K. (2013). Linking religion and spirituality with psychological well-being: Examining self-actualisation, meaning in life, and personal growth initiative. *Journal of Religion and Health, 52*, 915–929.

Jackson, B. R., & Bergeman, C. S. (2011). How does religiosity enhance well-being? The role of perceived control. *Psychology of Religion and Spirituality, 3*(2), 149–161.

Kashdan, T. B., & Nezlek, J. B. (2012). Whether, when, and how is spirituality related to well-being? Moving beyond single occasion questionnaires to understanding daily process. *Personality and Social Psychology Bulletin, 38*, 1523–1535.

Koenig, H. G. (1999). Religion and medicine. *The Lancet, 353*(9166), 1804.

Koenig, H. G. (2009). Research on religion, spirituality, and mental health: A review. *The Canadian Journal of Psychiatry, 54*(5), 283–291.

Koenig, H. G. (2015). Religion, spirituality, and health: A review and update. *Advances in Mind-Body Medicine, 29*(3), 19–26.

Koenig, H. G., King, D., & Carson, V. B. (2012). *Handbook of religion and health*. New York: Oxford University Press.

Koenig, H. G., McCollough, M. E., & Larson, D. B. (2001). *Handbook of religion and health*. Oxford: University Press.

Kok, B. E., & Fredrickson, B. L. (2010). Upward spirals of the heart: Autonomic flexibility, as indexed by vagal tone, reciprocally and prospectively predicts positive emotions and social connectedness. *Biological Psychology, 85*(3), 432–436.

Krause, N., Ellison, C. G., & Marcum, J. P. (2002). The effects of church-based emotional support on health: Do they vary by gender? *Sociology of Religion, 63*(1), 21–47.

Kroenke, K., Spitzer, R. L., Williams, J. B., & Löwe, B. (2009). An ultra-brief screening scale for anxiety and depression: The PHQ-4. *Psychosomatics, 50*(6), 613–621.

Lachman, M. E. (2004). Development in midlife. *Annual Review of Psychology, 55*, 305–331.

Lavretsky, H. (2010). Spirituality and aging. *Aging Health, 6*(6), 749–769.

Liam, C., & Putnam, R. D. (2010). Religion, social networks and life satisfaction. *American Sociological Review, 75*(6), 914–933.

Lyubomirsky, S., & Lepper, H. (1999). A measure of subjective happiness: Preliminary reliability and construct validation. *Social Indicators Research, 46*, 137–155.

MacKinlay, E. (2001). The spiritual dimension of caring: Applying a model for spiritual tasks of ageing. *Journal of Religious Gerontology, 12*(3/4), 151–166.

Martínez-Marti, M. L., & Ruch, W. (2014). Character strengths and well-being across the life span: Data from a representative sample of German-speaking adults living in Switzerland. *Frontiers in Psychology, 5*, 1253.

Maselko, J., & Kubzansky, L. D. (2006). Gender differences in religious practices, spiritual experiences and health: Results from the US general social survey. *Social Science & Medicine, 62*(11), 2848–2860.

Masten, A. S. (2001). Ordinary magic: Resilience processes in development. *American Psychologist, 56*(3), 227–238.

McCullough, M. E., Hoyt, W. T., Larson, D. B., Koenig, H. G., & Thoresen, C. (2000). Religious involvement and mortality: A meta-analytic review. *Health Psychology, 19*(3), 211–222.

McCullough, M. E., & Laurenceau, J. P. (2005). Religiousness and the trajectory of self-rated health across adulthood. *Personality and Social Psychology Bulletin, 31*(4), 560–573.

Miller, W. R., & Thoresen, C. E. (2003). Spirituality, religion, and health: An emerging research field. *American Psychologist, 58*(1), 24–35.

Moberg, D. O. (2005). Research in spirituality, religion, and aging. *Journal of Gerontological Social Work, 45*(1–2), 11–40.

Paloutzian, R. F., & Park, C. L. (Eds.). (2005). *Handbook of the psychology of religion and spirituality*. New York: Guilford Press.

Pargament, K. I. (1997). *The psychology of religion and coping*. New York: Guilford Press.

Park, C. L. (2007). Religiousness/spirituality and health: A meaning systems perspective. *Journal of Behavioral Medicine, 30*(4), 319–328.

Park, C. L., & Slattery, J. M. (2012). Spirituality, emotions, and physical health. In L. J. Miller (Ed.), *The Oxford handbook of psychology and spirituality* (pp. 379–387). New York: Oxford University Press.

Park, N., & Peterson, C. (2009). Character strengths: Research and practice. *Journal of College and Character, 10*(4).

Parsian, N., & Dunning, T. (2009). Developing and validating a questionnaire to measure spirituality: A psychometric process. *Global Journal of Health Science, 1*(1), 2–11.

Perrig-Chiello, P., & Höpflinger, F. (2012). *Pflegende Angehörige älterer Menschen. Probleme, Bedürfnisse, Ressourcen und Zusammenarbeit mit der ambulanten Pflege*. Bern, CH: Huber.

Perrig-Chiello, P., & Margelisch, K. (2017). Spiritual Care – eine psychologische Annäherung. In I. Noth, E. Schweizer, & G. Wenz (Eds.), *Seelsorge und Spiritual Care in interkultureller Perspektive* [Pastoral and spiritual care across religions and cultures] (pp. 44–56). Goettingen, DE: Vandenhoek & Ruprecht.

Perruccio, A. V., Katz, J. N., & Losina, E. (2012). Health burden in chronic disease: Multimorbidity is associated with self-rated health more than medical comorbidity alone. *Journal of Clinical Epidemioly, 65*, 100–106.

Peterson, C., & Seligman, M. E. P. (2004). *Character strengths and virtues: A handbook and classification*. New York: Oxford University Press.

Pinquart, M., & Sörensen, S. (2000). Influences of socioeconomic status, social network, and competence on subjective well-being in later life: A meta-analysis. *Psychology and Aging, 15*(2), 187–224.

Plante, T. G., & Boccaccini, M. (1997). The Santa Clara strength of religious faith questionnaire. *Pastoral Psychology, 45*, 375–387.

Ruch, W., Proyer, R. T., & Weber, M. (2010). Humor as a character strength among the elderly. Theoretical considerations. *Zeitschrift für Gerontologie und Geriatrie, 43*, 8–12.

Sadler, E., & Biggs, S. (2006). Exploring the links between spirituality and 'successful ageing'. *Journal of Social Work Practice, 20*(3), 267–280.

Shaw, R., Gullifer, J., & Wood, K. (2016). Religion and spirituality: A qualitative study of older adults. *Ageing International, 41*, 311–330.

Sheldrake, P. (2007). *A brief history of spirituality*. Oxford: Blackwell Publishing Ltd.

Silvestri, G. A., Knittig, S., Zoller, J. S., & Nietert, P. J. (2003). Importance of faith on medical decisions regarding cancer care. *Journal of Clinical Oncology, 21*(7), 1379–1382.

Smith, T. B., McCullough, M. E., & Poll, J. (2003). Religiousness and depression: Evidence for a main effect and the moderating influence of stressful life events. *Psychological Bulletin, 129*(4), 614–636.

Staton, J., Shuy, R., & Byock, I. (2001). *A few months to live. Different paths of life's end.* Washington, DC: Georgetown University Press.

Thoresen, C. E., & Harris, A. H. (2002). Spirituality and health: What's the evidence and what's needed? *Annals of Behavioral Medicine, 24*(1), 3–13.

Tomer, A., Eliason, G. T., & Wong, P. T. P. (Eds.). (2008). *Existential and spiritual issues in death attitudes.* New York: Lawrence Erlbaum Associates.

Trzebiatowska, M., & Bruce, S. (2012). *Why are women more religious than men?* Oxford: Oxford University Press.

Van Cappellen, P., & Rimé, B. (2014). Positive emotions and self-transcendence. In V. Saroglou (Ed.), *Religion, personality, and social behavior.* New York: Psychology Press.

Van Cappellen, P., Toth-Gauthier, M., Saroglou, V., & Fredrickson, B. L. (2016). Religion and well-being: The mediating role of positive emotions. *Journal of Happiness Studies, 17*(2), 485–505.

Van Ranst, N., & Marcoen, A. (2000). Structural components of personal meaning in life and their relationship with death attitudes and coping mechanisms in late life. In G. T. Reker & K. Chamberlain (Eds.), *Exploring existential meaning: Optimizing human development across the life span* (pp. 59–74). Thousand Oaks, CA: Sage.

Wilhelm, M. O., Rooney, P. M., & Tempel, E. R. (2007). Changes in religious giving reflect changes in involvement: Age and cohort effects in religious giving, secular giving, and attendance. *Journal for the Scientific Study of Religion, 46*(2), 217–232.

Williams, D. R., & Sternthal, M. J. (2007). Spirituality, religion and health: Evidence and research directions. *Medical Journal of Australia, 186*(10), S47–S50.

Wink, P., & Dillon, M. (2001). Religious involvement and health outcomes in late adulthood. In T. G. Plante & A. C. Sherman (Eds.), *Faith and health: Psychological perspectives* (pp. 75–106). New York: Guilford Press.

Yoon, D. P., & Lee, E. O. (2004). Religiousness/spirituality and subjective well-being among rural elderly whites, African Americans and Native Americans. *Journal of Human Behavior in the Social Environment, 10*(1), 191–211.

Zimmer, Z., Jagger, C., Chiu, C. T., Ofstedal, M. B., Rojo, F., & Saito, Y. (2016). Spirituality, religiosity, aging and health in global perspective: A review. *SSM-Population Health, 2*, 373–381.

Zinnbauer, B. J., & Pargament, K. I. (2005). Religiousness and spirituality. In R. F. Paloutzian & C. L. Park (Eds.), *Handbook of the psychology of religion and spirituality* (pp. 21–42). New York: Guilford Press.

Part III
Comparisons of Elements and Levels
of Hope Across Cultures

Chapter 7
Hope in the Indian Psychology Context: Philosophical Foundations and Empirical Findings

Andreas M. Krafft and Rajneesh Choubisa

Introduction

The experience of hope has been the focus of debate for hundreds and thousands of years in Western Philosophy and Theology. Just recently, mostly since the eighties of the twentieth century, it also has become a topic of enquiry for psychological research, especially in Anglo-Saxon countries. In the last 20–30 years, a huge number of theories and models have been developed, which base their conceptualizations of hope on very diverse scientific, philosophical and theological worldviews. In western psychology, the mainstream conceptualization of hope considers it an individual trait-like cognitive-behavioral phenomenon (Stotland, 1969). Snyder's theory, currently the most diffused cognitive approach on hope, has a self-centered character in that it refers to the person's perception in relation to his or her own will-power and efficacy to attain personal goals (Snyder, 2002). In the meantime, a variety of alternative and multidimensional concepts and models emerged, defining hope in cognitive, emotional, relational, spiritual and moral terms among others (Dufault & Martocchio, 1985; Farran, Herth, & Popovich, 1995; Scioli & Biller, 2009).

In recent years, authors in the new field of Positive Psychology (PP) have incorporated hope very prominently as one of the central positive emotions and character strengths, valuing it as an important source for achieving a good and fulfilling life (Fredrickson, 2004; Peterson & Seligman, 2004). In their comprehensive Handbook of Character Strengths and Virtues, Peterson and Seligman (2004) defined six core

A. M. Krafft (✉)
Institute of Systemic Management and Public Governance, University of St. Gallen, St. Gallen, Switzerland
e-mail: andreas.krafft@unisg.ch

R. Choubisa
Department of Humanities and Social Sciences, Birla Institute of Technology & Science (BITS), Pilani, Rajasthan, India

© Springer International Publishing AG, part of Springer Nature 2018　　　131
A. M. Krafft et al. (eds.), *Hope for a Good Life*, Social Indicators Research Series 72, https://doi.org/10.1007/978-3-319-78470-0_7

virtues that exist across cultures and included hope as belonging to the virtue of transcendence, entailing aspects of life that are beyond the human knowledge (e.g. Singh & Choubisa, 2010). In this sense, hope is intimately related to spirituality and religiosity, which means to beliefs and practices regarding the sacred, defined as a divine being, higher power, or ultimate reality. Religious and spiritual faith enables people to rely on a benevolent transcendent power, expecting the best in the future, committing oneself to attain it, and developing positive beliefs about one's higher life purpose and meaning as well as moral values for the pursuit of goodness. Hope, in this view, goes much beyond one's own cognitive capabilities because it is connected to something larger and bigger in the universe and within oneself, especially helping the person to overcome difficult moments of personal anxiety, suffering and despair (Scioli, 2007).

Several scientists in India have started to highlight the similarities and analyze the basic differences between the two young disciplines of Positive and Indian Psychology, the latter being a school that integrates social science and the ancient Indian philosophy and spirituality (Cornelissen, 2014; Dalal & Misra, 2010; Rao, 2014a, 2014b). Both schools of thought were born out of the reaction to mainstream psychology, with its traditional focus on pathologies and on curing illnesses, and adopted the mission to promote the good and uplifting aspects in life, in order to help people to develop their strengths, potentials and possibilities, to flourish and to live a happy and fulfilling life.

From the Indian Psychology (IP) standpoint, there exists a need to foster collaboration between IP and PP, since both, albeit sharing a common mission, have particular strengths and weaknesses that could complement each other. PP has developed a strong methodological basis of empirical research, but in theoretical terms, it lacks a coherent and unifying theoretical foundation, producing a proliferation of distinct definitions and models, often giving rise to conceptual ambiguity and confusion (Rao, 2014a). This is particularly true in the case of the concept of hope, since many researchers have developed so divergent definitions, leading to a multifaceted and essentially inconsistent picture of the construct (Eliott, 2005; Lopez, Snyder, & Pedrotti, 2003). On the other hand, it has been argued, that IP has its roots in a holistic and consistent body of philosophical, psychological and spiritual knowledge, comprising and integrating concepts such as happiness, subjective wellbeing, spirituality, positive emotions, wisdom and others (Dalal & Misra, 2010; Rao, 2014a). Conversely, the weakness of IP resides in the lack of solid scientific empirical data, at least in Western terms, to support its axioms and theories.

Indian Psychology claims to be a universal and applied psychology dealing with the essential human nature and does not describe only the psychology of Indian people (Dalal, 2010; Dalal & Misra, 2010). On the other hand, although hope is a universal phenomenon, its definition and experience can vary across cultures (Averill & Sundararajan, 2005). Since various cultures hold different norms and values, cross-cultural studies of hope can help to find similarities and particularities in order to replicate and validate empirical results and support the generalizability of a certain theory. Therefore, the objectives of our contribution are threefold: (1) To briefly outline the philosophical roots of IP; (2) to explore the notion of hope within the philosophical foundations of IP; and (3) to present cross-cultural empirical findings from the Hope-Barometer survey in India, aiming to examine the philosophical propositions of hope. Out of the scope of this contribution is to investigate the similarities and differences in the conceptualization of hope in Western and Eastern philosophical traditions, including Christian theology, Aristotelian philosophy and other philosophical works, an effort worth doing in future contributions.

Philosophical Roots of Indian Psychology

Indian Psychology has emerged as a new scientific discipline only recently, that is, at the beginning of this century, but its roots go back to thousands of years of Indian traditions, thoughts and the practices of yoga and meditation (Rao & Paranjpe, 2016). The ancient Vedic texts such as the *Upanishads* as well as later writings, e.g. *Shrimad Bhagavad Gita*, deliver a holistic philosophical system, which became part of the Indian and many other Eastern cultures and ethos. Several Indian thinkers, especially at the end of the nineteenth and the beginning of the twentieth century, contributed to the interpretation of these classical texts, integrating their spiritual, philosophical and psychological insights into one big and coherent corpus of knowledge (see for example, Aurobindo, 1990, 1997; Vivekananda, 2015). The philosophy and psychology rooted in this ancient Indian wisdom are characterized by many principles and axioms that largely differ from the common Western thinking. Differences can be found in the ontological and epistemological premises, in the conceptualization of the self and the psychic function, in the causes of illness, in the remedies to overcome suffering and in the necessary conditions to enjoy a good and fulfilling life. While Western science often claims to be value free, Indian philosophy is explicitly based on a normative worldview that focuses on the human virtues of love, altruism and compassion. All these elements have far-reaching consequences on how the phenomenon of hope is conceived and on the role it plays in human experience and existence.

Ontology, Epistemology, and Non-duality in Indian Philosophy

At the core of Indian Philosophy and Psychology, we can recognize a completely different understanding and conceptualization of reality, compared to the scientific mainstream in the West. In the Indian tradition, ontology and epistemology are closely interlinked, giving rise to a much wider and comprehensive view of the world and of human existence (Cornelissen & Ashram, 2001). In the Western world, there is a clear separation between the person as psychophysical entity and the material world in which he or she exists. The Western paradigm is basically characterized by its analytical, rational, logical and structured way of thinking, focusing its attention on what can be seen and measured (e.g. matter and behavior). This is also the basis for the individualistic and cognitive understanding of hope. In contrast, the Indian perspective is characterized by a non-dual paradigm. It tends to integrate different types of experiences and the inherent contradictions of fundamental phenomena such as continuity and transformation, self-identity and universal oneness, the manifest and the un-manifest, the given and the possible, the materialistic and the spiritual, the state of being and the process of becoming, etc. (Menon, 2005). The Indian way of thinking known as *Darsana*, constitutes the attempt to integrate the theoretical, experiential and transcendental issues in life, hence acknowledging the complex and emergent nature of reality.

Especially relevant to IP is the wider and holistic understanding of the person and the self and its connection to the others and the world in general. The Indian tradition differentiates between mind and consciousness, conceiving the person as a unique entity composed of body, mind and consciousness and making a clear distinction between the true Self and the superficial self, called ego (Rao, 2014a). The ego is of temporary nature and functions to establish our individuality, but the true inner Self of every person called *Aatman* is considered to be of divine nature, expressed by consciousness and being of unchangeable quality. Overall, the Indian worldview recognizes the existence of different levels of consciousness, from the lower to the highest universal and absolute consciousness known as *Brahman*, and maintains that these and not matter alone are the true basis of reality (Cornelissen & Ashram, 2001). One fundamental goal in life is to acquire higher levels of consciousness comprising the physical, the social and the metaphysical and moral levels of existence. The highest state is that of pure consciousness, in which our true Self is one with the divine and hence with the Self of all others, characterized by a condition of absolute truth, joy and bliss (Dalal, 2010).

This holistic and integrative view of the Self and the world has far-reaching consequences regarding the understanding of the constitution and functioning of our psychic system, about the different types of thinking and knowing as well as concerning the universal moral order in which we are embedded. Within the human psyche, the mind is regarded as the cognitive instrument and consciousness as the agentic function from which thought and action are generated (Rao, 2005). The interaction of mind and consciousness enables the person to acquire knowledge, to develop volition and to experience emotions. Sensory perception is only one way of thinking and acquiring knowledge. The Indian understanding of the human capacity of thinking is characterized by the integration of its dual function, on the one hand to represent what is considered to be given and observable and on the other hand, to transcend this sphere of representational perception, in order to apprehend what is latent but not perceivable by the common senses. The acquisition and generation of knowledge is therefore possible via three different forms of thinking and experience: the analytical, the reflective and the intuitive thinking (Menon, 2005). Above all, the main objective is to learn to distinguish the true spiritual Self we really are, from the surface self, as the conjunction of mind and body.

Whereas in the Western paradigm, knowledge is something that the person can possess, in the Indian tradition, knowledge is something that is linked to personal experience and that defines and transforms the person in who he/she is (Cornelissen & Ashram, 2001). The generation of higher level knowledge is intimately related with the different forms of experience that can be attained using the practices of yoga and meditation to enhance intuition and permit revelation. The different modes of knowing are of sensory, extra-sensory, holistic, insightful and ethical nature (Dalal & Misra, 2010). Accordingly, there are different ways of knowledge generation: Concentration in sensorial observation (*Dharana*); cognitive attention focus through meditation (*Dhyana*); and trans-cognitive meditative absorption (*Samadhi*) that results in self-transformation and self-realization (Rao, 2014a). Acquisition of knowledge by logical and rational reasoning is therefore only one but not the most important way of knowing. The most significant forms of knowledge are related to experiences of love, altruism, compassion, faith, gratitude, awe and beauty, which helps to widen our consciousness, to realize the divine and eternal of our true Self in ourselves and in every other person and to experience joy, happiness and bliss (Cornelissen & Ashram, 2001).

Moral Order, Sources of Illness and Ways to Healing

While Western life sciences are very much focused on the study and explanation of the natural order, especially when it comes to understand its disruption and the causes of illness, Indian philosophy acknowledges the existence of a universal moral order, which is closely interrelated with the natural order (Paranjpe, 1996). To understand this moral order, a distinction must be drawn between godlike and demonic qualities that is to say between the good and the evil, always present in our thoughts and actions. In the Indian philosophy, there is no neutral or amoral action, since every action has an intrinsic value. Every action has a cause and an effect and therefore a positive or negative consequence, making every person responsible for the results of his/her behavior.

The *law of Karma* precisely refers to the sequence of causes and effects of human actions: Good actions lead to good consequences and bad actions to bad consequences. What can be defined as good and what as evil was established by the universal moral order. Western philosophers like Schopenhauer and Nietzsche have misinterpreted the principle of *Karma*, conceiving it as deterministic and deducing from it a fatalistic and pessimistic worldview. On the contrary, in Indian philosophy the concept of *Karma* always implies human freedom and the possibility to choose, to change and to progress. Every person can transform the future course of events and free oneself from the negative imprints of the past by consciously and responsibly undertaking virtuous actions (Dalal & Misra, 2010). In this way, human beings can attain higher forms of existence until achieving the highest form of the divine.

Coming back to the distinction between the true Self and the superficial self, the ego, the cause of all illnesses and sufferings is the misconception of our true being, confounding the ego with our spiritual and transcendental Self, and therefore running behind the satisfaction of material desires, bodily needs, selfish wishes and all kind of pleasures known as hedonism (Rao, 2014a). The truly human is related to the divine natural and moral order, whereas the evil is connected to egoism and selfishness. Ultimately, the basic source of all sufferings is of mental nature, namely ignorance and wrong thoughts that bias and blinds the mind, which is present within the person as ego. Pathologies and all types of psycho-social problems including the sentiments of hate and aversion as well as their effects on depression, anxiety, deprivation, poverty and social conflicts emerge when the natural balance between thoughts, actions and feelings is being disturbed. This can be explained by the assumption that not only actions but also thoughts and emotions have a direct impact on bodily and even social processes (Dalal & Misra, 2010).

The only way to overcome suffering effectively is by deconstructing and overcoming the ego, which is possible by cultivating an attitude of altruism and compassion, practicing selfless activities and by doing so, gaining higher levels of consciousness and self-awareness (Salagame, 2014). The transcendence of the ego implies to detach oneself from excessive worldly desires, to seek the truth and the good, to regain one's own freedom, to strive for the common good, and to move towards moral perfection, which will result in psychological health and wellbeing. This attitude is also linked to Gandhi's principle of non-violence to avoid and resolve social conflicts positively. As Rao (2014b, p. 130) formulates it: "The goal therefore is to drive the devil out and experience the divine within".

Since the sources of most evils can be found within the person him−/herself, the first aim is to free the mind from all negative influences and thoughts. The practices of yoga and meditation are precisely directed to transcend the own ego by eliminating the internal biases, in order to discover the true Self and to achieve a state of pure consciousness called *Samadhi*, moving from the mundane and sensory to the intuitive and sublime (Dalal, 2010; Rao & Paranjpe, 2008). Experiences with yoga and meditation as well as scientific research in the field were able to confirm how effective these techniques are towards controlling anger, depression, and anxiety, and have demonstrated the power of the mind over the body (Menon, 2005).

These phenomena have been deemed as the process of personal healing, which is something completely different from the Western concept of cure. While therapies and treatments to cure an illness are basically conceived as external interventions on a more or less passive patient, healing in the *Ayurveda* practice presupposes and requires the active engagement of the person. Genuine healing is fundamentally self-healing and self-transformation of the own spirit, since the Self is the real agent. Mental health comes from reestablishing the internal balance, changing the own worldviews, creating a sense of communion with others, developing new visions and goals, and unfolding one's own potentials (Menon, 2005). By doing so, not only the mind but also the body and the entire society can heal and flourish.

Achieving a Good Life by Liberation and Self-Realization

The central matter of concern of Indian Philosophy and Psychology is to gain as much knowledge as possible about the true Self and the real nature of the world and by doing so, support liberation from personal suffering and social unrests to promote self-realization. The ultimate objective is to guide the person and society to the highest level of human perfection, realizing the divine within, achieving redemption, happiness, fulfillment and an all-embracing bliss (Rao, 2014a). The way to bliss requires the transcendence of the own ego, the avoidance of selfish actions and the psychological detachment from materialistic and self-centered wishes and pleasures (Rao, 1978). Healing is given by a harmonic balance between consciousness, mind and body, founded in positive thoughts and actions as well as in inner and outer peace. Harmony is a central pillar of self-realization: Harmony of the spirit, harmony in the human relations and harmony between the person and his/her wider natural and social environment. In this sense, the good and thriving life is characterized by an attitude of altruism, of un-selfishness, of violence-avoidance and the performance of virtuous actions such as helping others and cultivating friendly human relationships. Self-realization is the phenomenon of displaying all the positive human potentials, of personal inner growth and transformation to a higher level of evolution and consciousness resulting in the promotion of the common good. The cardinal virtues are those of love, altruism, and compassion instead of competition and the optimization for own benefit (Dalal & Misra, 2010).

Summarizing the previously mentioned, the scope and goal of Indian Psychology is in many aspects very close to that of Positive Psychology: Promotion of a happy and fulfilling life, unfolding the human potentials and possibilities and establishing a harmonious social order of peace, justice and respect. Within this framework, the satisfaction of personal desires and the acquisition of material possessions and wealth are not dismissed but considered to be legitimate goals to achieve prosperity. However, these goals should not be confounded with the highest good, the divine bliss, which is solely located in our inner Self (Paranjpe, 1996). The transformation towards mental and spiritual health and the ideal society comes not from outside but from within and comprises the following elements:

1. Knowing the true inner Self, its communion with the divine and attaining a higher level of consciousness.
2. Liberating the mind from negative influences and thoughts and bringing it to rest.
3. Detachment (*Anasakti*) from superfluous goals and pleasures to transcend one's own ego.
4. Adopting an attitude of love, altruism, unselfishness and compassion with others.
5. Performing meaning- and purposeful life duties and pursuits.
6. Living a harmonious, conflict- and violence-free life.

7. Nurturing one's own cognitive and spiritual potentials and possibilities for the good.
8. Achieving self-realization, happiness, fulfillment and bliss.
9. Transforming society by realizing the common good.

We examine the concept of hope against this backdrop that seems to be entwined in the framework of Indian Philosophy and explore its meaning by comparing a sample of Indians vis-á-vis German speaking Europeans.

Hope in the Context of Indian Philosophy

As far as we know, no formal and systematic theory of hope has been explicitly developed in Indian Psychology until now, though the concept of hope has a significant role in Indian Philosophy. In this section, our goal is to explore the concept of hope as it has been employed by two interpreters of the Vedantic scriptures, the *Upanishads* and the *Bhagavad Gita*, namely *Swami Vivekananda* and *Shri Aurobindo*. It is not our aim to formulate a systematic and comprehensive theory of hope based on Indian Philosophy, but to work out in a first step the basic elements and properties, the Indian concept of hope entails. Based on their interpretation of the Indian scriptures, German Philosophers like Schopenhauer and Nietzsche came to the conclusion, that in the face of the omnipresent pain and suffering on earth, hope and optimism are just a farce and an absurdity and that hope has to be considered "…the worst of all evils, because it protracts the torments of men." (Nietzsche, 1996, p. 45). On the contrary, in his lead article, Rao highlights Vivekananda's view on hope, saying: "We must love others because the others are no other than ourselves. Thus, love becomes the cardinal virtue, which, along with hope and optimism, guides our conduct. Altruism is the opposite of selfishness; it involves detachment as opposed to attachment *(Aasakti)*, which is the source of all misery. Hope is the driving force. 'Infinite hope begets infinite aspiration'. (*Vivekananda, vol. 3, p. 443*)" (Rao, 2014a, p. 101).

Exploring the Concept of Hope in Indian Philosophy

To understand the differentiated use of the term hope within Indian Philosophy, one cannot analyze a theoretical definition of the concept, but the context and the meaning of how this term has been employed, is certainly achievable. Therefore, to its right interpretation, the function, the targets and the sources of hope become relevant. At the core of the understanding of different types of hope is the basic differentiation between the superficial ego and *Maya (the illusionary world)* on the one hand and the true nature of the Self and the entire cosmos, on the other.

This distinction has fundamental consequences on the judgment of the quality of different categories of action, as described by Aurobindo in his reading of the Bhagavad Gita:

> *Tamasic* action is that done with a confused, deluded and ignorant mind, in mechanical obedience to the instincts, impulsions and unseeing ideas, without regarding the strength or capacity or the waste and loss of blind misapplied effort or the antecedent and consequence and right conditions of the impulse, effort or labor. *Rajasic* action is that which a man undertakes under the dominion of desire, with his eyes fixed on the work and it's hoped-for fruit and nothing else, or with an egoistic sense of his own personality in the action, and it is done with inordinate effort, with a passionate labor, with a great heaving and straining of the personal will to get at the object of its desire. *Satwic* action is that which a man does calmly in the clear light of reason and knowledge and with an impersonal sense of right or duty or the demand of an ideal, as the thing that ought to be done, whatever may be the result to himself in this world or another, a work performed without attachment, without liking or disliking for its spur or its drag, for the sole satisfaction of his reason and sense of right, of the lucid intelligence and the enlightened will and the pure disinterested mind and the high contented spirit. At the line of culmination of *sattva* it will be transformed and become a highest impersonal action dictated by the spirit within us and no longer by the intelligence, an action moved by the highest law of the nature, free from the lower ego and its light or heavy baggage and from limitation even by best opinion, noblest desire, purest personal will or loftiest mental ideal. There will be none of these impedimenta; in their place, there will stand a clear spiritual self-knowledge and illumination and an imperative intimate sense of an infallible power that acts and of the work to be done for the world and for the world's Master. (Aurobindo, 1997, p. 501)

Based on these fundamental distinctions, two opposite types of hope can be identified relating to the one or the other kind of action. Referring to the Vedic legend of *Satyavan* and *Savitri* as interpreted by Aurobindo, Sarcar exposes the different sorts of hope as follows:

> In material nature, life is interned but life in its higher glory expresses its joys in a nature evolved to a greater truth. Life there has hopes that are vaster and more splendid, although to the veiled human sight they lie hidden. But Aswapathy's visionary eyes see them:
> *He glimpsed the hidden wings of her songster hopes,*
> *A glimmer of blue and gold and scarlet fire.*
> Hopes are often glimmering shadows to which defeated and desperate men and women cling to be able to go on living. But these hopes in the greater life are not illusions; they sing joyfully like songster birds; their bright-hued glimmer is that of a burning fire that has light and force. (Sarkar, 2011, p. 94)

On the one hand, following the principle of detachment from one's actions and their results, there is nothing to hope for unless humankind detaches itself from all kind of superfluous worldly desires:

> The liberated man has no personal hopes; he does not seize on things as his personal possessions; he receives what the divine *will* brings him, covets nothing, is jealous of none: what comes to him he takes without repulsion and without attachment; what goes from him he allows to depart into the whirl of things without repining or grief or sense of loss. His heart and self are under perfect control; they are free from reaction and passion, they make no turbulent response to the touches of outward things. (Aurobindo, 1997, p. 180)... All its hope, action, knowledge are vain things when judged by the divine and eternal standard, for

it shuts out the great hope, excludes the liberating action, banishes the illuminating knowledge. It is a false knowledge that sees the phenomenon but misses the truth of the phenomenon, a blind hope that chases after the transient but misses the eternal, a sterile action whose every profit is annulled by loss and amounts to a perennial labor of Sisyphus. (Gita, IX. 11–12). (Ibid., p. 326)

On the other hand, hope is regarded as a cornerstone of the whole Indian Philosophy, without which the entire worldview would not make any sense at all. Vivekananda explains the importance of hope through an old Indian story:

There was a great king in ancient India who was once asked four questions, of which one was: "What is the most wonderful thing in the world?" "Hope", was the answer. This is the most wonderful thing. Day and nights, we see people dying around us, and yet we think we shall not die; we never think that we shall die, or that we shall suffer. Each man thinks that success will be his, hoping against hope, against all odds, against all mathematical reasoning. (Vivekananda, 2015, p. 373)

Vivekananda explains this understanding of hope relating it to the concept of faith:

To preach the doctrine of *Shraddha* (or genuine faith) is the mission of my life. Let me repeat to you that this faith is one of the potent factors of humanity and of all religions. First, have faith in yourselves. Know that, though one may be a little bubble and another may be a mountain-high wave, yet behind both the bubble and the wave there is the infinite ocean. Therefore, there is hope for everyone. There is salvation for everyone. Everyone must sooner or later get rid of the bonds of Maya. This is the first thing to do. Infinite hope begets infinite aspiration. (Ibid., p. 1340)

In a similar way, Aurobindo refers to the lessons and the ultimate goal of the Bhagavad Gita:

And this is how the Gita leads us: it lays down a firm and sure but very large way of ascent, a great *Dharma*, and then it takes us out beyond all that is laid down, beyond all dharmas, into infinitely open spaces, divulges to us the hope, lets us into the secret of an absolute perfection founded in an absolute spiritual liberty, and that secret, *"Guhyatamam"*, is the substance of what it calls its supreme word, that the hidden thing, the inmost knowledge. (Aurobindo, 1997, p. 527)

In one of his central works, The Life Divine, Aurobindo argues that suffering and pain can be transcended and that our hope should be directed to achieve the highest good in life:

But if we could grasp the essential nature and the essential cause of error, suffering and death, we might hope to arrive at a mastery over them which should be not relative but entire. We might hope even to eliminate them altogether and justify the dominant instinct of our nature by the conquest of that absolute good, bliss, knowledge and immortality which our intuitions perceive as the true and ultimate condition of the human being. (Aurobindo, 1990, p. 62–63)

But this can only be accomplished by his growing into a larger being and a larger consciousness: self-enlargement, self-fulfilment, self-evolution from what he partially and temporarily is in his actual and apparent nature to what he completely is in his secret self and spirit and therefore can become even in his manifest existence, is the object of his creation. This hope is the justification of his life upon earth amidst the phenomena of the cosmos. (Ibid., p. 711)

Now the crucial question before all of us is: Where should this hope come from? What are the roots and sources of hope? On the one hand, hope seems to have a purely individualistic nature. Everybody must count on him−/herself:

> Be free; hope for nothing from anyone. I am sure if you look back upon your lives you will find that you were always vainly trying to get help from others, which never came. All the help that has come was from within yourselves. You only had the fruits of what you yourselves worked for, and yet you were strangely hoping all the time for help. (Vivekananda, 2015, p. 758)

However, the lesson of hope goes far beyond this individualistic idea. The person alone is too weak to overcome pain and suffering by him−/herself. Self-confidence, patience and perseverance are very limited when the individual rely on his−/her own strengths only. The crucial element is that of the divine grace. Vivekananda says:

> Is there no hope then? True it is that we are all slaves of Maya, born in Maya, and live in Maya. Is there then no way out, no hope? That we are all miserable, that this world is really a prison, that even our so-called trailing beauty is but a prison-house, and that even our intellects and minds are prison-houses, have been known for ages upon ages. […] Is there no way out? We find that with all this, with this terrible fact before us, in the midst of sorrow and suffering, even in this world where life and death are synonymous, even here, there is a still small voice that is ringing through all ages, through every country, and in every heart: "This Maya is divine, made up of qualities, and very difficult to cross. Yet those that come unto me, cross the river of life." "Come unto me all ye that labor and are heavy laden and I will give you rest." This is the voice that is leading us forward. Man has heard it, and is hearing it all through the ages. This voice comes to men when everything seems to be lost and hope has fled, when man's dependence on his own strength has been crushed down and everything seems to melt away between his fingers, and life is a hopeless ruin. Then he hears it. This is called religion. (Vivekananda, 2015, p. 580)

In his Letters on Yoga, Aurobindo tells us, that there is no reason for hopelessness, as long as our will has decided to transit the right way. It does not make any sense to ruminate about the failures of the past. We have to direct our attention with patience, hope and trust towards the future (Aurobindo, 1970). This is the freedom we always have. The freedom to decide ourselves for the good and to trust God. As Vivekananda puts it:

> If we are not free, how can we hope to make the world better? We hold that human progress is the result of the action of the human spirit. What the world is, and what we ourselves are, are the fruits of the freedom of the spirit. We believe in one God, the Father of us all, who is omnipresent and omnipotent, and who guides and preserves His children with infinite love. We believe in a Personal God as the Christians do, but we go further: we below that we are He! That His personality is manifested in us, that God is in us, and that we are in God. (Vivekananda, 2015, p. 1597)

That hope for redemption is not only limited to a minority of enlightened people but that the grace of God reaches all people, becomes clear in the following passage of Aurobindo's essays on the Gita:

> This highest message is first for those who have the strength to follow after it, the master men, the great spirits, the God-knowers, God-doers, God-lovers who can live in God and for God and do their work joyfully for him in the world, a divine work uplifted above the

restless darkness of the human mind and the false limitations of the ego. At the same time, and here we get the gleam of a larger promise which we may even extend to the hope of a collective turn towards perfection, – for if there is hope for man, why should there not be hope for mankind? – the Gita declares that all can if they will, even to the lowest and sinfullest among men, enter into the path of this Yoga. (Aurobindo, 1997, p. 570)

In *The Life Divine*, he reinforces this idea of collective evolution based on the individual power of will:

Not individuals only, but in time the race also, in a general rule of being and living if not in all its members, can have the hope, if it develops a sufficient will, to rise beyond the imperfections of our present very undivine nature and to ascend at least to a superior humanity, to rise nearer, even if it cannot absolutely reach, to a divine manhood or supermanhood. At any rate, it is the compulsion of evolutionary Nature in him to strive to develop upward, to erect the ideal, to make the endeavor. (Aurobindo, 1990, p. 745)

Upon a careful observation of this discourse, we summarize that hope and hopelessness, optimism and pessimism, are equally present in Indian Philosophy but related to different targets and nurtured by different sources:

The Vedanta system begins with tremendous pessimism, and ends with real optimism. We deny the sense-optimism but assert the real optimism of the supersensuous. That real happiness is not in the senses but above the senses; and it is in every man. The sort of optimism which we see in the world is what will lead to ruin through the senses. (Vivekananda, 2015, p. 2246)

The Central Elements of Hope in Indian Philosophy

After having deliberated the core thoughts around the hope construct, our attempt now is to outline the main elements and dimensions that seem to entail in Indian Philosophy. We do this, without aspiring to formulate a holistic conceptualization of an Indian Psychology of Hope, but offering our interpretation and conclusions as a starting point for further scientific scrutiny, elaboration and debate.

1. The first obvious finding is the existence of two opposite types of hope, differentiated by the objects and aims they are directed to: On the one hand, ephemeral, illusive and detrimental hopes focused on materialistic and egoistic goals. On the other hand, a sublime and divine hope, aiming to achieve liberation and self-realization.
2. Hope is intimately related to spirituality and transcendence, and in particular to love and religious faith. Yet, transcendence does not denote an unknown spiritual world, which is far away from this material earth, but refers to the possibility to overcome the blinding illusions and the harmful desires of our ego in order to achieve higher levels (right here and now on this earth) of consciousness.

3. Consequently, hope is based on the acquisition of knowledge, but not in a purely rational and cognitive sense, but through personal, subjective and spiritual experience. The most important knowledge is not that about the material world, but about our true Self. In this sense, contemplation, meditative introspection and intuition become important sources of knowledge and therefore of hope.

4. Hope is mainly directed to existential aspects in life and has a transformative effect on men. In peoples' daily life, one primary hope is to overcome pain and suffering, to liberate oneself from negative constrains, in order to be able to live a healthy, harmonious, happy, and fulfilling life.

5. Hope has an agentic character. It drives the person to act. However, the agent is not located in the rational and self-centered mind, but in the divine Self within oneself. The will-power stemming from the divine Self is the fundamental condition for the possibility of liberation and self-realization.

6. Although hope is associated with action, it is fundamentally based on feelings of inner peace, calm, tranquility, and persistence. The inner force to hope and persevere comes from an attitude of humility, not demanding and expecting anything but being prepared to exhume the highest bliss.

7. Anchored in a natural and moral order, true hope must be understood as a moral virtue. In this sense, we are asked to hope only for the good and never for something evil. If thoughts have an effect on other persons including ourselves, following the principle of *Karma* (of cause and effect), negative hopes (or wishes) will have negative effects on us and our environment as well. Therefore, hope must be attached to an attitude of charity, altruism and compassion.

8. According to the principle of non-duality, hope and hopelessness, like optimism and pessimism, must not be considered opposites but the two sides of the same coin. Both experiences come often together, have a fundamental value in itself and help the person to become aware of his/her true nature. Hopeless suffering is sometimes the best way to discover the need for inner transformation, liberation and self-realization, which in turn gives rise to a new quality of hope.

9. The scope of hope is both located at the individual and at the collective level. Point of departure is the single individual but the final goal is the common good and the transformation of the human race to a higher level of evolution. Personal harmony will lead to harmonious human relations as well as to harmony between humanity and the natural environment.

10. Notably, it stands out that the social dimension as an important source of hope has apparently been neglected in Indian Philosophy. This is even more surprising because the main virtues to attain self-realization are that of helping other people in an unselfish way. If altruism, charity and compassion were expected to have a positive effect on others' life, particularly helping them in turn to achieve liberation and self-realization, the consequence would be to believe that altruistic and supportive people would be able to engender hope in others.

Empirical Findings from the Hope-Barometer Survey

The number of studies on hope in the Indian context has increased rapidly during the last years. Especially in the Indian Journal of Positive Psychology, empirical results have been published on the relation of hope and spirituality (Budhiraja & Midha, 2015), hope and faith (Chaudhary, Chadha, & Seth, 2017), hope and personal growth (Sharma & Garg, 2016), hope and well-being (Singh, Singh, Singh, & Srivastava, 2013), hope and life satisfaction (Thakre, 2013; Yadav & Thingujam, 2015), hope and meaning in life (Vidwans & Raghvendra, 2016), hope, mindfulness and happiness (Singh & Devender, 2015), hope and self-esteem (Yadav & Thingujam, 2015), and hope, self-efficacy and procrastination (Tripathi, Kochar, & Dara, 2015), mostly addressing young adults at university. Remarkably, all these studies endorse and employ the cognitive concept of Dispositional Hope developed by Snyder (2002) to assess the level of general hope of the Indian participants. Exponents of Indian Psychology have already noticed and regretted, that psychological research in India has mainly focused on adopting and replicating Western concepts blindly, without judging their theoretical and practical appropriateness (Dalal, 2010; Rao, 2014a). To our knowledge, only one study in India did not take the cognitive definition of hope as granted, and explored the concept of hope as perceived by people, using a phenomenological research methodology (Behrani & Jadeja, 2016). The authors came to the conclusion, that hope is a vast, abstract and sometimes irrational phenomenon and that it "is beyond our immediate reality, experience and thus limitless" (Ibid, p. 107). One major limitation of this study, although appropriate for the chosen research approach, is the small number of participants (N = 12) that have been examined.

The goals of our empirical study are the exploration of the concept of hope as perceived by a sample of about 300 Indians aged 18–29, the assessment of the correlations of perceived hope with other psychological constructs, the identification of the targets and sources of hope and comparing these results with a similar sample of European participants so as to identify cultural similarities and differences. In addition, one further objective is to evaluate as to how far the empirical findings help to support the concept of hope, which is duly endorsed by Indian Philosophy as outlined in the previous sections.

Procedure and Samples

Data collection for Indian respondents was done by the second author through distribution of the Hope-Barometer questionnaire via e-mail and social media in November 2015 and 2016. The sample of 2015 includes a total of 130 respondents and that of 2016 a total of 183. For data analysis, we merged both samples, obtaining the following demographic distribution: From the 313 participants living in

India, 247 (78.9%) were males and 66 females (21.1%). All respondents were between 18 and 29 years old (M = 20.9; SD = 2.6). Regarding their occupation, 295 participants (94.2%) were still in education, 12 had a fulltime job (3.8%), one a part-time job (0.3%) and five were jobless (1.6%). Concerning their religious denomination, 217 (69.3%) declared to be Hinduist, 10 (3.2%) belonged to a Christian faith, six (1.9%) were Islamic, one (0.3%) Buddhist, 31 (9.9%) considered themselves to be spiritual persons outside the traditional world religions, 30 (9.6%) affirmed to be without religion or confession, and 18 (5.8%) were of another religious faith.

In order to compare the Indian data with a similar homogeneous group of European people, we employed a subsample of 384 respondents of Christian denomination aged 18–29, who answered the questionnaire in Germany (n = 95; 24.7%) and German speaking Switzerland (n = 289; 75.3%). This sample is constituted by 244 (63.5%) women and 140 (36.5%) men, 154 (40.1%) people still in education, 186 (48.4%) with a fulltime job, 28 (7.3%) with part-time employment, and 16 (4.2%) without any occupation. In the current chapter, we refer to this sample as the German group or the Germans, not in terms of nationality, but in the ethnic and cultural sense. In both samples all participants were singles (unmarried and without a partnership).

Methods

Instruments to Measure Hope

Perceived Hope Scale   To measure the general level of hope, we used the unidimensional six-items Perceived Hope Scale (PHS) (Krafft, Martin-Krumm, & Fenouillet, 2017) with a response scale ranging from 0 (strongly disagree) to 5 (strongly agree). Cronbach's alpha in the Indian sample was 0.83 and it was 0.88 for the German sample.

Agency   Dispositional hope is defined as a trait-like cognitive mindset involving two basic components: Agency and Pathways (Snyder et al., 1991). Agency is the basic perception of one's determination and motivation to initiate and sustain actions (will-power) to reach defined personal goals. The four items were scored on a 6-point scale from 0 (strongly disagree) to 5 (strongly agree). Alpha coefficients were satisfactory in both, the Indian (α = 0.73) and the German (α = 0.80) sample.

Pathways   Snyder's theory of hope has a self-centered character, in that it refers to the person's perception in relation to his or her own efficacy to attain personal goals (Snyder et al., 1991). Pathways represents the belief in one's own capabilities to create alternative routes in case of facing obstacles and setbacks (way-power). The four items were also scored on a 6-point scale from 0 (strongly disagree) to 5 (strongly agree). Cronbach's alphas were satisfactory (Indian sample α = 0.78 and German sample α = 0.75).

Personal Hopes for the Coming Year in Different Life Domains In order to evaluate the importance of different targets of hope, we used a self-constructed scale with 15 life domains in terms of people's hopes for the coming year. The 15 life domains belong to six basic dimensions: (1) Wellbeing, (2) social relations, (3) hedonic experiences, (4) work and material goods, (5) religiosity/spirituality, and (6) meaning and purpose. The items were rated on a 4-point scale from 0 (not important) to 3 (very important).

Activities to Fulfil One's Own Hopes A further pool of items includes ten activities people perform in order to fulfil their own hopes. These activities together constituted: (1) The cognitive-rational dimension, (2) the social-relational dimension, (3) the spiritual-religious dimension, and (4) the motivational dimension. The Likert scale for rating the single items was ranging between 0 (not at all) to 3 (very often).

Hope Providers A scale with ten items was also developed to evaluate the people or categories of people that are considered to be hope providers. The ten items cover six basic dimensions: (1) The self-centered category of oneself, (2) the inner circle of people in the closer social environment, (3) a group of people in the work environment, (4) people in the wider social environment that are usually known personally, (5) people in the general social environment, and (6) the transcendent environment (i.e. "God"). The items are rated on a Likert scale from 0 (not at all) to 3 (yes, definitely).

Instruments for Comparison of Mean Values and Correlation Coefficients

A couple of relevant standardized scales were also employed to assess the relation of hope to other constructs representing five basic dimensions relevant to Indian and Positive Psychology. These include measures on Social Relations (Attachment, Loneliness), Transcendence (Religious Faith, Spiritual Beliefs), Virtuous Thoughts and Actions (Generativity, Compassion, Helping Others), Fulfillment (Meaning and Harmony in Life), and Subjective Well-being (Positive Affects, Life-satisfaction, Happiness).

Social Relations

Attachment The intensity of social relations was measured with the Attachment subscale of the Comprehensive Trait Hope Scale of Scioli and his colleagues (Scioli, Ricci, Nyugen, & Scioli, 2011). This subscale is composed of four items measuring basic trust in others and four items to assess openness towards other people and the larger community. The items are rated on a 4-point Likert scale from 0 (not me) to 3 (exactly like me). Cronbach's alphas for the composed scores were 0.69 for the Indian and 0.80 for the German sample.

Loneliness The Short Loneliness Scale was developed by Hughes, Waite, Hawkley, and Cacioppo (2004). The scale measures the perception of social isolation using three items to be rated from 1 (never) to 5 (all of the time). The Cronbach's alpha in the present study was 0.87 for the Indian and 0.82 for the German sample.

Transcendence

Religious Faith We used the short form of the Santa Clara Strength of Religious Faith Questionnaire (Plante & Boccaccini, 1997; Storch, Roberti, Bravata, & Storch, 2004) with 5 items scored on a 4-point scale (1 = strongly disagree to 4 = strongly agree). Cronbach's alpha in the Indian sample was 0.93 and it was 0.92 for the German sample.

Spiritual Beliefs We employed the four items of the Importance of Spiritual Beliefs in Life, a subscale of the Spirituality Questionnaire (Parsian & Dunning, 2009) which is rated on a 4-point scale (1–4). The scale revealed a very good internal consistency of $\alpha = 0.96$ for both the samples.

Virtuous Thoughts and Actions

Generativity Generativity has been defined as the creation of things of lasting value and for future generations (Schnell, 2009). Six items of the Sources of Meaning and Meaning in Life Questionnaire (Schnell & Becker, 2007) are dedicated to score generativity on a 6-point scale from 0 (strongly disagree) to 5 (strongly agree). The alpha coefficients were 0.90 for the Indian and 0.82 for the German sample.

Compassion We used the Brief Santa Clara Compassion Scale developed by Hwang, Plante and Lackey (2008) as a short version of the Compassionate Love Scale from Sprecher and Fehr (2005). Compassion has been defined as an attitude toward others, containing feelings, cognition, and behavior that are focused on caring, concern, tenderness, and a pro-social orientation toward supporting, helping, and understanding others. The five items, scored on a Likert scale from 1 (not at all true for me) to 7 (very true for me), revealed a very good internal consistency at $\alpha = 0.89$ for the Indian and $\alpha = 0.86$ for the German sample.

Helping Others Helping others is a pro-social attitude and behavior that positively correlates with altruism, empathy and social responsibility, and negatively correlates with selfishness. We measured this attitude with a short-form of the Helping Attitude Scale (Nickell, 1998), employing seven items with a 5-point scale from 1 (not at all true of me) to 5 (very true of me). Cronbach's alpha reliability was high, both in the Indian ($\alpha = .92$) as well as in the German sample ($\alpha = .88$).

Fulfillment

Meaning in Life Meaning in Life was measured with four items measuring the presence of meaning in life from the Meaning in Life Questionnaire (Steger, Frazier, Oishi, & Kaler, 2006) using a 7-point scale from 1 (strongly disagree) to 7 (strongly agree). Internal consistency was very good at $\alpha = 0.95$ for the Indian and $\alpha = 0.89$ for the German sample.

Harmony in Life The recently developed Harmony in Life Scale (Kjell, Daukantaité, Hefferon, & Sikström, 2016) measures psychological experiences of inner balance, peace of mind, calm and unity. The five items are scored on a 7-point scale ranging from 1 (strongly disagree) to 7 (strongly agree). The authors highlight the concept of harmony in life as being related to a holistic world-view that incorporates a more balanced and flexible approach to personal well-being. Cronbach's alphas in our samples were 0.89 for the Indian and 0.87 for the German group.

Subjective Well-Being

Positive Affects We applied the six items designed by Diener et al. (2010) to assess pleasant emotional experiences and feelings. The participants were asked to think about what they have been doing and experiencing during the past 4 weeks and to score feelings such as "good", "pleasant" and "joyful" on a 5-point scale from 1 (very rarely or never) to 5 (very often or always). The alpha coefficients were 0.89 for the Indian and 0.92 for the German sample.

Life Satisfaction Life satisfaction is one of the cognitive components of subjective well-being and according to Diener and his colleagues (Diener, Emmons, Larsen, & Griffin, 1985) it is the result of comparing one's life circumstances to one's expectations, also predicting people's future behavior (Pavot & Diener, 2008). The Satisfaction with Life Scale (SLS) consists of five items scored on a 7-point scale from 1 (strongly disagree) to 7 (strongly agree). Cronbach's alpha in the Indian sample was 0.87 and it was 0.88 for the German sample.

Happiness The four items of the Subjective Happiness Scale (SHS) represent a subjective and global judgment about the extent to which people feel happy or unhappy (Lyubomirsky & Lepper, 1999). The possible scores go from 1 to 7. In the Indian sample the alpha coefficient was 0.84 and it was found to be 0.83 for the German sample.

Data Analysis

Invariance Between Groups In order to be able to compare the results of the Indian and the German samples accurately, we firstly tested the measurement invariance of the Perceived Hope Scale. Measurement invariance can be tested using confirmatory factor analysis in a stepwise incremental way, going from a least restricted solution to models that entail increasingly restrictive constraints (Brown, 2006). When researchers want to compare scores between groups, a strong (scalar) invariance is needed. The resulting CFA models were evaluated using the following goodness-of-fit indices: Root-Mean-Square Error of Approximation (RMSEA), Standardized Root Mean Residual (SRMR), Comparative Fit Index (CFI) and the Tucker-Lewis Index (TLI). To evaluate the invariance tests, the recommended threshold values for comparing the baseline model (equal form) and the nested models are a decrease in CFI and TLI equal or lower than .01, a change in RMSEA of .015 or less, a maximum change in SRMR of .03 for metric variance and of 0.01 for scalar variance (Chen, 2007).

Comparison of Mean Values via t-Test for Independent Samples In order to find out the main commonalities and differences between the Indian and the German participants, we compared the mean values of the employed variables. Since two different samples were being compared, we presumed that the survey conditions of the two groups of participants in India (via e-mail and social media) and German speaking Europe (via internet) could have been perceived differently, hence we chose to compare the mean values of the variables employing the *t*-test for independent samples.

Comparison of Pearson's Correlation Coefficients To analyze the relation between hope and other variables in the Indian and the German group and for being able to find similarities and significant differences between both groups, the correlation comparison procedure of Fisher was performed, calculating the z-values to evaluate the significance of the difference between two correlation coefficients.

Linear Multiple Regression Analysis Defining perceived hope as dependent variable (criterion), several multiple regression analyses were performed, defining the personal hopes, the activities to fulfill one's hopes, and the hope providers alternatively as independent variables (predictors).

Data was computed using SPSS and AMOS v.23 software (Arbuckle, 2014; IBM, 2014).

Results

Invariance of the PHS Across the Indian and the German Groups

To be able to compare scores between groups accurately, the first analysis aims to measure the invariance of the Perceived Hope Scale across the Indian and the German group of participants. The overall fit indices exhibited in Table 7.1 reveal that the one-factor model for the total sample achieves good model fit. All freely estimated factor loadings were statistically significant ($p < .001$), and completely standardized loadings ranged from 0.635 to 0.847. The equal form provided a good

Table 7.1 Measurement invariance of the PHS (Indian & German sample)

Model	χ^2	df	RMSEA	SRMR	CFI	TLI
Total sample	52.18	9	.083	.0304	.976	.961
Configurational invariance	93.21	18	.068	.0306	.971	.952
Metric (weak) invariance	93.68	23	.058	.0306	.973	.962
Scalar (strong) invariance	134.18	29	.063	.0309	.961	.958
Full invariance	175.72	36	.065	.0395	.946	.955

Indicators: *PHS* Perceived Hope Scale; *df* degrees of freedom, *RMSEA* root mean square error of approximation, *SRMR* standardized root mean residual, *CFI* comparative fit index, *TLI* Tucker-Lewis Index

fit to the data, suggesting reasonable support for configurational invariance across the two groups. Using the equal form as baseline model, the equal factor loading solution to measure metric (weak) invariance produced acceptable goodness-of-fit indices (ΔRMSEA = .01; ΔSRMR = 0; ΔCFI = .002; ΔTLI = $-$.01). The equal intercepts model to measure scalar (strong) invariance was also found to have a good fit to the data (ΔRMSEA = $-$.005; ΔSRMR = .0003; ΔCFI = $-$.01; ΔTLI = .007). Strict invariance (full uniqueness) was achieved for the indices ΔRMSEA = $-$.003, ΔSRMR = $-$.003 and ΔTLI = .003, but not for ΔCFI = $-$.025. This means that the PHS reveals strong invariance, and that comparison of scores between the Indian and the German groups is possible.

Descriptive Analysis, Bivariate Pearson Correlations and Value Comparisons

Table 7.2 exhibits the mean values, standard deviations and bivariate correlation values between the different variables and perceived hope. The first analysis is dedicated to compare the mean values of the list of variables between the Indian and the German sample, using the *t*-Test for independent groups. In the following paragraphs, we report the full data of *t*-values (*t*), degrees of freedom (*df*), significance levels (*p*), standard errors (*SE*) and effect sizes (*ES*) only for cases where the differences between the Indian and the German groups are significant. The differences in degrees of freedom are the consequence of assuming equal variances or not, following the results of Levene's Test. Effect sizes around 0.10 are considered to be small, around 0.30 medium and around 0.50 large (Cohen, 1992).

The differences of Indians and Germans in mean values of the hope variables perceived hope, agency and pathways reflect low effect sizes ($ES < .07$) and are statistically not significant ($p > .05$). With regard to the variables to measure social relations, Indians reveal significantly lower levels of social attachment ($M = 2.00$, $SE = .04$; t (575) = -3.98, p < .001; $ES = .16$) and higher levels of loneliness ($M = 2.96$, $SE = .08$; t (695) = 4.57, p < .001; $ES = .14$) than the German participants (attachment: $M = 2.20$, $SE = .03$; loneliness: $M = 2.59$; $SE = .03$). Inversely, the Indian group is significantly higher in those variables belonging to the dimension of

Table 7.2 Means, standard deviations and partial correlation coefficients with perceived hope

Constructs	Indian			German		
	M	SD	PHS, r	M	SD	PHS, r
Hope						
Perceived hope	3.36	0.94		3.29	0.86	
Agency	3.27	0.92	.433*	3.31	0.86	.581*
Pathways	3.63	0.85	.392*	3.54	0.74	.626*
Social relations						
Attachment	2.00	0.51	.199*	2.20	0.57	.487*
Loneliness	2.96	0.92	−.255*	2.59	0.84	−.403*
Transcendence						
Religious faith	2.36	0.87	.352*	1.74	0.82	.204*
Spiritual beliefs	2.34	0.94	.263*	1.77	0.88	.239*
Virtues thoughts and actions						
Generativity	3.77	1.08	.397*	3.27	0.91	.344*
Compassion	4.87	1.36	.275*	4.68	1.32	.164*
Helping others	4.06	0.76	.418*	4.14	0.63	.325*
Fulfillment						
Meaning in life	4.42	1.69	.449*	4.77	1.27	.502*
Harmony in life	4.72	1.32	.330*	4.63	1.14	.622*
Subjective well-being						
Positive affects	3.52	0.78	.281*	3.66	0.78	.583*
Life satisfaction	4.02	1.41	.553*	4.77	1.27	.616*
Happiness	4.58	1.39	.479*	4.62	1.30	.645*

PHS Perceived Hope Scale
*$p < .001$

transcendence, namely religious faith ($M = 2.36$, $SE = .08$; $t (695) = 8.05$, p < .001; $ES = .24$) and spiritual beliefs ($M = 2.34$, $SE = .08$; $t (695) = 6.91$, p < .001; $ES = .21$) compared to the German group (religious faith: $M = 1.74$, $SE = .03$; spiritual beliefs: $M = 1.77$; $SE = .03$).

In the field of virtuous thoughts and actions, Indian participants are notably and significantly higher in generativity ($M = 3.77$, $SE = .09$; $t (155) = 5.03$, p < .001; $ES = .37$) vis-á-vis their German counterparts ($M = 3.27$; $SE = .03$). Not significant are the differences in compassion and helping others. While the German group is slightly higher in life meaning and the Indian group in harmony, these differences are also statistically not significant. In the dimension of Subjective Well-being, the German sample manifests significantly higher values of positive affects ($M = 3.66$, $SE = .04$; $t (695) = 2.02$, p < .05; $ES = .08$) and especially of life satisfaction ($M = 4.77$, $SE = .04$; $t (695) = 6.21$, p < .001; $ES = .19$) than the Indian sample (positive affects: $M = 3.52$, $SE = .06$; life satisfaction: $M = 4.02$; $SE = .12$). Not significant and of low effect is the difference in happiness.

The next analysis focuses on the Pearson correlation coefficients between the single variables and perceived hope and furthermore on the comparisons of these values between the Indian and the German groups using Fischer's test. As control variables, we included gender and main occupation (in education, fulltime, part-time job, etc.) in the analysis. The first glance at this analysis suggests that all correlation coefficients are highly significant at $p < .001$.

The motivational and cognitive dimensions of hope, agency and pathways, display moderate to large correlation values with perceived hope, significantly higher for the German than for the Indian sample (agency: $z = -2.26$; $p < .05$; pathways: $z = -3.61$; $p < .001$). Of medium size but significantly higher for the German group are the correlation values of perceived hope with social attachment ($z = -3.72$; $p < .001$) and (in negative terms) with loneliness ($z = 1.76$; $p < .05$). Indians, to the contrary, display higher correlation values of hope with religious faith ($z = 1.70$; $p < .05$) and with spiritual beliefs (not significant). Of medium size and larger than the German values, though statistically not significant, are the correlation coefficients of generativity, compassion and helping others in the Indian group. The two constructs covering the dimension of fulfillment, namely meaning and harmony in life, reveal moderate to large correlation values with hope, especially for the German group. Remarkably, harmony in life displays in relation with hope a significantly higher correlation coefficient for the German than for the Indian group ($z = -4.34$; $p < .001$). The variables to assess positive emotions show moderate to large correlation values with hope, especially for the German sample. Statistically significant are the differences for positive affects ($z = -4.26$; $p < .001$) and happiness ($z = -2.59$; $p < .01$).

Exploring Hope: Personal Hopes, Hope Activities and Hope Providers

This section is dedicated to explore the phenomenon of hope, as experienced by people in their daily life. It includes the enquiry of the main objects of hope, the activities people perform in order to get their hopes fulfilled and the people envisioned as hope providers. The three pools of items will be analyzed in three similar ways: (1) Computing the mean value of every single item and defining the rank order within the list; (2) comparing the rank orders and the mean values between the Indian and the German groups performing t-tests for independent samples; (3) running a linear multiple regression with perceived hope as dependent variable and the list of items as predictors.

The goals of these analyses were mainly: (1) to examine the aspects people consciously and explicitly connect in different degrees with their experience of hope; (2) to detect similarities and differences between two groups of people living in diverse cultural and religious environments; and (3) to assess the relation between the single hope targets, activities and providers with the general experience and level of hope so as to recognize the possible value of singular life aspects with respect to hope.

Table 7.3 Personal hopes. Mean values, rank orders and *t*-tests (N = 697)

	Indian		German					
	R	M	R	M	t	df	p	d
Success at work, university, etc.	1	2.54	4	2.45	1.65	695	.099	.13
Personal independence	2	2.52	7	2.29	4.22	689	.000	.32
Personal health	3	2.44	1	2.64	−3.62	627	.000	.29
Meaningful and satisfying task	4	2.39	8	2.28	1.99	695	.047	.15
Good and trustful relationships	5	2.35	2	2.59	−4.34	612	.000	.34
Harmony in life	6	2.18	5	2.38	−3.38	695	.001	.25
Happy partnership, family, marriage	7	2.13	3	2.56	−6.61	587	.000	.52
More fun with friends	8	2.10	6	2.32	−3.62	695	.000	.28
Helping other people	9	1.98	13	1.88	1.50	695	.135	.11
Secure job	10	1.95	9	2.25	−4.01	584	.000	.31
More money	11	1.81	14	1.59	3.05	624	.002	.23
More sex, romantic experiences	12	1.64	10	2.01	−4.67	605	.000	.37
More spare time	13	1.60	11	1.98	−5.28	620	.000	.41
More time to relax	14	1.58	12	1.96	−5.20	625	.000	.40
Religious and spiritual experiences	15	1.48	15	0.75	9.16	630	.000	.71

Contrary to normative standards, negative sign of *t*-test values are reported for a quick comparison

Personal Hopes

In Table 7.3, we report the mean values (*M*), rank orders (R), *t*-values (*t*), degrees of freedom (*df*), probability levels (*p*), and Cohen's effect sizes (*d*) of the list of personal hopes in terms of their perceived importance. If we split the list (somewhat arbitrarily) in three segments with five items each, we can recognize the relative importance of the single items for the two groups of participants. Looking at the upper segment of the two lists, the rank order of the first five items indicates that while for the Indian group, personal achievements (e.g. success) seem to be more important than personal health and the social dimension (e.g. good social relationships). Whereas for the German people, it appears to be the other way round (social relations and personal health more important than success). Drawing the attention to the bottom of the list, it becomes evident that materialistic (e.g. more money) and hedonic hopes (e.g. more sex), as well as religious and spiritual experiences are less important for both groups.

Comparing the single items across both groups, the following striking results become evident: The Indian group scores the item 'success at work, university, etc.', on the one hand, and the item 'to help other people', on the other hand, slightly but in statistical terms not significantly higher than the German group. The mean value for 'personal independence' is significantly higher for the Indian group, whereas the score for 'personal health' is stronger for the German participants. While a 'meaningful and satisfying task' is more important for the Indian people, the item 'secure job' is higher for the German group. In all three items belonging to the social dimension (happy partnership, good social relationships and fun with friends) the German group scores significantly higher than the Indian group. Although relatively less important in the rank list, Indians hope for 'money' more intensely than Germans, whereas Germans are more wishful compared to Indians regarding 'more sex', 'more spare time' and 'more time to relax'. Especially interesting is the least valued item for both groups i.e. the relevance of 'religious and spiritual experiences'. It seems evident that the difference between the Indian and the German groups is the largest; the score of the Indian group is much higher than that of the Germans.

The relation of the individual hope items with the general level of perceived hope was assessed by a multiple stepwise regression analysis. For the Indian sample, the regression model was significant [F (3,309) = 15.397; $p < 0.001$; Adjusted $R^2 = .12$], with only three items displaying significant regression coefficients, namely: (1) Meaningful and satisfying task ($\beta = .215$; $p < .001$); (2) religious and spiritual experiences ($\beta = .139$; $p < .05$); and (3) helping other people ($\beta = .141$; $p < .05$). The regression coefficients of all other items were not significant.

The German sample generated a significant regression model [F (7,376) = 12.897; $p < 0.001$; Adjusted $R^2 = .18$], with seven coefficients resulting to be significant predictors: (1) Personal health ($\beta = .208$; $p < .001$); (2) meaningful and satisfying task ($\beta = .178$; $p < .001$); (3) religious and spiritual experiences ($\beta = .166$; $p < .001$); (4) to help other people ($\beta = .129$; $p < .01$); (5) success at work, etc. ($\beta = .108$; $p < .05$); (6) more money ($\beta = -.165$; $p < .001$) and (7) secure job ($\beta = -.157$; $p < .01$). It is worth to be noted that the facets of importance of 'more money' and of a 'secure job' correlated negatively with perceived hope.

Hope Activities

The next question was concerned with the activities people may undertake in order to accomplish their targets of hope. Table 7.4 exhibits ten items belonging to the cognitive, motivational, social, and religious/spiritual dimensions, which were ranked according to their mean values. For the Indian sample, among the first five activities with the highest scores, four can be counted as the cognitive and motivational dimensions and one as the social dimension ('I motivate my friends'). In the German group, the highest score was achieved by the item 'I motivate my friends', followed by three cognitive-motivational activities and one additional social item. In both samples, the four items with the lowest scores include the three religious-spiritual activities as well as the giving activity of donating money. In general, the Indian participants scored all items significantly higher than the German group, with exception of the items 'I motivate my friends' (significantly higher for Germans) and 'I motivate my family' (not significant). The largest differences are those related to the cognitive items 'I inform myself…' and 'I think a lot…', to the item 'I donate money…', as well as to the religious/spiritual items 'I go to church…' and 'I trust God'.

Table 7.4 Activities to fulfil hope. Mean values, rank orders and t-tests ($N = 697$)

	Indian		German		t	df	p	d
	R	M	R	M				
I think a lot and analyze circumstances	1	2.45	2	2.06	6.85	695	.000	.52
I inform myself (read, use internet, ...)	2	2.27	6	1.29	14.38	695	.000	1.08
I take responsibility and commit myself	3	2.21	3	1.93	4.87	695	.000	.37
I motivate my friends	4	1.95	1	2.13	−2.81	595	.005	.22
I save money	5	1.91	5	1.57	4.82	687	.000	.36
I motivate my family	6	1.87	4	1.86	0.23	695	.817	.01
I trust God	7	1.86	7	1.10	8.75	695	.000	.67
I donate money ...	8	1.38	9	0.61	11.27	610	.000	.86
I pray, meditate	9	1.33	8	0.86	6.25	695	.000	.47
I go to church/other place of warship	10	1.23	10	0.57	9.00	613	.000	.69

The linear multiple regression analysis for the Indian sample resulted in a significant model [$F (4,308) = 11.603$; $p < 0.001$; Adjusted $R^2 = .12$], including four items with significant predictor coefficients: (1) I pray, meditate ($\beta = .171$; $p < .01$); (2) I motivate my friends ($\beta = .127$; $p < .05$); (3) I take responsibility and commit myself ($\beta = .125$; $p < .05$); and (4) I motivate my family ($\beta = .123$; $p < .05$). No item belonging to the cognitive dimension (e.g. 'I think a lot...' and 'I inform myself...') was a significant predictor of perceived hope.

A very similar picture emerges when analyzing the German sample. A significant model [$F (3,380) = 34.657$; $p < 0.001$; Adjusted $R^2 = .21$] includes three predictors with significant coefficients: (1) I take responsibility and commit myself ($\beta = .359$; $p < .001$); (2) I motivate my family ($\beta = .161$; $p \leq .001$); and (3) I pray, meditate ($\beta = .119$; $p \leq .01$). All other items turned out to be not significant.

Summarizing, whereas in the Indian sample 'to pray and to meditate' is the strongest predictor of perceived hope and to take responsibility is the third largest, in the German sample it is the other way round: to 'take responsibility and to commit oneself' is the main predictor and 'to pray and to meditate' appears on the third place.

Hope Providers

The last pool of items is comprised of a list of people from whom the participants of the survey might expect the transmission of hope. On the top of the Indian list (see Table 7.5) stands the self-centered item 'I give myself hope- it's the responsibility of every person him-/herself', followed by the items 'parents/grandparents' and 'friends'. These three items are also at the top of the German list, but with the items 'friends' and 'parents, grandparents' ranking first and second, followed by 'I give myself hope' as third item. Moreover, the mean score of the item 'friends' is significantly higher in the German compared to the Indian group. Conversely, the item 'I give myself hope' displays a significantly higher score in the Indian group vis-á-vis

Table 7.5 Hope providers. Mean values, rank orders and t-tests (N = 697)

	Indian		German					
	R	M	R	M	t	df	p	d
I give myself hope …	1	2.34	3	2.06	4.53	695	.000	.35
Parents, grandparents	2	2.27	2	2.31	−0.59	695	.553	.05
Friends	3	2.05	1	2.37	−4.81	603	.000	.37
Teachers, educators, professors, …	4	1.95	4	1.55	5.44	682	.000	.42
God	5	1.58	8	1.09	5.57	695	.000	.42
Experts, scientists, researchers, …	6	1.34	7	1.22	1.66	648	.098	.12
Physicians, therapists, etc.	7	1.28	6	1.41	−1.72	695	.087	.12
Entrepreneurs, businessmen, managers	8	1.21	9	0.86	4.84	632	.000	.38
Priests, spiritual leaders, gurus, …	9	1.05	10	0.64	5.50	613	.000	.42
Politicians, the government	10	0.93	5	1.48	−6.99	674	.000	.53

the German sample. The religious/spiritual items 'God' and 'Priests, spiritual leaders, gurus' ranks at the center and at the end of the list in both samples respectively. The mean values of both items are significantly higher for the Indian group.

The multiple regression analysis performed with the Indian sample, generated a significant model [F (3,309) = 21.311; $p < 0.001$; Adjusted R^2 = .16] with three predictors achieving a significant regression coefficient: (1) I give myself hope (β = .240; $p < .001$); (2) entrepreneurs, businessmen, managers (β = .237; $p < .001$); and (3) God (β = .140; $p < .01$).

For the German sample, a significant model resulted [F (3,380) = 23.098; $p < 0.001$; Adjusted R^2 = .15] that also includes three significant predictors namely (1) Priests, spiritual leaders, gurus (β = .269; $p < .001$); (2) I give myself hope (β = .224; $p < .001$); and (3) parents, grandparents (β = .125; $p < .01$).

Discussion

The mainstream theory of hope in Western psychology, largely adopted by many psychology researchers in India, has been that of Snyder, who understands hope as an individual, self-centered cognitive and motivational trait and experience, related to the attainment of personal goals. As he formulated it: "Hope is the essential process of linking oneself to potential success" (Snyder, 1994, p. 18). The emphasis in Snyder's hope theory is put on achievement, performance, self-efficacy, resilience and coping (Snyder, 2000a). Very hopeful people perceive themselves in control of their lives and having a sense of self-direction. Hope is related to perceptions of personal mastery, individual will-power and the ability to solve problems. Hopeful people are ambitious because they tend to have a greater number and more difficult goals than average people do. The process of hoping is seen as a universal phenomenon largely neutral about the moral value of the goals (Snyder, 2002). Thoughts and actions have predominance over feelings. Relationships to other people are important, however, primarily in taking into consideration the goals and perspectives of others to pursue one's own goals (Snyder, 2000b).

Although hope is an important concept in Indian Philosophy, until now, as far as we know, Indian Psychology does not maintain any formal theory of hope. Reverting to interpretations of ancient Indian scriptures by Aurobindo and Vivekananda, we attempted to identify the central meanings and attributes of hope in Indian Philosophy. Basically, there are two distinct types of hope: Those superfluous hopes directed to materialistic and egoistic goals, on the one hand, and the uplifting hope related to spiritual inner growth and self-realization, on the other. This latter hope refers to existential life domains. The main goal is to overcome suffering and to be able to live a healthy, harmonious, happy, and fulfilling life. Key aspects of this kind of hope are spirituality and religious faith, connected to the wish and to concrete practices that transcend one's own ego. Sources of hope can be found in cognitive but even more in intuitive forms of knowledge rooted in the divine within ourselves. Furthermore, hope has an agentic character based on the will-power of higher consciousness. Hope can be nourished by feelings of inner peace, calm, tranquility, humility and persistence. This kind of hope is in essence a moral virtue, comprising values of charity, altruism and compassion, transforming the person for the better. The ultimate goal is to lead the human race to a higher level of peace, harmony and bliss. Surprisingly, the social dimension of hope, seen in terms of the importance of other people, especially family members and friends, as relevant hope providers, seems to have been considered less significant in the Indian philosophical system.

Many Western authors have integrated into their conceptualization of hope several dimensions, such as the cognitive, the spiritual, the relational and the existential (Dufault & Martocchio, 1985; Farran et al., 1995; Scioli & Biller, 2009). Particularly in Positive Psychology, the spiritual and transcendent dimension of hope has started to gain more attention (Peterson & Seligman, 2004; Scioli, 2007). The results of the Hope-Barometer survey can contribute to add new insights into the nature and the quality of hope, particularly from and in the Indian context. Comparing the Indian sample of young adults with the European group, the first striking findings are related to the levels of different psychological experiences: Indians enjoy similar levels of perceived hope, agency, pathways and overall happiness as their German-speaking counterparts. Differences, nonetheless, can be found in other psychological phenomena: Indians express lower levels in their quality of social relations, in positive emotions and in life satisfaction. On the contrary, Indians reveal higher levels of religious faith, spirituality and generativity. Whereas when it comes to differences in the levels of compassion, helping others, meaning and harmony in life, the differences between the two groups are not significant.

When we look at the several dimensions in more detailed manner and from many different angles, we are able to find further similarities and distinctions between the two groups of participants. The correlation values of the cognitive, goal and achievement oriented constructs, agency and pathways, with perceived hope are moderate and significantly lower for the Indian sample. Yet, for the Indian group, personal success and self-determination are located at the top of the personal hopes, whereas for the European sample the top three personal hopes are related to personal health, good social relations and a happy family. In general, the importance of hope concerning good social relations is higher for Europeans than for Indians. Interestingly, the hopes regarding personal success and self-determination are not significant predictors of the general perception of hope neither for Indians nor for Europeans. Conversely, the hope for a meaningful and satisfying task is positively related with perceived hope in both groups. Many Indians consider the self-centered attitude of giving oneself hope the supreme source of hope, and indeed, this item is one of the major predictors of hope in both samples. However, Europeans, on average, consider parents, grandparents and friends as more worthy sources of hope than merely to trust in one's own capabilities. Parents and grandparents are in fact a significant predictor of perceived hope only for the German group. Looking at the concrete activities people perform to attain their personal hopes, Indians consequently deem the cognitive activities (to think a lot, to analyze circumstances and inform oneself widely) as the mostly valued. For the German group, the social activities to motivate friends and to motivate family members are at the top of the list instead, which turns out to be significant predictors of general hope in both groups. Remarkably, no item describing a cognitive activity appeared to be a significant predictor of perceived hope in neither of the two groups.

Guiding the attention to the religious, spiritual, transcendent and altruistic dimensions, Indians reveal to have significantly higher correlation values of perceived hope with religious faith but similar levels in relation to spiritual beliefs, compassion, generativity and altruism. Germans hold a stronger correlation value between hope and harmony in life. In both groups, materialistic and hedonic hopes are located far below in the ranking list and have significantly lower mean scores in the Indian sample. The altruistic wish to help other people is in general terms less relevant than personal success and good social relations but more important than the materialistic and hedonic desires in both groups. Interestingly, the attitude of wishing to help other people is a significant positive predictor for the overall level of hope and is similar for Indians as well as Germans.

The hope for spiritual and religious experiences is the least important among all life domains hoped for, both for Germans and Indians alike, but Indians have significantly and notably higher values than Germans. In both cases, the hope for religious experiences is a significant predictor of the general level of hope. Accordingly, religious and spiritual practices, such as to pray, to meditate and to visit a church or temple are the least relevant for Indians and Germans. However, the Indian participants exhibit considerably higher levels at these religious and spiritual activities and for them the practice of prayer and meditation turned out to be the most significant predictor of perceived hope. Finally, priests and spiritual leaders are barely considered to be hope providers, both in India and in Europe, and God is located in the middle of the list. Indians scores God as well as priests and spiritual leaders much higher than Germans. Furthermore, to believe in God is a significant predictor of hope for the Indian group and the item 'priests, spiritual leaders' is the second largest predictor of hope in the German sample.

Summing up, the main findings of the Hope-Barometer lead us to following conclusions:

1. Materialistic and hedonic goals are the least important for both groups and not significant at all in terms of predictors of the general level of hope.
2. An altruistic attitude in life is not highly valued by the participants neither in India nor in German speaking Europe, however, this attitude displays a significant positive connection to the general perception of hope.
3. For Indians as well as for Germans, religious faith and spiritual beliefs seems to be the least relevant life aspects compared to other cognitive, relational and materialistic life domains. Yet, Indians revealed to have significantly higher values in the religious and spiritual sphere than Germans.
4. Remarkably, religious and spiritual attitudes and practices, although barely valued, turned out to stand among the most relevant factors in terms of general hope for both groups and principally for Indians.
5. Indian participants value most of all the cognitive activities to achieve personal goals, but the relation between these activities and perceived hope is relatively low.
6. To take responsibility for one's own hopes is very significant mainly in terms of personal will and commitment.
7. Whereas Indians exhibit particularly low scores in all aspects related to social relations with family members and friends, Germans recognize the social domain as the most important in life.
8. Good relations to family members and friends turned out to be of exceptional importance in terms of the individual level of general hope for both groups, but notably more for Germans.
9. Although Indians seem to be less satisfied with their lives and experience fewer positive affects, they enjoy similar levels of happiness, harmony and meaning in life compared to their German counterparts.

Conclusion

Following the results of the Hope-Barometer, we come to the conclusion that although the cognitive dimension of hope is highly valued, especially in India, its relevance in terms of hope has been largely overestimated. And conversely, that the spiritual dimension, although generally neglected, has been mostly underestimated in both cultures. Furthermore, there is an interesting parallel between the apparently low relevance of personal social relations with regard to hope in Indian Philosophy and the results of the Hope-Barometer that show that Indians are less concerned with and less aware of the value of social relations as an essential source of hope. Therefore, we want to encourage particularly the young Indian generation to become aware of their cultural and spiritual heritage and to find a harmonious balance between the cognitive, the social and the spiritual practices to nourish hope. The Western society can learn from the Indian worldview in terms of spirituality and altruism as much as the Indians could learn from the Western performance and coping techniques.

To conclude we want to remark that we cannot maintain that the Indian understanding of hope is better than the Western worldview or vice-versa. Both are describing a certain portion of human experience and both have clear strengths but weaknesses are also evident. With this presentation of the Indian notion of hope, we want to offer an additional perspective to the currently maintained in mainstream Positive Psychology. This will eventually enrich the concept of the multifaceted experience people may have regarding the phenomenon of hope. In a largely secularized society (also like in India), the spiritual understanding of hope may spark many doubts. However, since many psychological and philosophical theories and concepts of hope have already underlined the importance of the spiritual dimension, we hope to have contributed to the understanding of its foundations. The overall final goal of the many existing theories of hope, and equally our own goal, is to support the realization of a happy, fulfilling and flourishing life for oneself and for others.

We are aware of the many limitations of our contribution and of the results of our study. To outline the philosophical concept of hope in the Indian tradition, we only referred to two interpreters of the ancient scriptures, namely *Vivekananda* and *Aurobindo*. For an exhaustive and comprehensive theoretical research, many other relevant sources (for instance, an especially dedicated website- https://www.gitasupersite.iitk.ac.in/ contains text interpretations of different epic texts by various thinkers) must be included in the future. Our empirical survey has focused on a small segment of the total population, namely young adults between 18 and 29, singles and many of them well educated or still in education, so we cannot claim at all that our findings are representative for the entire Indian and German speaking society. In order to be able to generalize our findings and conclusions, further research will be necessary to include the whole range of socio-economic, religious and ethnic groups. A further limitation is the cross-sectional nature of our study, which does not permit any statement and conclusion in terms of causality. If we would like to explain in how far and in which way the cognitive, the hedonic, the social, the spiritual and the moral dimensions have a concrete impact on the level of hope and moreover, how the experience and the cultivation of hope can contribute to a happy and fulfilling life, longitudinal studies would be an indispensable necessity. Quantitative studies using self-report instruments are considered to be a powerful, scientifically sound and well-established research practice. However, they lack the possibility to explore in depth the cultural nuances, a subjective phenomenon like hope, may embrace for different people in distinct cultural settings. For this, qualitative research is better suited to differentiate the many aspects of a specific construct. Our findings and conclusions at this juncture serves as stimulating and thought provoking points of departure to develop new research questions and set up further inter-cultural research projects. We hope that such endeavors will help researchers to comprehend, understand and propagate scientific knowledge about hope to societies and communities in more fruitful manner.

References

Arbuckle, J. (2014). *IBM SPSS Amos 23 User's guide*. Chicago: IBM Corp.

Aurobindo, S. (1970). *Letters on yoga* (Vol. 1). Lotus Press.

Aurobindo, S. (1990). *The life divine*. Lotus Press.

Aurobindo, S. (1997). *Essays on Gita. The complete works of Sri Aurobindo* (Vol. 19). Pondicherry, India: Sri Aurobindo Ashram Publication Department.

Averill, J. R., & Sundararajan, L. (2005). Hope as rhetoric: Cultural narratives of wishing and coping. In: Eliott, J. (Hrsg.), *Interdisciplinary perspectives on hope* (pp. 133–165). New York: Nova Science Publishers

Behrani, P., & Jadeja, M. (2016). An exploratory study of hope and its process using focus groups and phenomenological analysis. *Indian Journal of Positive Psychology, 7*(1), 107.

Brown, T. A. (2006). *Confirmatory factor analysis for applied research*. New York: The Guildford Press.

Budhiraja, A., & Midha, P. (2015). Hope and spirituality as portals to subjective well-being among geriatrics. *Indian Journal of Positive Psychology, 6*(2), 175.

Chaudhary, N., Chadha, N. K., & Seth, S. (2017). Hope: Faith in what will be. *Indian Journal of Positive Psychology, 8*(2), 203–207.

Chen, F. F. (2007). Sensitivity of goodness of fit indexes to lack of measurement invariance. *Structural Equation Modeling, 14*(3), 464–504.

Cohen, J. (1992). Statistical power analysis. *Current Directions in Psychological Science, 1*(3), 98–101.

Cornelissen, M., & Ashram, S. A. (2001). Introducing Indian psychology: The basics. In 12th annual NAOP conference, Kerala, India. Accessed at www. infinityfoundation.com

Cornelissen, R. M. (2014). A commentary on "positive psychology and Indian psychology: In need of mutual reinforcement". *Psychological Studies, 59*(2), 103–104.

Dalal, A. K. (2010). A journey back to the roots: Psychology in India. *Foundations of Indian psychology, Volume 1: Theories and concepts*, 27.

Dalal, A. K., & Misra, G. (2010). The core and context of Indian psychology. *Psychology and Developing Societies, 22*(1), 121–155.

Diener, E. D., Emmons, R. A., Larsen, R. J., & Griffin, S. (1985). The satisfaction with life scale. *Journal of Personality Assessment, 49*(1), 71–75.

Diener, E. D., Wirtz, D., Tov, W., Kim-Prieto, C., Choi, D. W., Oishi, S., & Biswas-Diener, R. (2010). New well-being measures: Short scales to assess flourishing and positive and negative feelings. *Social Indicators Research, 97*(2), 143–156.

Dufault, K., & Martocchio, B. C. (1985). Symposium on compassionate care and the dying experience. Hope: Its spheres and dimensions. *The Nursing Clinics of North America, 20*(2), 379–391.

Eliott, J. A. (2005). What have we done with hope? A brief history. In: J. A. Eliott (Hrsg.), *Interdisciplinary perspectives on hope* (pp. 3–45) New York: Nova Publishers.

Farran, C. J., Herth, K. A., & Popovich, J. M. (1995). *Hope and hopelessness: Critical clinical constructs*. Thousand Oaks, CA: Sage.

Fredrickson, B. L. (2004). The broaden-and-build theory of positive emotions. *Philosophical Transactions-Royal Society of London Series B Biological Sciences, 359*, 1367–1378.

Hughes, M. E., Waite, L. J., Hawkley, L. C., & Cacioppo, J. T. (2004). A short scale for measuring loneliness in large surveys results from two population-based studies. *Research on Aging, 26*(6), 655–672.

Hwang, J. Y., Plante, T., & Lackey, K. (2008). The development of the Santa Clara brief compassion scale: An abbreviation of Sprecher and Fehr's compassionate love scale. *Pastoral Psychology, 56*(4), 421–428.

IBM. (2014). *IBM SPSS advanced statistics 23*. Chicago: IBM Corp.

Krafft, A. M., Martin-Krumm, C., & Fenouillet, F. (2017). Adaptation, further elaboration, and validation of a scale to measure hope as perceived by people: Discriminant value and predictive utility vis-à-vis dispositional hope. *Assessment*, 1–16. https://doi.org/10.1177/1073191117700724

Kjell, O., Daukantaité, D., Hefferon, K., & Sikström, S. (2016). Harmony in life scale complements the satisfaction with life scale: Expanding the conceptualization of the cognitive component of subjective well-being. *Social Indicators Research, 126*, 893–919.

Lopez, S. J., Snyder, C. R., & Pedrotti, J. T. (2003). Hope: Many definitions, many measures. In: S. J. Lopez & C. R. Snyder (Hrsg.), *Positive psychological assessment: A handbook of models and measures, 1* (pp. 91–107). Washington, DC: American Psychological Association.

Lyubomirsky, S., & Lepper, H. S. (1999). A measure of subjective happiness: Preliminary reliability and construct validation. *Social Indicators Research, 46*(2), 137–155.

Menon, S. (2005). What is Indian psychology: Transcendence in and while thinking. *Journal of Transpersonal Psychology, 37*(2).

Nickell, G. S. (1998) *The Helping Attitude Scale: A new measure of prosocial tendencies*. Paper presented at the American Psychological Association, San Francisco, CA.

Nietzsche, F. (1996). *Human, all too human: A book for free spirits*. Cambridge University Press.

Paranjpe, A. C. (1996). Some basic psychological concepts from the intellectual tradition of India. *Psychology and Developing Societies, 8*(1), 7–27.

Parsian, N., & Dunning, T. A. (2009). Developing and validating a questionnaire to measure spirituality: A psychometric process. *Global Journal of Health Science, 1*(1), 2–11.

Pavot, W., & Diener, E. (2008). The satisfaction with life scale and the emerging construct of life satisfaction. *The Journal of Positive Psychology, 3*(2), 137–152.

Peterson, C., & Seligman, M. E. (2004). *Character strengths and virtues: A handbook and classification*. Oxford University Press.

Plante, T. G., & Boccaccini, M. (1997). The santa clara strength of religious faith questionnaire. *Pastoral Psychology, 45*, 375–387.

Rao, K. R. (1978). Psychology of transcendence: A study in early Buddhistic psychology. *The Journal of Individual Psychology, 1*(1), 1–21.

Rao, K. R. (2005). Perception, cognition and consciousness in classical Hindu psychology. *Journal of Consciousness Studies, 12*(3), 3–30.

Rao, K. R. (2014a). Positive psychology and Indian psychology in need of mutual reinforcement. *Psychological Studies, 59*(2), 94–102.

Rao, K. R. (2014b). Indian psychology in prospect. *Psychological Studies, 59*(2), 124–134.

Rao, K. R., & Paranjpe, A. C. (2008). Yoga psychology: Theory and application. In K. R. Rao, A. C. Paranjpe, & A. K. Dalal (Eds.), *Handbook of Indian psychology* (pp. 186–216). New Delhi, India: Cambridge University Press India.

Rao, K. R., & Paranjpe, A. C. (2016). Applied Indian Psychology. In *Psychology in the Indian tradition* (pp. 205–227). New Delhi, India: Springer India.

Salagame, K. K. (2014). Positive psychology and Indian psychology: Birds of the same feather. *Psychological Studies, 59*(2), 116–118.

Sarkar, R. (2011). The Bird-Image. In *Savitri. Sraddha – A Quarterly devoted to an exposition of the teachings of The Mother and Sri Aurobindo* (Vol. 2 No. 4, Special issue on Savitri, part II, pp, 73–97). Kolkata, India: Sri Aurobindo Centre for Research in Social Sciences

Schnell, T. (2009). The sources of meaning and meaning in life questionnaire (SoMe): Relations to demographics and well-being. *The Journal of Positive Psychology, 4*(3), 483–499.

Schnell, T., & Becker, P. (2007). *Fragebogen zu Lebensbedeutungen und Lebenssinn: LeBe*. Göttingen, Germany: Hogrefe.

Scioli, A. (2007). Hope and spirituality in the age of anxiety. In *Advancing quality of life in a turbulent world* (pp. 135–150). Dordrecht, The Netherlands: Springer.

Scioli, A., & Biller, H. (2009). *Hope in the age of anxiety*. New York: Oxford University Press.

Scioli, A., Ricci, M., Nyugen, T., & Scioli, E. R. (2011). Hope: Its nature and measurement. *Psychology of Religion and Spirituality, 3*(2), 78–97.

Sharma, M., & Garg, D. (2016). Personal growth as a correlate of gratitude, hope and curiosity among college students. *Indian Journal of Positive Psychology, 7*(2), 201.

Singh, A. K., Singh, S., Singh, A. P., & Srivastava, A. (2013). Hope and well-being among students of professional courses. *Indian Journal of Community Psychology, 9*(1), 109–119.

Singh, K., & Choubisa, R. (2010). Empirical validation of values in action-inventory of strengths (VIA-IS) in Indian context. *Psychological Studies, 55*(2), 151–158. https://doi.org/10.1007/s12646-010-0015-4

Singh, S., & Devender, S. (2015). Hope and mindfulness as correlates of happiness. *Indian Journal of Positive Psychology, 6*(4), 422.

Snyder, C. R. (1994). *The psychology of hope: You can get there from here.* New York: Simon and Schuster.

Snyder, C. R. (2000a). Hypothesis: There is hope. In C. R. Snyder (Ed.), *Handbook of hope: Theory, measures, and applications* (pp. 3–21). San Diego, CA: Academic.

Snyder, C. R. (2000b). Genesis: Birth and growth of hope. In C. R. Snyder (Ed.), *Handbook of hope: Theory, measures, and applications* (pp. 25–57). San Diego, CA: Academic.

Snyder, C. R. (2002). Hope theory: Rainbows in the mind. *Psychological Inquiry, 13*(4), 249–275.

Snyder, C. R., Harris, C., Anderson, J. R., Holleran, S. A., Irving, L. M., Sigmon, S. T., et al. (1991). The will and the ways: Development and validation of an individual-differences measure of hope. *Journal of Personality and Social Psychology, 60*(4), 570–585.

Sprecher, S., & Fehr, B. (2005). Compassionate love for close others and humanity. *Journal of Social and Personal Relationships, 22*(5), 629–651.

Steger, M. F., Frazier, P., Oishi, S., & Kaler, M. (2006). The meaning in life questionnaire: Assessing the presence of and search for meaning in life. *Journal of Counseling Psychology, 53*(1), 80–93.

Storch, E. A., Roberti, J. W., Bravata, E. A., & Storch, J. B. (2004). Strength of religious faith: A comparison of intercollegiate athletes and non-athletes. *Pastoral Psychology, 52*(6), 485–489.

Stotland, E. (1969). *The psychology of hope.* San Francisco: Jossey-Bass.

Thakre, N. (2013). Satisfaction with life and hope in youth. *Indian Journal of Positive Psychology, 4*(2), 347–349.

Tripathi, S. R., Kochar, A., & Dara, P. (2015). Role of self-efficacy and hope in academic procrastination among undergraduate students. *Indian Journal of Positive Psychology, 6*(4), 376.

Vidwans, S. S., & Raghvendra, P. (2016). A study of meaningful work, hope and meaning in life in young professional artists. *Indian Journal of Positive Psychology, 7*(4), 469.

Vivekananda, S. (2015). *The complete works of Swami Vivekananda.* Manonmani Publishers.

Yadav, K. V., & Thingujam, N. S. (2015). Hope's relation with self-esteem, optimism, and life satisfaction in engineering students. *Indian Journal of Positive Psychology, 6*(3), 283.

Chapter 8
Psychosocial Correlates and Predictors of Perceived Hope Across Cultures: A Study of Czech and Maltese Contexts

Alena Slezáčková, Carmel Cefai, and Tomáš Prošek

Introduction

This chapter discusses the new concept of perceived hope in relation to other positive psychology variables. It explores the correlates and predictors of perceived hope among two different samples, Czech and Maltese, and the similarities and differences between the two samples. Although both the Czech Republic and Malta are developed European countries, they differ in terms of history, socio-economic background, culture and language. Thus, we assume that there might also be differences between Czech and Maltese populations in the psychosocial determinants of perceived hope.

As the concept of perceived hope is relatively new, we were interested in whether perceived hope is more related to (a) social resources, i.e. the quality and quantity of social relationships in terms of positive relations and loneliness, (b) internal, dispositional characteristics such as optimistic mindset, or (c) to self-transcendence (spirituality and generativity), and whether the role of the resources varies across countries.

A. Slezáčková (✉) · T. Prošek
Faculty of Arts, Department of Psychology, Masaryk University, Brno, Czech Republic
e-mail: alena.slezackova@phil.muni.cz

C. Cefai
Department of Psychology, Faculty for Social Wellbeing, University of Malta, Msida, Malta

© Springer International Publishing AG, part of Springer Nature 2018
A. M. Krafft et al. (eds.), *Hope for a Good Life*, Social Indicators Research
Series 72, https://doi.org/10.1007/978-3-319-78470-0_8

Perspectives on Hope

Snyder (2000) defined hope as a positive motivational state that comprises both goal-directed energy (the agency component) and planning to meet goals (the pathways component). Hope can be viewed either as a changeable phenomenon dependent on the individual's experiences (state hope), or as a relatively stable personality trait (dispositional hope). Drawing on his research on the correlates of dispositional hope, Snyder (2000) came to distinguish between low-hopers and high-hopers. While the latter see obstacles as challenges, trying to seek alternative goal attainment solutions, low-hopers view obstacles as "traps" they prefer to avoid. It is typical of low-hopers to hold onto a single goal; high-hopers, on the other hand, are ready to create alternative goals when the need arises. The two groups also differ with respect to their stress-coping capacity, intensity of negative emotions, and time needed for recovery (Snyder, 2000).

Krafft (Krafft, Martin-Krumm, & Fenouillet, 2017; Krafft & Walker, 2018) developed the concept of perceived hope that seeks to assess the general level of hope independently from pre-established dimensions such as cognitive, motivational, emotional, social or spiritual. In comparison to Snyder's (2000) dispositional hope, perceived hope is a broader concept, since it relates not only to the cognitive but also to the relational and spiritual aspects of hope, and accounts especially for phenomena that is beyond human control. According to Krafft, perceived hope refers to the sense of deep trust that things will turn out well. Because the concept is most prominent in difficult life situations that one cannot control, it is seen as being closely related to experiencing meaning in life, helping other people, enjoying close and trusted relationships, and to spiritual or religious experience (Krafft et al., 2017; Krafft & Walker, 2018).

Hope and Optimism

The concept of hope needs to be distinguished from related phenomena such as optimism (Magaletta & Oliver, 1999; Snyder, Rand, & Sigmon, 2002).

Dispositional optimism is considered to be a relatively stable personality trait, as confirmed by numerous studies (Atienza, Stephens, & Townsend, 2004; Carver & Scheier, 2002; Carver, Scheier, & Segerstrom, 2010; Lucas, Diener, & Suh, 1996; Scheier & Carver, 1985). Optimists and pessimists differ particularly in their approach to life's challenges and in their ways of coping with difficult life situations. While optimists tend to believe that good things are awaiting them and that they will be successful in their activities, pessimists typically expect a negative course of events and a lack of success in their activities (Hefferon & Boniwell, 2011; Scheier & Carver, 1992). Optimistic expectations produce positive emotions;

pessimistic expectations, on the other hand, result in anger, sadness and anxiety (Brissette, Scheier, & Carver, 2002; Carver et al., 1993; Carver, Scheier, & Segerstrom, 2010). When obstacles occur, optimists and pessimists differ in chosen coping strategies (Scheier, Carver, & Bridges, 2001).

Optimism and pessimism do not only determine the individual's success in coping with adversities to a large extent, but they also affect the overall mental and physical well-being (Baker, 2007; Carver & Scheier, 2002; Forgeard & Seligman, 2012; Peterson, 2000; Schweizer, Beck-Seyffer, & Schneider, 1999). Gallagher, Lopez, and Pressman's study (2013) on a sample of over 150 thousand respondents from 142 countries, revealed positive relations among optimism, positive emotions and life satisfaction, and a significant, albeit less strong, negative correlation between optimism and negative emotions.

Although both optimism and hope are related to positive future expectations, the two concepts are not identical (Alarcon, Bowling, & Khazon, 2013). In several studies (Bailey, Eng, Frisch, & Snyder, 2007; Gallagher & Lopez, 2009), dispositional hope and optimism were found to serve as unique predictors of subjective well-being. While optimism can be viewed as context-independent, hope is mostly related to situations that are personally important (Arnau, Rosen, Finch, Rhudy, & Fortunato, 2007; Bruininks, Malle, Johnson, & Bryant, 2005).

Hope and Subjective Well-Being

According to Diener (Diener, 1984; Diener, Oishi, & Lucas, 2003; Pavot & Diener, 2008), subjective well-being (SWB) contains an affective element (the presence of positive emotions and lack of negative emotions; a related concept is happiness) and a cognitive element (cognitive evaluation of one's life, comparing reality with own expectations; a related concept is life satisfaction). Several studies have established a positive relationship between dispositional hope and subjective well-being (Alarcon et al., 2013; Bailey et al., 2007; Bailey & Snyder, 2007; Ciarrochi, Parker, Kashdan, Heaven, & Barkus, 2015; Demirli, Türkmen, & Arik, 2015; O'Sullivan, 2010).

Slezáčková and Krafft (2016) reported significant positive interrelationships among life satisfaction, perceived hope, dispositional hope and perceived meaning in life among Czech adults. Both types of hope (along with meaningfulness) served as independent predictors of life satisfaction, with perceived hope being the strongest predictor. Similarly, in a study on Swiss and German populations conducted by Krafft et al. (2017), perceived hope had stronger predictive power with respect to life satisfaction and happiness than dispositional hope.

Hope and Social Relationships

The quality and quantity of social relationships affect both mental and physical health (Smith & Christakis, 2008; Umberson & Montez, 2010). The basic aspects of social relationships include (a) social networks, which refer to the web of social relationships of an individual; (b) social integration, i.e. overall level of involvement with formal and informal social relationships; (c) social isolation, which refers to the relative absence of social relationships; and (d) quality of relationships, which includes positive aspects of social relationships (Umberson & Montez, 2010).

The quality of social relationships significantly affects psychological well-being and flourishing (Berscheid & Reis, 1998; Diener & Seligman, 2002; Seligman, 2011). Good social relations are a source of social support, which can be described as support accessible to an individual through social ties to other individuals, groups, and the larger community (Lin, Simeone, Ensel, & Kuo, 1979). Social support as an interpersonal transaction can be expressed through emotional concern, instrumental aid, information, or appraisal (House, 1981). Social support mitigates the negative consequences of stress, reduces feelings of loneliness and improves social well-being (Hombrados-Mendieta, García-Martín, & Gómez-Jacinto, 2013; Yildirim & Kocabiyik, 2010).

The importance of social relationships has been confirmed also in relation to hope (Horton & Wallander, 2001; Morse & Doberneck, 1995). Lopez (2013) believed that the individual's level of dispositional hope determines his or her success both in relationships and career. Significant relationships between positive relations with others and perceived hope were also reported in previous studies (e.g. Krafft et al., 2017; Slezáčková, 2017; Slezáčková & Krafft, 2016).

Loneliness

Low quality and quantity of social relationships can lead to loneliness (Betts & Bicknell, 2011), a state which needs to be distinguished from solitude. One can feel lonely even when surrounded by people, and conversely solitude does not necessarily imply loneliness (Page & Scanlan, 1994).

Loneliness is defined as a set of feelings resulting from the individual's perceived lack of satisfactory social and intimate relationships (Cacioppo et al., 2006; Cacioppo & Patrick, 2008). It is characterised by feelings of sadness, boredom and isolation (Roberts & Quayle, 2001, as cited in Betts & Bicknell, 2011). Loneliness has been identified as a key predictor of mental and physical health (Cacioppo et al., 2002) and one of the significant factors leading to depression (Golden et al., 2009; Green et al., 1992). Numerous studies have focused on the health effects of social isolation on the elderly (Heikkinen, Berg, & Avland, 1995; Stek et al., 2005).

The research attention has been also drawn to loneliness in adolescence and early adulthood (Mahon, Yarcheski, Yarcheski, Cannella, & Hanks, 2006). The results of a recent study by Goosby, Bellatorre, Walsemann, and Cheadle (2013) indicate that loneliness in adolescence results in depression, poorer adult self-rated health, and increased cardiovascular risks.

Hope and Self-Transcendence

Spirituality

Spirituality can be perceived as a significant, self-transcendent phenomenon establishing a deep connection between the inner self, other people and the universal whole (Marcel, 2010; Reich, 2000). Pargament and Mahoney (2002, p. 647) see spirituality as "a search for the sacred", while Garssen, Visser, and de Jager Meezenbroek (2016, p. 1) define spirituality as "one's striving for and experience of connection with the essence of life", encompassing three main dimensions: connectedness with oneself, connectedness with others and nature, and connectedness with the transcendent.

In Peterson and Seligman's (2004) view, spirituality is a character strength that falls under the transcendence virtue that creates connections to the higher universe and provides meaning. A spiritual person has coherent beliefs about his or her place in the order of universe and about the purpose of human life, and the beliefs function as a source of spiritual guidance and consolation.

Research shows that spirituality is related to higher well-being (Sawatzky, Ratner, & Chiu, 2005; Visser, Garssen, & Vingerhoets, 2010). According to Parsian and Dunning (2009), spirituality is a significant factor that contributes to health and well-being in people with chronic health issues. Also, they view spirituality as a crucial element aiding the search for meaning and inner peace, which facilitates coping with difficult life situations.

There is evidence that spiritual beliefs and practices are associated with better mental health and life satisfaction (Anand, 2013; Brillhart, 2005; Zullig, Ward, & Horn, 2006). Increased spiritual well-being was found to be negatively correlated with depressive symptoms and also to have a preventive effect (Bekelman et al., 2007; Cotton, Larkin, Hoopes, Cromer, & Rosenthal, 2005). However, several studies do not support the above findings (Baetz, Bowen, & Jones, 2006; Leurent et al., 2013).

Nevertheless, many researchers view spirituality as an important component or correlate of hope (Dufault & Martocchio, 1985; Hong, Hodge, & Choi, 2015; Scioli, Ricci, Nyugen, & Scioli, 2011). A longitudinal study by Marques, Lopez, and Mitchell (2013) found that hope and spirituality, but not religious practice, were strongly linked to life satisfaction amongst adolescents.

Generativity

According to Erikson's theory of psychosocial development (Erikson & Erikson, 1998), generativity versus stagnation is the key topic of the seventh stage which takes place during middle adulthood and can span across over 30 years. During this time, adults strive to create something that will outlast them; this can involve parenting or positive contributions to society (McAdams & de St. Aubin, 1992).

There has been a surge of interest in research into how generativity is related to subjective well-being, personality, mental health, and spirituality (Millová & Blatný, 2016; Sandage, Hill, & Vaubel, 2011; Schnell, 2009).

Schnell (2009) views generativity as one of the dimensions of self-transcendence, which can be defined as commitment to objectives beyond one's immediate needs. While vertical self-transcendence encompasses orientation towards an immaterial, cosmic power, the horizontal self-transcendence concerns taking responsibility for worldly affairs beyond one's immediate concerns.

McAdams and de St. Aubin (1992) claimed that generativity can be shaped by spirituality and religion. Dillon, Wink, and Fay (2003) found a positive relationship between spirituality seeking and various aspects of generativity, while a significant relationship between generativity and spirituality was also reported in a study by Brady and Hapenny (2010).

Numerous studies have found a positive relationship between generativity and psychological well-being (An & Cooney, 2006; Grossbaum & Bates, 2002; Peterson & Duncan, 2007; Rothrauff & Coney, 2008). The question as to whether the relationship between generativity and life satisfaction is affected by age was addressed by McAdams, St. Aubin, and Logan (1993), with no significant differences found between three age groups (22–27 years, 37–42 years, and 67–72 years).

Huta and Zuroff (2007) attempted to explain the mechanism behind the correlation between generativity and life satisfaction. They found that the relationship is mediated by a specific variable called symbolic immortality, suggesting that life satisfaction associated with generative behaviour springs from the person's feeling that they made a lasting and/or valuable contribution to the lives of the other people, and thus a part of themselves will live on.

Several studies focused on the relationship between generativity and volunteering. Generativity was found to be closely related to prosocial behaviour and engagement in voluntary activities in adolsecents and young adults (Frensch, Pratt, & Norris, 2007; Lawford, Pratt, Hunsberger, & Pancer, 2005). Cox, Wilt, Olson, and McAdams (2010) found that generativity in midlife adults was more strongly associated with positive societal engagement than dispositional personality traits within the Big Five taxonomy. De Espanés, Villar, Urrutia, and Serrat (2015) studied motivation and commitment to volunteering in a sample of adults aged between 18 and 86. They found that generative concern, unlike sociodemographic variables, predicted all the motives for volunteering that were considered in the study.

Generativity was also studied with respect to gender. In women, life satisfaction and satisfaction with self were both significantly affected by generativity, and the effect was stronger in women who were particularly devoted to motherhood

(Rittenour & Colaner, 2012). In men, generativity was positively correlated with job satisfaction (Clark & Arnold, 2008).

Millová and Blatný (2016) point out that so far there is not enough attention to the cultural context of generativity. Previous studies have focused primarily on manifestation of generativity depending on the degree of individualism and collectivism of the culture (de St. Aubin, 2004; Hofer, Busch, Chasiotis, Kärtner, & Campos, 2008). However, studies examining generativity with regard to other dimensions of culture, such as power distance, uncertainty avoidance, and masculinity vs. femininity (Hofstede, 2001; Hofstede & Bond, 1984) are still missing.

Background: The Czech Republic and Malta

In this study, we have set out to compare the correlates and predictors of perceived hope in two different national samples – Czech and Maltese.

The Czech Republic (CZ) is a developed Central European state with a parliamentary democracy. It covers an area of 78,866 km^2 and has over 10.5 milion inhabitants (population density 134/km^2). The majority of the inhabitants are Czechs, followed by Moravians and Slovaks (IndexMundi, 2017). Most people (88.5%) identify themselves as non-religious (also undeclared religion or spiritual but not religious); over 10% are Roman Catholics.

The Republic of Malta (M) is a Southern European island country with a parliamentary democracy. The country has a small population of approx. 450,000. It covers around 316 km^2 and has a population density of 1410/km^2, which makes it one of the world's smallest and most densely populated countries. The majority of the people are Maltese, but, there are relatively small minorities such as British, North and sub-Saharan Africans and East Europeans. The official religion is Catholicism; over 90% of the inhabitants are Roman Catholics (IndexMundi, 2017).

To obtain culture-related data, we used a six-dimensional model of national culture by Hofstede (2001). The six dimensions include Power Distance (PD), Individualism vs. Collectivism (IDV), Masculinity vs. Femininity (MAS), Uncertainty Avoidance (UA), Long Term Orientation vs. Short Term Normative Orientation (LTO), and Indulgence vs. Restraint (IND).

According to Hofstede (2001), the Czech Republic and Malta both scored relatively high on Individualism (CZ: 58; M: 59) and Power Distance (CZ: 57; M: 56). The results suggest that both countries have individualist societies whose members are expected to take care of themselves and their immediate families only. The PD score reflects the degree to which the less powerful members of the society accept unequal distribution of power.

The Czech Republic scores higher than Malta on Masculinity (CZ: 57; M: 47) and Long Term Orientation (CZ: 70, M: 47). The high Masculinity score indicates that achievement, assertiveness and material rewards for success are valued highly in Czech society. The Long Term Orientation dimension is a "pragmatic" one, with the high score implying that Czech society encourages thrift and other means of preparation for the future. Both countries received high scores on Uncertainty Avoidance (CZ: 74; M: 96), with Malta scoring extremely high, suggesting that both societies tend to maintain strict codes of belief and behaviour and that the people are uncomfortable with ambiguity and uncertainty.

The greatest difference between the Czech and Maltese cultures is in Indulgence (CZ: 26; M: 66). The high score received by Malta reflects the inhabitants' tendency towards optimism and willingness to enjoy life. Czechs, on the other hand, were found to be much less indulgent and to have a tendency towards pessimism and cynicism.

In view of the globalised nature of today's world in which many cultural differences are fading away, we find it interesting to explore whether and to what extent there are differences between two nationalities that are culturally relatively similar, yet differ in many respects.

Objectives

The main aim of our study was to explore the determinants of perceived hope among Czech and Maltese populations and to investigate possible differences between the two populations. Although both the Czech Republic and Malta are developed European countries, they differ in terms of history, socio-economic background, culture and language. Thus, we assume that there might also be differences between Czech and Maltese populations in the psychosocial determinants of perceived hope.

As the concept of perceived hope is relatively new, we were interested in whether it is more related to social factors (variables measured: Positive Relations, Loneliness), internal, dispositional characteristics such as positive mindset (variable measured: Dispositional Optimism), or self-transcendent resources (variables measured: Spirituality, Generativity), and whether the role of these resources varies across the two countries.

More specifically, the objectives of the study were fourfold:

Firstly, it was to measure the participants' level of satisfaction with the past year (2015) and their outlook on personal, political, economical, environmental and social issues for the coming year (2016). We also aimed to explore the respondents' personal wishes and hopes, and to identify what steps they take to achieve their wishes and whom they expect to boost their hope.

Secondly, it was to examine the levels of perceived hope, optimism, life satisfaction, positive relations, loneliness, generativity, and spirituality among Czech and Maltese populations, and to investigate whether there are significant differences between the two samples in these variables.

Thirdly, we aimed to explore the relationships among the variables of interest in both Czech and Maltese samples. Based on previous research we expected significant intercorrelations among perceived hope, optimism, life satisfaction, positive relations, spirituality, and generativity. We also expected significant negative relationships between loneliness and perceived hope and generativity. Subsequently, we focused on examining the independent predictors of perceived hope, assuming that they will be different for each sample. Based on studies claiming that the essence of true spirituality is an affection and concern for others, which is expressed in altruistic and compassionate behaviour (Neusner & Chilton, 2005), we also expected an association between spirituality, generativity, and the engagement in volunteering activities.

Fourthly, we addressed the question of whether there are any significant differences in the measured variables related to gender, age, family status, education level, religious beliefs, and engagement in voluntary activities.

Method

Sample

The research sample consisted of 267 respondents (108 male, 159 female, aged 18 to 79). The Czech sample comprised 177 respondents, 48 (27.1%) male and 129 (72.9%) female. The Maltese sample comprised 90 respondents, 60 (66.7%) male and 30 (33.3%) female.

The respondents were divided into several age groups: 18–29 years (CZ: 62.7%; M: 21.1%), 30–39 years (CZ: 11.3%; M: 25.6%), 40–49 years (CZ: 14.1%; M: 21.1%), 50–59 years (CZ: 9%; M: 17.8%), 60–69 years (CZ: 2.8%; M: 11.1%), and 70–79 years (CZ: 0%; M: 3.3%).

Most participants were married (CZ: 24.3%; M: 51.1%) or living with a partner (CZ: 33.9%; M: 15.5%); the rest were single (CZ: 36.2%; M: 26.8%), and divorced or widowed (CZ: 5.6%; M: 6.6%).

Most respondents had a university degree (CZ: 62.1%; M: 72.2%) or had completed standard secondary education (CZ: 36.2%; M: 27.8%); the rest had primary education only (CZ: 1.7%; M: 0%).

The majority of participants were Christian (CZ: 37.3%; M: 74.4%); the remaining were spiritual but not religious (CZ: 30.5%; M: 6.7%), atheists (CZ: 23.2%; M: 15.6%) or members of a different religion (such as Buddhism or Judaism; CZ: 9%; M: 3.3%).

70.6% of Czech respondents and 75.6 % Maltese participants did not participate in any voluntary activities, while 29.4 % Czechs and 24.4 % Maltese indicated they were actively involved in voluntary activities.

Measures

Variables measured and respective measures:

Perceived Hope *The Perceived Hope Scale, PHS* (Krafft, Martin-Krumm, & Fenouillet, 2017) is a six-item tool covering aspects such as level of hope, effect of hope, fulfillment of hope, hope/anxiety duality, and the special situations in which hope arises. The scale employs a five-point Likert-type response scale (0 – strongly disagree, 5 – strongly agree). The Cronbach's α coefficient for the scale in the present study was .87 for the Czech sample and .90 for the Maltese sample.

Optimism *Life Orientation Test – Revised, LOT-R* (Scheier, Carver, & Bridges, 1994) contains 10 items, three of which focus on dispositional optimism, three on dispositional pessimism and four are fillers. A six-point Likert-type response scale is used (1 – strongly disagree, 6 – strongly agree). The measure shows high internal consistency and stability over time. The authors report Cronbach's α of .78; in our study it was .80 for the Czech sample and .87 for the Maltese one.

Positive Relations *Positive Relations with Others* is one of the sub-scales of Ryff's Psychological Well-Being Scale (PWBS; Ryff, 1989). Each of the nine items is answered using a six-point response scale (1 – strongly disagree, 6 – strongly agree). Low scores indicate a lack of close and trustful relationships, problems with expressing warmth in relationships, social frustration, isolation and unwillingness to make compromises to sustain important ties with others. By contrast, high scores indicate that the person is involved in warm and satisfying relationships with others, is concerned about the welfare of others and is capable of strong empathy, affection and intimacy (Ryff & Keyes, 1995). The Cronbach's α coefficient for the scale in the present study was .82 for the Czech sample and .85 for the Maltese sample.

Loneliness *The Loneliness Scale, LS* (Hughes, Waite, Hawkley, & Cacioppo, 2004) contains three items (1. How often do you feel starved for company; 2. How often do you feel shut out and excluded by others; 3. How often do you feel isolated), each of which is answered using a five-point scale (1 – never, 2 – hardly ever, 3 – sometimes, 4 – often, 5 – all of the time). The authors report a satisfactory Cronbach's α of .72 (Hughes et al., 2004); in our study, it was .86 for both populations.

Spirituality *Spirituality Questionnaire, SQ* (Parsian & Dunning, 2009) includes four subscales, namely Self-Awareness, Spiritual Practices, Spiritual Needs, and Importance of Spiritual Beliefs in Life, of which only the last one was used in our study. The subscale contains four items that are answered using a Likert-type response scale (1 – strongly disagree, 4 – strongly agree). The total score is reflective of how important spirituality is for the respondent. In our study the subscale showed very good internal consistency (α = .97 for the Czech sample and .95 for the Maltese sample).

Generativity *Sources of Meaning and Meaning in Life Questionnaire, SoMe* (Schnell, 2009; Schnell & Becker, 2007) comprises 151 items arranged into 4 dimensions and 26 subscales focusing on sources of meaning and meaningfulness and on the crisis of meaning. In our study, we used a six-item Generativity subscale only (Self-Transcendence dimension). The subscale uses a six-point Likert-type response scale (0 – strongly disagree, 5 – strongly agree). The internal consistency in our study was Cronbach's α = .87 for the Czech sample and α = .71 for the Maltese sample.

Life Satisfaction *Satisfaction with Life Scale, SWLS* (Diener, Emmons, Larsen, & Griffin, 1985) was designed to assess global life satisfaction defined as a subjective evaluation of the overall conditions of existence based on a comparison between one's aspirations and actual achievements. The scale contains five items, each of which is answered using a seven-point response scale (1 – strongly disagree, 7 – strongly agree). Diener et al. (1985) report a Cronbach's α of .87; in our study, it was .87 for the Czech sample and .92 for the Maltese sample.

Basic demographic data (gender, age, family status, education level, and religious belief) were also collected. We were also interested in whether the respondents were engaged in any voluntary activities.

In addition to the questionnaire, the study employed a set of questions related to hope and personal wishes developed by Krafft (2013, 2014).

With respect to personal wishes and hope, the respondents were asked to indicate:

1. How satisfied they were in the last year in terms of personal, political, economical, environmental and social issues (1 = very unsatisfied, ..., 5 = very satisfied)
2. What was their outlook on the coming year in terms of personal, political, economical, environmental and social issues (1 = very pessimistic, ..., 5 = very optimistic)
3. What their personal wishes were and how they rated their subjective importance (0 = not important, 1 = slightly important, 2 = important, 3 = very important);
4. What steps they were taking towards fulfilling their hopes and how often (0 = not at all, 1 = rarely, 2 = sometimes, 3 = very often);
5. Who they expected to boost their hope and to what extent (0 = not at all, 1 = a little bit, 2 = pretty much, 3 = yes, definitely).

Procedure and Data Analysis

Data were obtained through an anonymous, self-administered questionnaire in November 2015. A convenience sampling technique was employed to recruit the potential respondents. A link to the questionnaire was distributed through e-mails, social networks, and websites. Varying types of media (newspapers, radio etc.) were also used to invite people to participate in the research. The collected data were processed using IBM SPSS, version 23.

We used descriptive statistics methods to describe the variables as well as the characteristics of the research sample, and a histogram to estimate the probability distribution of the variables. The relationships between the variables were determined using Pearson's correlation and multiple linear regression analysis. An independent-samples t-test and one-way ANOVA were employed to determine the differences between the two research samples and between the selected categories of demographic variables. The significant differences among particular groups within a sample were determined using Welch test, Tukey's test, Hochberg GT2 or Games-Howell post-hoc test. A two-way Anova was used to examine the effect of country and gender on the differences between the variables of interest in the two samples, and to examine possible interaction between gender and country. The internal consistency of the instruments used was measured with Cronbach's alpha.

Throughout both data collection and processing we strictly observed the principles of research ethics. Participation in the research was strictly voluntary. All participants were informed of the research focus of the study and of the estimated amount of time needed to complete the questionnaires. It was also made clear to the respondents that they could withdraw from the research at any time.

Results

Satisfaction with the Last Year and Expectations for the Next Year

The respondents were asked to indicate how satisfied they were during the last year with regards to personal, political, economical, environmental and social issues. The results showed that both Czech and Maltese respondents reported the highest level of satisfaction with their personal life. While Czechs were the least satisfied with national politics, Maltese showed the lowest satisfaction with climate and environmental issues (see Table 8.1). Significant differences between the two samples were found in satisfaction with national politics ($t(265) = 2.26$; $p < 0.05$; $d = 0.29$; 95% CI [0.024; 0.557]), national economy ($t(265) = 3.16$; $p < 0.01$; $d = 0.41$; 95% CI [0.148; 0.692]), and climate and the environment ($t(197.23) = 7.52$; $p < 0.001$; $d = 0.95$; 95% CI [0.791; 0.135]). While Czech respondents reported higher satisfaction with national politics and climate issues, Maltese showed higher satisfaction with the national economy.

The Czech and Maltese groups were both most optimistic about their personal life for the forthcoming year (2016). The lowest levels of optimism were in national

Table 8.1 Mean scores for satisfaction of both groups during the last year

	Czech Republic		Malta	
Satisfaction with…	*M*	*SD*	*M*	*SD*
Personal life	3.82	1.17	3.58	1.19
National politics	2.16	0.99	1.87	1.07
National economy	2.77	0.98	3.19	1.11
Social issues	2.18	0.90	2.29	1.06
Climate and the environment	2.90	1.17	1.83	1.05

Table 8.2 Mean scores for expectations for both groups for the forthcoming year

	Czech Republic		Malta	
Expectations for the coming year	*M*	*SD*	*M*	*SD*
Personal life	4.11	0.86	3.64	1.05
National politics	2.50	1.00	2.08	1.02
National economy	3.03	0.99	3.11	1.03
Social issues	2.50	1.06	2.36	0.93
Climate and the environment	3.11	1.13	2.03	0.94

politics and social issues for the Czechs, and climate and environmental issues and national politics for the Maltese (see Table 8.2). The Czech respondents showed significantly higher optimistic expectations in personal life ($t(150.68) = 3.65$; $p < 0.001$; $d = 0.51$; 95% CI [0.217; 0.723]), national politics ($t(265) = 3.22$; $p < 0.01$; $d = 0.42$; 95% CI [0.162; 0.678]), and climate and environment ($t(210.2) = 8.22$; $p < 0.001$; $d = 1.01$; 95% CI [0.822; 1.337]) than the Maltese respondents.

Hope Objects, Activities and Providers Among Czech and Maltese Samples

The respondents were asked what their personal wishes were and to rate their subjective importance. For most Czech and Maltese respondents, personal wishes involved relationships with the other people. The most important wishes for both groups were related to happy family relationships, good personal health, harmonious life, high-quality relationships with other people, and personal autonomy and self-determination. The least popular wishes amongst the Czech cohort, were related to money, spiritual and religious experiences, and secure job. For the Maltese, the least popular wishes were spiritual and religious experiences, fun with friends, and money.

We also examined what actions the respondents were taking to achieve their hopes. In most cases, both Czech and Maltese respondents analysed circumstances, did plenty of reading and gathered information, and took responsibility for their actions. The other frequently listed activities were motivating the family or friends, and saving money. The least frequent activities were entrepreneurial engagement, going to church or praying and donating money.

Most Czech and Maltese respondents viewed hope as something for which everyone was responsible for himself or herself; thus seeing themselves as their own primary hope providers. The runner-up source of hope was a life partner, husband or wife; followed by friends. Another valuable source of hope were the people who the respondents found inspiring in finding solutions in difficult life situations. Some of the participants listed parents and grandparents as their source of hope. The least popular hope providers for both samples were businessmen and managers, bankers and financial advisors, politicians and the government.

Table 8.3 Descriptive statistics of the investigated variables (for both samples)

	Mean		SD		Minimum		Maximum	
	CZ	M	CZ	M	CZ	M	CZ	M
Perceived hope	22.36	18.72	5.27	6.22	5	0	30	30
Optimism	25.59	23.17	5.38	6.68	6	6	35	36
Posit. Relations	41.18	37.92	7.74	8.73	19	13	54	54
Loneliness	7.57	7.89	2.56	2.62	3	3	15	15
Spirituality	10.95	9.51	4.27	3.88	4	4	16	16
Generativity	23.06	23.78	5.46	4.21	0	9	30	30
Life satisfaction	24.97	22.38	6.05	7.45	5	6	35	34

Note: CZ = Czech Republic, M = Malta

Comparison of the Czech and Maltese Samples

We examined the levels of perceived hope, optimism, life satisfaction, positive relations, loneliness, generativity, and spirituality among the Czech and Maltese samples, and compared the two samples on these variables. Means and standard deviations for the variables of interest are shown in Table 8.3.

As the distribution of gender in Czech and Maltese samples was uneven, we wanted to clarify whether the gender differences significantly influenced the dependent variables. We used two-way Anova to examine the effect of country and gender on the differences between the variables of interest in the two samples, and to explore possible interaction between country and gender.

Czech respondents showed a significantly higher level of perceived hope than Maltese participants [$F(1,263) = 17.53$; $p < 0.001$; $\eta_p^2 = 0.062$; $d = 0.65$]. No significant main effect of gender [$F(1,263) = 1.34$; $p = 0.248$; $\eta_p^2 = 0.05$] nor interaction between gender and country [$F(1,263) = 0.15$; $p = 0.697$; $\eta_p^2 = 0.001$] were found.

The Czech participants also attained a significantly higher level of optimism than the Maltese [$F(1,263) = 5.87$; $p < 0.05$; $\eta_p^2 = 0.022$; $d = 0.41$]. Interaction between country and gender was not statistically significant [$F(1,263) = 0.60$; $p = 0.441$; $\eta_p^2 = 0.002$] and neither was main effect of gender [$F(1,263) = 2.21$; $p = 0.138$; $\eta_p^2 = 0.008$].

A significant difference between the two samples was found in the level of spirituality [$F(1,263) = 5.03$; $p < 0.05$; $\eta_p^2 = 0.019$; $d = 0.35$]. Czech respondents showed a higher spirituality level than Maltese. Main effect of gender [$F(1,263) = 0.88$; $p = 0.349$; $\eta_p^2 = 0.003$] and interaction between gender and country [$F(1,263) = 3.55$; $p = 0.06$; $\eta_p^2 = 0.013$] were not significant.

Czech participants also displayed significantly a higher level of life satisfaction as compared to Maltese respondents [$F(1,263) = 7.06$; $p < 0.01$; $\eta_p^2 = 0.026$; $d = 0.40$]. No significant results were found for main effect of gender [$F(1,263) = 0.23$; $p = 0.634$; $\eta_p^2 = 0.001$] and interaction between gender and country [$F(1,263) = 0.35$; $p = 0.556$; $\eta_p^2 = 0.001$].

The results did not reveal any significant difference between Czech and Maltese samples in positive relationships [$F(1,263) = 3.65$; $p = 0.057$; $\eta_p^2 = 0.014$; $d = 0.40$].

There was a significant main effect of gender [$F(1,263) = 6.53$; $p = 0.011$; $\eta_p^2 = 0.024$] showing that females reported a higher level of positive relationships. However, the interaction between gender and country was non-significant [$F(1,263) = 0.123$; $p = 0.73$; $\eta_p^2 = 0.000$].

No significant differences between the two samples were found neither in the level of loneliness [$F(1,263) = 0.44$; $p = 0.508$; $\eta_p^2 = 0.002$, $d = 0.12$]. Results also showed non-significant gender and country interaction [$F(1,263) = 0.47$; $p = 0.496$; $\eta_p^2 = 0.002$] and non-significant main effect of gender [$F(1,263) = 0.43$; $p = 0.515$; $\eta_p^2 = 0.002$].

The Czech sample also did not differ from Maltese in the level of generativity [$F(1,263) = 2.52$; $p = 0.11$; $\eta_p^2 = 0.009$; $d = 0.14$]. Interaction between gender and country was non-significant [$F(1,263) = 0.31$; $p = 0.58$; $\eta_p^2 = 0.001$] and there was also no significant main effect of gender [$F(1,263) = 1.90$; $p = 0.17$; $\eta_p^2 = 0.007$].

To sum up, Czech respondents scored significantly higher in perceived hope, optimism, spirituality, and life satisfaction when compared to Maltese participants. No significant differences between the two samples were found in positive relations, loneliness and generativity. The differences in the variables examined between Czech and Maltese samples were not affected by the interaction between country and gender.

Correlates and Predictors of Perceived Hope

We also examined whether there were any significant relationships between perceived hope and the other investigated variables.

Table 8.4 shows the relationships among all the measured variables in the Czech sample. In addition to the hypothesised strong correlations among perceived hope, optimism, and life satisfaction, we also found significant positive relationships among perceived hope and positive relations, spirituality, and generativity. Perceived hope was significantly negatively correlated with loneliness; the latter was also closely related to less positive relations with other people. However, no relationship was found between spirituality and either life satisfaction or loneliness; nor did the

Table 8.4 Pearson's correlation coefficients for all variables in the Czech sample (N = 177)

	Variable	1	2	3	4	5	6
1	Perceived hope	1					
2	Optimism	.72***	1				
3	Positive relations	.54***	.59***	1			
4	Generativity	.42***	31***	.27***	1		
5	Spirituality	.30***	.23**	.18*	.34***	1	
6	Life satisfaction	.62***	.57***	.47***	.17*	.09	1
7	Loneliness	−.51***	−.54***	−.68***	−.11	−.05	−.55***

Note: *$p < 0.05$; **$p < 0.01$; ***$p < 0.001$

Table 8.5 Pearson's correlation coefficients for all variables in the Maltese sample (N = 90)

	Variable	1	2	3	4	5	6
1	Perceived Hope	1					
2	Optimism	**.61*****	1				
3	Positive Relations	**.47*****	**.51*****	1			
4	Generativity	**.34****	**.21***	**.43*****	1		
5	Spirituality	**.33****	.14	**.28****	**.45*****	1	
6	Life Satisfaction	**.54*****	**.67*****	**.57*****	.19	**.28****	1
7	Loneliness	**−.36****	**−.55*****	**−.76*****	**−.25***	**−.22***	**−.65*****

Note: $^*p < 0.05$; $^{**}p < 0.01$; $^{***}p < 0.001$

Table 8.6 Multicollinearity diagnostic – Czech sample

Variable	Tolerance	VIF
Positive relations	.457	2.190
Generativity	.809	1.237
Loneliness	.496	2.018
Optimism	.577	1.733
Spirituality	.854	1.171

Table 8.7 Multicollinearity diagnostic – Maltese sample

Variable	Tolerance	VIF
Positive relations	.355	2.816
Generativity	.689	1.452
Loneliness	.381	2.624
Optimism	.674	1.483
Spirituality	.787	1.271

results confirm the hypothesised negative relationship between generativity and loneliness.

Table 8.5 shows the relationships among all the measured variables in the Maltese sample. Similarly to the Czech sample, significant correlations were found among perceived hope, optimism, and life satisfaction, though here the correlations were less strong. We also found significant correlations between perceived hope and positive relations, spirituality, and generativity, and a significant negative correlation between perceived hope and loneliness. However, unlike the Czech sample, the Maltese group showed no significant relationship either between spirituality and optimism, or between life satisfaction and generativity. They did exhibit, however, a significant negative correlation between loneliness and spirituality/generativity. Spirituality was also found to be positively related to life satisfaction.

In view of the high correlations in some of the variables (e.g. positive relationships and loneliness) we used the multicollinearity diagnostics for both Czech and Maltese samples before doing a regression analysis. All the values of tolerance and variance inflation factors (VIF) are displayed in Tables 8.6 and 8.7. The results for

Table 8.8 Regression model predicting Perceived Hope (PHS) for the Czech and Maltese samples

Predictors of perceived hope	Czech Republic				Malta			
	B	SE	β	p	B	SE	β	p
Positive relations	.039	.049	.057	.431	.181	.095	.254	.060
Generativity	.185	.052	**.192**	**.001**	.117	.141	.079	.411
Optimism	.506	.063	**.516**	**.000**	.509	.090	**.547**	**.000**
Loneliness	−.342	.143	**−.166**	**.018**	.468	.305	.198	.128
Spirituality	.115	.065	.093	.078	.297	.143	**.186**	**.041**

the Czech sample do not indicate problematic multicollinearity as the values of VIF are below 5 and no variable reached critical tolerance value below 0.2 (Table 8.6). In the Maltese sample the VIF values are higher in positive relations and loneliness, but this does not indicate a serious problem of multicollinearity as the values are not higher than 5. Neither do the tolerance values in the Maltese sample drop below critical value of 0.2 (Table 8.7).

Two separate regression analyses were then performed to determine which of the examined variables were independent predictors of perceived hope and whether there were any differences between the two samples. The results are presented in Table 8.8.

The first regression analysis showed that in the Czech sample perceived hope was strongly predicted by optimism (*beta* = 0.516; $p < 0.001$) and moderately predicted by generativity (*beta* = 0.192; $p < 0.001$) and loneliness (*beta* = −0.166; $p < 0.05$). Positive relations and spirituality were not found to be significant predictors of perceived hope. The linear regression model for the Czech sample was significant [$F(5,171) = 50.001$; $p < 0.001$] and explained 59.4% of the variance of perceived hope ($R = 0.771$; $R^2 = 0.594$; R^2 *adjusted* = 0.582).

The second regression analysis identified optimism (*beta* = 0.547; $p < 0.001$) and spirituality (*beta* = 0.186; $p < 0.05$) as the independent predictors of perceived hope in the Maltese sample. Positive relations, generativity and loneliness were not found to be significant predictors of perceived hope. The model was significant [$F(5,84) = 14.907$; $p < 0.001$] and explained 47% of the variance of perceived hope ($R = 0.686$; $R^2 = 0.470$; R^2 *adjusted* = 0.439).

The Effect of Demographic Variables

Finally we investigated whether perceived hope and the other variables of interest are affected by age, gender, family status, level of education, religious beliefs, and engagement in voluntary activities.

Age

Due to the weak representation of the last three age groups (50–59, 60–69, and 70–79) in both samples, these were merged together into a single "50+ group" for each of the two samples.

One-way ANOVA showed statistically significant age-related differences in loneliness [$F(3,173) = 3.531$; $p < 0.05$; $\eta_p^2 = 0.058$] in the Czech sample. The highest level of loneliness was among the youngest group aged 18–29 years ($M = 8.04$; $SD = 2.48$), while the lowest level was found among the 40–49 years ($M = 6.6$; $SD = 2.80$). The 30–39 age group ($M = 6.8$; $SD = 2.17$) showed similar results to the 50+ group ($M = 7.0$; $SD = 2.53$). However, Tukey's post-hoc test did not confirm any significant differences between age groups in Czech sample.

One-way ANOVA carried out on the Maltese sample showed statistically significant age-related differences in perceived hope [$F(3,86) = 2.98$; $p < 0.05$; $\eta_p^2 = 0.094$], spirituality [$F(3,86) = 4.20$; $p < 0.05$; $\eta_p^2 = 0.127$], optimism [$F(3,86) = 2.85$; $p < 0.05$; $\eta_p^2 = 0.9$], and generativity [$F(3,86) = 3.17$; $p < 0.05$; $\eta_p^2 = 0.1$]. The Tukey's post-hoc test confirmed significant difference in perceived hope between the youngest age group (18–29 years), which was the least hopeful ($M = 16$; $SD = 6.29$; $p = 0.045$; $d = 0.73$), and the 50+ age group, which was the most hopeful ($M = 20.72$; $SD = 6.62$). The oldest age group (50+) also reported significantly higher spirituality ($M = 11.14$; $SD = 3.96$; $p = 0.006$; $d = 0.97$) than the youngest group ($M = 7.47$; $SD = 3.47$), which was the lowest in spirituality. The highest level of optimism ($M = 26.0$; $SD = 6.35$) was found among the age group of 40–49 years, while the youngest group exhibited the lowest optimism ($M = 20.95$; $SD = 5.86$). The oldest age group also displayed significantly higher level of generativity ($M = 25.28$; $SD = 3.62$; $p = 0.025$; $d = 0.78$) when compared to the 30–39 age group ($M = 22$; $SD = 4.88$).

Gender

An independent samples t-test did not reveal any significant gender-related differences in the variables in the Czech sample.

On the other hand, significant gender-related differences were found in the Maltese group in spirituality ($t(74.268) = 2.095$; $p = 0.040$; $d = 0.43$; 95% CI [0.081, 3.179]), with males ($M = 8.97$; $SD = 4.13$) exhibiting significantly lower levels of spirituality than females ($M = 10.6$; $SD = 3.11$).

Marital Status

The respondents in both samples were grouped into four categories: single, living in a partnership, married, and divorced/widowed.

While the respondents' marital status was found to exert a significant impact on most variables related to the Czech sample, no such differences were found in the Maltese sample.

One-way ANOVA and Hochberg GT2 post-hoc test identified significant inter-group differences in perceived hope [$F(3,173) = 5.654$; $p < 0.05$; $\eta_p^2 = 0.089$], optimism [$F(3,173) = 3.937$; $p < 0.05$; $\eta_p^2 = 0.064$], positive relations [$F(3,173) = 3.645$; $p < 0.05$; $\eta_p^2 = 0.06$] and loneliness [$F(3,173) = 5.895$; $p < 0.01$; $\eta_p^2 = 0.093$] in the Czech sample. A Welch test of variance also revealed signifiant differences in life satisfaction (asymptotic distribution $F (3; 40.04) = 8.813$; $p < 0.01$).

Czech participants who were single exhibited significantly lower levels of perceived hope ($M = 20.30$; $SD = 5.66$) than those living with a partner ($M = 23.23$; $SD = 4.15$; $p = 0.009$; $d = 0.59$) or married ($M = 23.88$; $SD = 5.32$; $p = 0.003$; $d = 0.65$). The single respondents also reported significantly lower optimism ($M = 23.81$; $SD = 5.54$) than those living with a partner ($M = 26.7$; $SD = 4.94$; $p = 0.015$; $d = 0.55$) or married ($M = 26.65$; $SD = 5.44$; $p = 0.039$; $d = 0.52$).

The participants who were single reported significantly lower level of positive relations with others ($M = 38.69$; $SD = 7.49$) than those who had a partner ($M = 42.55$; $SD = 7.81$; $p = 0.03$; $d = 0.51$); unsurprisingly, they also showed higher loneliness ($M = 8.52$; $SD = 2.46$; $p = 0.001$; $d = 0.8$) than married participants ($M = 6.6$; $SD = 2.40$). In addition, they scored significantly lower in life satisfaction ($M = 22.23$; $SD = 6.48$) compared to those who were married ($M = 27.35$; $SD = 5.27$; $p = 0.001$; $d = 0.86$) or living with a partner ($M = 26.18$; $SD = 5.17$; $p = 0.001$; $d = 0.68$).

Education

The participants with an elementary level education were excluded from both of the samples due to their isufficient representation and education-related differences were examined only with respect to secondary and university levels of education. While no significant differences were found between the two education categories in the Czech sample, the Maltese sample did exhibit education-related differences in the level of loneliness ($t(88) = 2.668$; $p = 0.009$; $d = 0.63$; 95% CI [0.337, 2.843]). The participants with secondary education ($M = 9.04$; $SD = 2.76$) reported higher loneliness than those with university education ($M = 7.45$; $SD = 2.45$).

Religion

The Czech sample showed significant religion-related differences in spirituality [$F(2,158) = 90.44$; $p < 0.001$; $\eta_p^2 = 0.53$], a variable reflecting the perceived importance of spiritual beliefs in one's life. A Tukey's test revealed that the participants without a religion ($M = 5.78$; $SD = 2.95$) exhibited lower spirituality in comparison with those who were Christian ($M = 13.24$; $SD = 2.65$; $p < 0.001$; $d = 2.33$) or spiritual but not religious ($M = 12.2$; $SD = 3.16$; $p < 0.001$; $d = 2.09$).

A Welch test revealed also differences in generativity (asymptotically distributed $F(2; 84,955) = 5.47$; $p < 0.01$). A Games-Howell post-hoc test showed that Czech respondents without a religion ($M = 20.49$; $SD = 6.66$) exhibited lower generativity than those who were Christian ($M = 24.30$; $SD = 3.96$; $p < 0.01$; $d = 0.74$) or spiritual but not religious ($M = 23.67$; $SD = 5.31$; $p < 0.05$; $d = 0.54$).

In the Maltese sample, a Welch test revealed that the only differences were related to spirituality (asymptotically distributed $F(2; 13,085) = 33.527$; $p < 0.001$). A Games-Howell test showed that the respondents without a religion ($M = 4.86$; $SD = 1.99$; $p < 0.001$; $d = 1.72$) had lower level of spirituality than those who were Christians ($M = 10.58$; $SD = 3.53$). However, no statistically significant difference in the level of spirituality was found between Christians and those who were spiritual but not religious.

Volunteering

Of the 177 Czech respondents, 52 (29.4%) were engaged in voluntary activites which is in accordance with the 30% rate of volunteering given by Dekker and Halman (2003). No significant difference in perceived hope and the other variables was found between volunteers and non-volunteers.

Twenty-two Maltese participants (24.4%) were engaged in volunteering. Significant differences between the two groups were found in perceived hope ($t(88) = 2.480$; $p = 0.015$; $d = 0.62$), spirituality ($t(88) = 2.946$; $p = 0.004$; $d = 0.73$), and generativity ($t(88) = 3.103$; $p = 0.003$; $d = 0.77$). Volunteers showed higher perceived hope ($M = 21.5$; $SD = 4.99$) than non-volunteers ($M = 17.82$; $SD = 6.34$), and scored higher in spirituality ($M = 11.55$; $SD = 3.73$) than non-volunteers ($M = 8.85$; $SD = 3.73$). Maltese volunteers also reported higher generativity ($M = 26.09$; $SD = 3.16$) in comparison with non-volunteers ($M = 23.03$; $SD = 4.26$).

Discussion

The first objective of the present study was to assess the participants' satisfaction with the foregoing year (2015) and their outlook on the forthcoming year (2016) on issues related to personal, political, economical, environmental and social matters. Of the five domains, both the Czech and Maltese respondents were most satisfied with their personal life, while their satisfaction with matters beyond one's control was the lowest. The Czech respondents were the least satisfied with national politics and social issues, reflecting the perceived low quality of political culture and predominantly negative reactions to the current migration crisis. The Maltese were even less satisfied with their national politics than the Czechs. Their lowest satisfaction was with climate and environmental issues, reflecting the salience of these matters in the daily life of a small, densely populated island nation. However, they were relatively satisfied with the economy, underling the economic boom of the current year with a record low rate of unemployment in contrast to other Mediterranean countries hard hit by the recent recession such as Italy, Greece, Spain and Portugal.

The participants' satisfaction with the foregoing year probably affected their expectations for the future as well. Both groups of respondents were the most optimistic about their personal life in 2016, and predominantly pessimistic about national politics. While the Czech respondents showed low optimism about social issues, the Maltese were rather pessimistic about future developments related to the climate and the environment. The above results appear to be related to the specific issues that each country is dealing with and as well as to the citizens' lack of trust in public institutions.

Since both the Czech and Maltese respondents were apparently able to retain hope about their personal life despite the perceived socio-political issues, we were interested in the content of their hopes and personal wishes, what they do to fulfil their hopes and whom they expect to provide them with hope.

The majority of both Czech and Maltese respondents expressed personal desires involving social relationships (particularly their relationships with significant others). For both nationalities the most important hopes were related to happy family relationships, good personal health, harmonious life, high-quality relationships with other people, and personal autonomy and self-determination. These findings are in line with the results obtained in previous studies on larger samples of Czech, German, and Swiss respondents (Krafft & Walker, 2018; Slezáčková, 2017; Slezáčková & Krafft, 2016).

The finding that the least popular wishes of the Czech respondents are related to money and secure job is reflective of the very low rate of unemployment in the country and the very few people in material need, thus making the above values of low importance. Similarly, the low importance of spiritual and religious experiences is not surprising because in the predominantly secular Czech society, spirituality and religion are marginalised. In the Maltese sample, the least popular wishes were spiritual and religious experiences, fun with friends, and money. While Maltese participants appreciated the importance of relationships and friendships, they did not necessarily see these as sources of fun, but more as avenues of support and connectedness. The low desire for spiritual and religious experience in the coming year could be a reflection of the growing trend towards secularisation in the past decades in Malta, with organised religion holding less influence on the daily life of the people, particularly the younger generations.

Both the Czech and Maltese respondents exhibited a rational, active and individualistic approach to pursuing their goals. Their view of hope is congruent with Snyder's (2000) cognitive theory of hope rather than with the more transcendental phenomenon of perceived hope (Krafft et al., 2017). The respondents in both samples analysed circumstances, gathered information and did plenty of reading, and took responsibility for their actions. The other frequently listed activities were motivating family members or friends, and saving money. The least frequent activities in both the samples included setting up one's own business, donating money, going to church and praying or meditating. The results are in line with the above mentioned low religiosity of the Czech society, and the increasing secularisation in Maltese society, though it must be mentioned that two thirds of Maltese participants in the study were under 50.

The majority of both Czech and Maltese participants saw themselves as their primary hope providers, suggesting an internal locus of hope (Bernardo, 2010). Other important sources of hope were a life partner, parents, grandparents, and friends, as well as people who inspired the respondents in finding solutions in difficult life situations. Similar results were obtained by Krafft and Walker (2018), who conducted a study on German and Swiss samples. The least popular "hope providers" in both the samples in our study were politicians and the government, businessmen and managers, bankers and financial advisors, which can be related to the above mentioned low satisfaction with national politics and low perceived importance of finance-related hopes and wishes.

A comparative analysis showed that the two samples differed on most of the investigated variables, with the exception of positive relations, loneliness, and generativity. The Czech respondents showed significantly higher levels of perceived hope, optimism, spirituality, and life satisfaction than their Maltese counterparts. Given that in international studies focusing on happiness, Malta usually ranks similar to the Czech Republic or even higher (Helliwell, Layard & Sachs, 2017; Veenhoven, 2016a, 2016b) and that it scores significantly higher than the Czech Republic on Hofstede's Indulgence Dimension (Hofstede, 2001) (which measures people's tendency towards optimism and willingness to enjoy life), our results on life satisfaction can be viewed as sample-specific. They might have been due to the differences in age distribution, as well as the relatively small sample of Maltese respondents which might not be representative of the population as a whole. For instance, the Czech sample contained more younger respondents than the Maltese cohort, which might have skewed the results because, as Arnett (2004) has argued, young adults tend to think positively about their future.

The significant relationships among perceived hope, life satisfaction, and positive relations with others in both samples are congruent with the results of previous studies (Krafft et al., 2017; Slezáčková, 2017; Slezáčková & Krafft, 2016). The positive relationship between hope (in the sense of Snyder's dispositional hope) and subjective well-being was found also in the studies by Demirli et al. (2015), Kato and Snyder (2005), and Werner (2012). The close relationship between life satisfaction and optimism reported in this study is in line with the results of a study conducted by Gallagher et al. (2013), and Schweizer et al. (1999). Significant correlations between hope and positive relations with others were also reported by Slezáčková (2017), Westburg (2001), and Windsor (2009). Since the concept of perceived hope is close to a transcendental conception of hope, it is not surprising that it is significantly correlated to spirituality (Scioli et al., 2011) and generativity (Damásio, Koller, & Schnell, 2013). We also confirmed an expected direct association between spirituality and generativity (Neusner & Chilton, 2005). Loneliness was found to be closely connected to a low level of life satisfaction and positive relations with other people, which had already been reported in earlier studies (Cacioppo & Patrick, 2008; Hansson, Jones, Carpenter, & Remondet, 1987).

We have also found, however, various differences between the two samples. We have already mentioned the low importance of spirituality for the Czech respondents; this finding was also reflected in the lack of relationship between spirituality and life satisfaction. By contrast, the Maltese sample exhibited a significant relationship between the two concepts, perhaps suggesting that despite increasing secularisation, spirituality is still a primary life goal. Similarly, while no relationships were found among loneliness, generativity and spirituality in the Czech sample, the relationships were significant in the Maltese sample. The negative correlations between loneliness and generativity and spirituality may be taken to indicate that cultivating spirituality in the sense of connectedness to others, God or the Universe, along with developing a generative concern, might serve as protective factors against feelings of loneliness. However, these effects may be bidirectional, meaning that less lonely people (i.e. those who have good and trustful relations with others) may show a greater propensity for generative behaviour and may have more opportunities to develop their spirituality thanks to the support of like minded people.

Further differences between the two samples are related to the relationships between life satisfaction and generativity, and between spirituality and optimism. While these relationships were significant in the Czech sample, they were not in the Maltese sample. Nevertheless, the fact that spirituality was found to be related to perceived hope but unrelated to optimism indicates that the two constructs are not identical (Krafft & Walker, 2018).

In the regression model for the Czech sample, the significant predictors of perceived hope were optimism, generativity, and loneliness. The predictive effects of positive relations and spirituality were entirely insignificant. The significant relationship between dispositional optimism and dispositional hope and perceived hope respectively, have already been reported in earlier studies (Gallagher & Lopez, 2009; Krafft et al., 2017; Magaletta & Oliver, 1999). The relationship between loneliness and hope is in line with a finding by Snyder that high-hope young adults report less loneliness (Snyder, 1994). The connection between basic hope (as conceptualised by Erickson) and generativity was established by Wojciechowska (2011). A possible explanation for our findings may be that hopeful feelings depend not only on positive expectations for one's own future, but also on the individual's propensity to create things of lasting value for others, and, last but not least, on the ability to maintain social relationships which protect us from loneliness.

In the Maltese-sample model, the strongest predictor of perceived hope was optimism, while spirituality had also a significant predictive effect. On the other hand, positive relations, loneliness, and generativity were not found to be significant predictors of perceived hope. It is interesting to observe that while the Maltese respondents, who are predominantly Christian, showed a significantly lower level of perceived importance of spirituality than the Czech respondents, they still considered spirituality as important in helping them to retain hope.

The youngest Maltese group (aged 18–29 years) exhibited the lowest levels on many of the investigated variables (perceived hope, optimism, and spirituality) of all the age groups. While there is evidence suggesting that hope levels can change with age (Benzein & Berg, 2005) and that people aged between 55 and 64 years tend to exhibit lower dispositional hope (Bailey & Snyder, 2007), this is different with regards to perceived hope. Earlier studies show that young adults (18–29 years) tend to have the lowest level of perceived hope, with the highest levels found in individuals aged 50–59 years (Slezáčková, 2017). The low levels of perceived hope among young adults may be explained by the previously reported close link between perceived hope and meaningfulness (Slezáčková & Krafft, 2016). The perception that one's life is meaningful has been repeatedly shown to be lower in adolescence and early adulthood than in late adulthood (Halama, 2015; Schnell, 2009), and low perceived hope in young adults can thus be reflective of low meaningfulness. The oldest age group of Maltese respondents displayed significantly higher levels of perceived hope, spirituality, and generativity, which can be considered to be keys to successful ageing (Bowling & Dieppe, 2005).

In the Czech sample, the youngest group showed also the highest level of loneliness, which is in line with recent findings on an increasing incidence of loneliness in adolescence and early adulthood (Goosby et al., 2013).

No significant gender-related differences were found in the Czech sample. On the other hand, Maltese females exhibited higher levels of perceived importance of spirituality in life than males, which is a reflection of international studies showing such gender differences in spirituality (Bryant, 2007; Hammermeister, Flint, El-Alayli, Ridnour, & Peterson, 2005).

Marital status had already been shown to be closely related to hope. In a study by Bailey and Snyder (2007), those who were divorced or widowed showed much lower dispositional hope than those who were in a long-term partnership or married relationship. The close relationship that marital status bore to hope and the rest of the investigated variables was reflected in our own results, too. Single Czech respondents reported significantly lower levels of perceived hope, optimism, positive relations and life satisfaction, and a higher level of loneliness, than those who had a partner or were married. Similar results on the positive impact of marriage on subjective wellbeing have been reported in other studies (Diener, Gohm, Suh, & Oishi, 2000; Lucas, Clark, Georgellis, & Diener, 2003). Most respondents identified their significant others as their primary objects of hope and main hope providers, reflecting the importance of close relationships for hope. Interestingly, no differences related to marital status were found in the Maltese sample, possibly suggesting that they make use of other sources of social support such as friends and family of origin.

No significant differences were found between respondents with secondary education and those with university education in the Czech sample. The fact that the participants with elementary education were excluded from the sample due to their isufficient representation, might have acted as a limitation. In another study conducted on a larger Czech sample (Slezáčková, 2017), respondents with a university degree showed higher perceived hope than both with elementary or secondary education. In this study, Maltese respondents with higher education reported less loneliness than those with secondary education, which is in line with the results of other studies focusing on the predictors and risk factors of loneliness (e.g. Savikko, Routasalo, Tilvis, Strandberg, & Pitkälä, 2005; Victor, Scambler, Bowling, & Bond, 2005).

An analysis of religion-related differences showed that the Czech respondents who were Christian or spiritual but not religious perceived spiritual beliefs as more important and showed greater generativity than the participants without a religion. The above finding supports the claim that generativity, one of the dimensions of self-transcendence (Schnell, 2009), is associated with greater spirituality and religiosity (Cox et al., 2010; Dillon et al., 2003). In the Maltese sample, the participants who were Christian also scored higher in spirituality than those without a religion.

Lastly, no significant differences were found between volunteering and any of the variables in the Czech sample. This is in contrast with the results of earlier studies in which volunteers were found to exhibit higher levels of perceived hope (Slezáčková & Krafft, 2016), generativity (Frensch et al., 2007), or life satisfaction (Heo, Chun, Lee, & Kim, 2016; Piliavin, 2003). However, the results of the Maltese sample show that volunteers exhibit higher perceived hope, spirituality, and generativity in comparison with non-volunteers. This is in congruence with earlier studies investigating the effects of volunteering on perceived hope (Slezáčková, 2017), and the relationships between volunteering, meaningfulness (Schnell & Hoof, 2012), and generativity (Brady & Hapenny, 2010).

These differences between Czech and Maltese samples might be explained to some extent by Hofstede's model of culture dimensions (Hofstede, 2001), which shows that Czech Republic scores higher than Malta on the dimensions Masculinity and Long Term Orientation, and lower on Indulgence. High value of achievement and material rewards for success in Czech society, along with its pragmatic future orientation and tendency towards cynicism and pessimism, may be related to rather extrinsic motivation for volunteering activites especially in younger generation (for instance, gaining new experience which can be useful at work, increasing the chance for future employment, etc.) which might not be related with transcendental phenomena such as perceived hope, spirituality, and generativity.

Conclusion

In our work we aimed to investigate the psychosocial aspects of perceived hope among two national samples, Czech and Maltese. Since perceived hope is a relatively novel construct, we were interested in examining whether it is more affected by social factors (quantity and quality of relationships with others), dispositional characteristics (such as dispositional optimism), or self-transcendent resources (spirituality and generativity). We also wanted to find out whether and to what extent the importance of these resources is culture-dependent.

In both samples, the most important independent predictor of perceived hope was dispositional optimism, a characteristic responsible for one's positive outlook on life. However, the predictive capability of the varying predictors in relation to perceived hope was found to be culturally-dependent. While in the Czech sample, higher perceived hope was predicted by higher generativity and lower loneliness, in the Maltese sample an important role was played by spirituality, which was found to be the second independent predictor of perceived hope.

In view of the above, our primary research question cannot be unequivocally answered. Perceived hope seems to be related predominantly to dispositional characteristics such as an optimistic and positive mindset, but, an important role is also played by self-transcendent resources and ability to maintain social relationships. In general, though, our results support the conceptualisation of hope suggested by Krafft et al. (2017), that is, perceived hope.

Further studies on the topic could devote more attention to overcoming the limits of the present study. The principal limitation of our study consists in the use of convenience sampling resulting in different age and gender distribution in each of the research samples. However, it turned out that the differences between Czech and Maltese samples in the variables measured were not affected by the interaction between country and gender. Moreover, the distribution of all the other demographic factors in both research samples was fairly even. Further bias might have been caused by factors such as self-presentation and decreased introspection. The samples, particularly the Maltese one, were also relatively small.

In addition, we are aware of the specific issues related to cross-cultural comparative research (Brislin, 1983). Mathews (2012) stresses that language differences (e.g. different expressions and concepts of happiness) and cultural distinctions can considerably affect the results. Because our study is only a correlational one, a longitudinal study that would include other psychosocial variables, would provide a deeper insight into the investigated phenomena and the dynamics and the direction of causality of the relations between the investigated variables.

Because the concepts of hope, optimism and spirituality have been repeatedly found to constitute important components of an individual's optimal development and flourishing, our findings can be applied both in educational and clinical contexts.

References

Alarcon, G., Bowling, N., & Khazon, S. (2013). Great expectations: A meta-analytic examination of optimism and hope. *Personality and Individual Differences, 54*(7), 821–827. https://doi.org/10.1016/j.paid.2012.12.004

An, J. S., & Cooney, T. M. (2006). Psychological well-being in mid to late life: The role of generativity development and parent-child relationships across the lifespan. *International Journal of Behavioral Development, 30*, 410–421.

Anand, H. (2013). Prayer and meditation: Way of improving psychological wellbeing. In S. K. Srivastava, N. Singh, & S. Kant (Eds.), *Psychological interventions of mental disorders* (pp. 215–226). New Delhi: Sarup Book Publishers.

Arnau, R., Rosen, D., Finch, J., Rhudy, J., & Fortunato, V. (2007). Longitudinal effects of hope on depression and anxiety: A latent variable analysis. *Journal of Personality, 75*(1), 43–64. https://doi.org/10.1111/j.1467-6494.2006.00432.x

Arnett, J. J. (2004). *Emerging adulthood: The winding road from the late teens through the twenties.* New York: Oxford University Press.

Atienza, A. A., Stephens, M. A. P., & Townsend, A. L. (2004). Role stressors as predictors of changes in women's optimistic expectations. *Personality and Individual Differences, 37*, 471–484. https://doi.org/10.1016/j.paid.2003.09.016

Baetz, M., Bowen, R., & Jones, G. (2006). How spiritual values and worship attendance relate to psychiatric disorders in the Canadian population. *Canadian Journal of Psychiatry, 51*, 654–661.

Bailey, T. C., Eng, W., Frisch, M. B., & Snyder, C. R. (2007). Hope and optimism as related to life satisfaction. *The Journal of Positive Psychology, 2*(3), 168–175.

Bailey, T. C., & Snyder, C. R. (2007). Satisfaction with life and hope: A look at age and marital status. *The Psychological Record, 57*(2), 233–240.

Baker, S. R. (2007). Dispositional optimism and health status, symptoms and behaviours: Assessing idiothetic relationships using a prospective daily diary approach. *Psychology & Health, 22*(4), 431–455. https://doi.org/10.1080/14768320600941764

Bekelman, D. B., Dy, S. M., Becker, D. M., Wittstein, I. S., Hendricks, D. E., Yamashita, T. E., & Gottlieb, S. H. (2007). Spiritual well-being and depression in patients with heart failure. *Journal of General Internal Medicine, 22*, 470–477.

Benzein, E. G., & Berg, A. C. (2005). The level of and relation between hope, hopelessness and fatigue in patients and family members in palliative care. *Palliative Medicine, 19*(3), 234–240.

Bernardo, A. B. I. (2010). Extending hope theory: Internal and external locus of trait hope. *Personality and Individual Differences, 49*(8), 944–949.

Berscheid, E., & Reis, H. T. (1998). Attraction and close relationships. In D. Gilbert, S. T. Fiske, & G. Lindzey (Eds.), *The handbook of social psychology* (pp. 193–281). New York: Mc Graw-Hill.

Betts, L. R., & Bicknell, A. S. A. (2011). Experiencing loneliness in childhood: Consequences for psychosocial adjustment, school adjustment, and academic performance. In S. J. Bevinn (Ed.), *Psychology of loneliness* (pp. 1–28). New York: Nova Science Publishers.

Bowling, A., & Dieppe, P. (2005). What is successful ageing and who should define it? *BMJ: British Medical Journal, 331*(7531), 1548–1551.

Brady, L. L. C., & Hapenny, A. (2010). Giving back and growing in service: Investigating spirituality, religiosity, and generativity in young adults. *Journal of Adult Development, 17*, 162–167.

Brillhart, B. (2005). A study of spirituality and life satisfaction among persons with spinal cord injury. *Rehabilitation Nursing, 30*, 31–34. https://doi.org/10.1002/j.2048-7940.2005.tb00353.x

Brislin, R. W. (1983). Cross-cultural research in psychology. *Annual Revue of Psychology, 34*, 363–400.

Brissette, I., Scheier, M. F., & Carver, C. S. (2002). The role of optimism in social network development, coping, and psychological adjustment during a life transition. *Journal of Personality and Social Psychology, 82*, 102–111.

Bruininks, P., Malle, B., Johnson, J., & Bryant, F. (2005). Distinguishing hope from optimism and related affective states. *Motivation and Emotion, 29*(4), 324–352. https://doi.org/10.5040/9781472594662.ch-015

Bryant, A. N. (2007). Gender differences in spiritual development during the college years. *Sex Roles, 56*(11–12), 835–846. https://doi.org/10.1007/s11199-007-9240-2

Cacioppo, J. T., Hawkley, L. C., Crawford, L. E., Ernst, J. M., Burleson, M. H., Kowalewski, R. B., ... Berntson, G. G. (2002). Loneliness and health: Potential mechanisms. *Psychosomatic Medicine, 64*, 407–417.

Cacioppo, J. T., Hawkley, L. C., Ernst, J. M., Burleson, M., Berntson, G. G., Nouriani, B., & Spiegel, D. (2006). Loneliness within a nomological net: An evolutionary perspective. *Journal of Research in Personality, 40*, 1054–1085.

Cacioppo, J. T., & Patrick, W. (2008). *Loneliness: Human nature and the need for social connection.* New York: Norton.

Carver, C. S., Pozo, C., Harris, S. D., Noriega, V., Scheier, M. F., Robinson, D. S., ... Clark, K. C. (1993). How coping mediates the effect of optimism on distress: A study of women with early stage breast cancer. *Journal of Personality and Social Psychology, 65*, 375–390.

Carver, C. S., & Scheier, M. F. (2002). Optimism. In C. R. Snyder & S. J. Lopez (Eds.), *Handbook of positive psychology* (pp. 231–243). New York: Oxford University Press.

Carver, C. S., Scheier, M. F., & Segerstrom, S. C. (2010). Optimism. *Clinical Psychology Review, 30*, 879–889.

Ciarrochi, J., Parker, P., Kashdan, T. B., Heaven, P. C., & Barkus, E. (2015). Hope and emotional well-being: A six-year study to distinguish antecedents, correlates, and consequences. *The Journal of Positive Psychology, 10*(6), 520–532. https://doi.org/10.1080/17439760.2015.1015154

Clark, M., & Arnold, J. (2008). The nature, prevalence and correlates of generativity among men in middle career. *Journal of Vocational Behavior, 73*, 473–484.

Cotton, S., Larkin, E., Hoopes, A., Cromer, B., & Rosenthal, S. (2005). The impact of adolescent spirituality on depressive symptoms and health risk behaviors. *Journal of Adolescent Health, 36*(6), 529.

Cox, K. S., Wilt, J., Olson, B., & McAdams, D. P. (2010). Generativity, the Big Five, and psychosocial adaptation in midlife adults. *Journal of Personality, 78*(4), 1185–1208.

Damásio, B. F., Koller, S. H., & Schnell, T. (2013). Sources of Meaning and Meaning in Life Questionnaire (SoMe): Psychometric properties and sociodemographic findings in a large Brazilian sample. *Acta De Investigación Psicológica, 3*(3), 1205–1227.

De Espanés, G. M., Villar, F., Urrutia, A., & Serrat, R. (2015). Motivation and commitment to volunteering in a sample of Argentinian adults: What is the role of generativity? *Educational Gerontology, 41*(2), 149–161. https://doi.org/10.1080/03601277.2014.946299

de St. Aubin, E. (2004). The propagation of genes and memes: Generativity through culture in Japan and the United States. In E. de St. Aubin, D. P. McAdams, & T. C. Kim (Eds.), *The generative society* (pp. 63–82). Washington, DC: American Psychological Association Press.

Dekker, P., & Halman, L. (2003). *The values of volunteering: Cross-cultural perspectives.* New York: Kluwer Aacademic/Plenum Publishers.

Demirli, A., Türkmen, M., & Arık, R. (2015). Investigation of dispositional and state hope levels' relations with student subjective well-being. *Social Indicators Research, 120*(2), 601–613. https://doi.org/10.1007/s11205-014-0607-9

Diener, E. (1984). Subjective well-being. *Psychological Bulletin, 95*(3), 542–575.

Diener, E., Emmons, R. A., Larsen, R. J., & Griffin, S. (1985). The Satisfaction with life scale. *Journal of Personality Assessment, 49*(1), 71–75.

Diener, E., Gohm, C. L., Suh, M., & Oishi, S. (2000). Similarity of the relation between marital status and subjective well-being across cultures. *Journal of Cross-Cultural Psychology, 31*, 419–436.

Diener, E., Oishi, S., & Lucas, R. E. (2003). Personality, culture, and subjective well-being: Emotional and cognitive evaluation of life. *Annual Review of Psychology, 54*(1), 403–425.

Diener, E., & Seligman, M. E. P. (2002). Very happy people. *Psychological Science, 13*, 81–84.

Dillon, M., Wink, P., & Fay, K. (2003). Is spirituality detrimental to generativity? *Journal for the Scientific Study of Religion, 42*, 427–444.

Dufault, K., & Martocchio, B. (1985). Hope: Its spheres and dimensions. *Nursing Clinics of North America, 20*(2), 379–391.

Erikson, E. H., & Erikson, J. M. (1998). *The life cycle completed: Extended version.* New York: W. W. Norton.

Forgeard, M. J. C., & Seligman, M. E. P. (2012). Seeing the glass half full: A review of the causes and consequences of optimism. *Pratiques Psychologiques, 18*, 107–120. https://doi.org/10.1016/j.prps.2012.02.002

Frensch, K. M., Pratt, M. W., & Norris, J. E. (2007). Foundations of generativity: Personal and family correlates of emerging adults' generative life-story themes. *Journal of Research in Personality, 41*(1), 45–62. https://doi.org/10.1016/j.jrp.2006.01.005

Gallagher, M. W., & Lopez, S. J. (2009). Positive expectancies and mental health: Identifying the unique contributions of hope and optimism. *The Journal of Positive Psychology, 4*(6), 548–556. https://doi.org/10.1080/17439760903157166

Gallagher, M. W., Lopez, S. J., & Pressman, S. D. (2013). Optimism is universal: Exploring the presence and benefits of optimism in a representative sample of the world. *Journal of Personality, 81*(5), 429–440.

Garssen, B., Visser, A., & de Jager Meezenbroek, E. (2016). Examining whether spirituality predicts subjective well-being: How to avoid tautology. *Psychology of Religion and Spirituality, 8*(2), 141–148. https://doi.org/10.1037/rel0000025

Golden, J., Conroy, R. M., Bruce, I., Denihan, A., Greene, E., Kirby, N., & Lawlor, B. A. (2009). Loneliness, social support networks, mood and wellbeing in community-dwelling elderly. *International Journal of Geriatric Psychiatry, 24*(7), 694–700. https://doi.org/10.1002/gps.2181

Goosby, B. J., Bellatorre, A., Walsemann, K. M., & Cheadle, J. E. (2013). Adolescent loneliness and health in early adulthood. *Sociological Inquiry, 83*(4), 505–536. https://doi.org/10.1111/soin.12018

Green, B. H., Copeland, J. R., Dewey, M. E., Sharma, V., Saunders, P. A., Davidson, I. A., … McWilliam, C. (1992). Risk factors for depression in elderly people: A prospective study. *Acta Psychiatrica Scandinavica, 86*(3), 213–217.

Grossbaum, M. F., & Bates, G. W. (2002). Correlates of psychological well-being at midlife: The role of generativity, agency and communion, and narrative themes. *International Journal of Behavioral Development, 26*(2), 120–127.

Halama, P. (2015). Maintaining meaning in life in old age: Personality and social factors. In M. Blatny (Ed.), *Personality and well-being across the life-span* (pp. 160–178). London, UK: Palgarve Macmillan.

Hammermeister, J., Flint, M., El-Alayli, A., Ridnour, H., & Peterson, M. (2005). Gender differences in spiritual well-being: Are females more spiritually-well than males? *American Journal of Health Studies, 20*(2), 80–84.

Hansson, R. O., Jones, W. H., Carpenter, B. N., & Remondet, J. H. (1987). Loneliness and adjustment to old age. *International Journal of Human Development, 27*(1), 41–53.

Hefferon, K., & Boniwell, I. (2011). *Positive psychology: Theory, research and applications.* Berkshire, UK: Open University Press.

Heikkinen, R., Berg, S., & Avland, K. (1995). Depressive symptoms in late life. *Journal of Cross-Cultural Gerontology, 10*, 315–330.

Helliwell, J., Layard, R., & Sachs, J. (2017). *World happiness report 2017.* New York: Sustainable Development Solutions Network.

Heo, J., Chun, S., Lee, S., & Kim, J. (2016). Life satisfaction and psychological well-being of older adults with cancer experience: The role of optimism and volunteering. *International Journal of Aging & Human Development, 83*(3), 274–289.

Hofer, J., Busch, H., Chasiotis, A., Kärtner, J., & Campos, D. (2008). Concern for generativity and its relation to implicit prosocial power motivation, generative goals, and satisfaction with life: A cross-cultural investigation. *Journal of Personality, 76*, 1–30.

Hofstede, G. (2001). *Culture's consequences: Comparing values, behaviors, institutions, and organizations across nations.* Thousand Oaks, CA: Sage Publications.

Hofstede, G., & Bond, M. (1984). Hofstede's culture dimensions: An independent validation using Rokeach's value survey. *Journal of Cross-Cultural Psychology, 15*, 417–433.

Hombrados-Mendieta, I., García-Martín, M. A., & Gómez-Jacinto, L. (2013). The relationship between social support, loneliness, and subjective well-being in a Spanish sample from a multidimensional perspective. *Social Indicators Research, 114*(3), 1013–1034. https://doi.org/10.1007/s11205-012-0187-5

Hong, P. Y. P., Hodge, D. R., & Choi, S. (2015). Spirituality, hope, and self-sufficiency among low-income job seekers. *Social Work, 60*(2), 155–164.

Horton, T. V., & Wallander, J. L. (2001). Hope and social support as resilience factors against psychological distress of mothers who care for children with chronic physical conditions. *Rehabilitation Psychology, 46*(4), 382–399. https://doi.org/10.1037/0090-5550.46.4.382

House, J. S. (1981). *Work stress and social support*. Reading, MA: Addison-Wesley Educational Publishers.

Hughes, M. E., Waite, L. J., Hawkley, L. C., & Cacioppo, J. T. (2004). A short scale for measuring loneliness in large surveys. Results from two population-based studies. *Research on Aging, 26*(6), 655–672.

Huta, V., & Zuroff, D. C. (2007). Examining mediators of the link between generativity and well-being. *Journal of Adult Development, 14*, 47. https://doi.org/10.1007/s10804-007-9030-7

IndexMundi. 2017. Retrieved from http://www.indexmundi.com/

Kato, T., & Snyder, C. (2005). Relationship between hope and subjective well-being: Reliability and validity of the Dispositional Hope Scale, Japanese version. *Shinrigaku Kenkyu: The Japanese Journal of Psychology, 76*(3), 227–234.

Krafft, A. (2013). *Hope, optimism, positive attributes and life-satisfaction across the lifespan in Germany and Switzerland: An internet study among 11,400 participants*. In the 3rd World Congress on Positive Psychology, Los Angeles, USA, June 2013.

Krafft, A. (2014). *Distinguishing hope measures: Manifold determinants and predictors in the Swiss and German sample*. The 7th European Conference on Positive Psychology, Amsterdam, The Netherlands, June 2014.

Krafft, A. M., & Walker, A. M. (2018). *Positive Psychologie der Hoffnung: Grundlagen aus Psychologie, Philosophie, Theologie und Ergebnisse aktueller Forschung*. Berlin: Springer.

Krafft, A. M., Martin-Krumm, C., & Fenouillet, F. (2017). Adaptation, further elaboration, and validation of a scale to measure hope as perceived by people: Discriminant value and predictive utility vis-à-vis dispositional hope. *Assessment, 24*, 1–16. https://doi.org/10.1177/1073191117700724

Lawford, H., Pratt, M. W., Hunsberger, B., & Pancer, S. M. (2005). Adolescent generativity: A longitudinal study of two possible contexts for learning concern for future generations. *Journal of Research on Adolescence, 15*(3), 261–273. https://doi.org/10.1111/j.1532-7795.2005.00096.x

Leurent, B., Nazareth, I., BellónSaameño, J., Geerlings, M. I., Maaroos, H., Saldivia, S., … King, M. (2013, January). Spiritual and religious beliefs as risk factors for the onset of major depression: An international cohort study. *Psychological Medicine*, 1–12. https://doi.org/10.1017/S0033291712003066

Lin, N., Simeone, R. S., Ensel, W. M., & Kuo, W. (1979). Social support, stressful life events, and illness: A model and an empirical test. *Journal of Health and Social Behavior, 20*(2), 108–119.

Lopez, S. J. (2013). *Making hope happen: Create the future you want for yourself and others*. New York: Atria Books.

Lucas, R. E., Clark, A. E., Georgellis, Y., & Diener, E. (2003). Reexamining adaptation and the set point model of happiness: Reactions to changes in marital status. *Journal of Personality and Social Psychology, 84*(3), 527–539. https://doi.org/10.1037/0022-3514.84.3.527

Lucas, R. E., Diener, E., & Suh, E. (1996). Discriminant validity of well-being measures. *Journal of Personality and Social Psychology, 71*, 616–628.

Magaletta, P. R., & Oliver, J. M. (1999). The hope construct, will, and ways: Their relations with self-efficacy, optimism, and general well-being. *Journal of Clinical Psychology, 55*(5), 539–551. https://doi.org/10.1002/(sici)1097-4679(199905)55:53.3.co;2-7

Mahon, N. E., Yarcheski, A., Yarcheski, T. J., Cannella, B. L., & Hanks, M. M. (2006). A meta-analytic study of predictors for loneliness during adolescence. *Nursing Research, 55*(5), 308–315.

Marcel, G. (2010). *Homo Viator: Introduction to the metaphysic of hope*. South Bend, IN: St. Augustine's Press.

Marques, S. C., Lopez, S. J., & Mitchell, J. (2013). The role of hope, spirituality and religious practice in adolescents' life satisfaction: Longitudinal findings. *Journal of Happiness Studies, 14*, 251. https://doi.org/10.1007/s10902-012-9329-3

Mathews, G. (2012). Happiness, culture, and context. *International Journal of Wellbeing, 2*(4), 299–312.

McAdams, D. P., & de St. Aubin, E. (1992). A theory of generativity and its assessment through self-report, behavioral acts, and narrative themes in autobiography. *Journal of Personality and Social Psychology, 62,* 1003.

McAdams, D. P., de St. Aubin, E., & Logan, R. L. (1993). Generativity among young, midlife, and older adults. *Psychology and Aging, 8,* 221–230.

Millová, K., & Blatný, M. (2016). Generativita v současném empirickém výzkumu. [Generativity in contemporary empirical research]. *Czechoslovak Psychology, 60*(6), 609–621.

Morse, J. M., & Doberneck, B. (1995). Delineating the concept of hope. *Image – the Journal of Nursing Scholarship, 27*(4), 277–285.

Neusner, J., & Chilton, B. D. (Eds.). (2005). *Altruism in world religions.* Washington, DC: Georgetown University Press.

O'Sullivan, G. (2010). The relationship between hope, eustress, self-efficacy, and life satisfaction among undergraduates. *Social Indicators Research, 101*(1), 155–172. https://doi.org/10.1007/s11205-010-9662-z

Page, R. M., & Scanlan, A. (1994). Childhood loneliness and isolation: Implications and strategies for childhood educators. *Child Study Journal, 24*(2), 107–118.

Pargament, K. I., & Mahoney, A. (2002). Spirituality: Discovering and conserving the sacred. In C. R. Snyder & S. J. Lopez (Eds.), *Handbook of positive psychology* (pp. 646–659). New York: Oxford University Press.

Parsian, N., & Dunning, T. (2009). Developing and validating a questionnaire to measure spirituality: A psychometric process. *Global Journal of Health Science, 1*(1), 2–11.

Pavot, W., & Diener, E. (2008). The Satisfaction With Life Scale and the emerging construct of life satisfaction. *The Journal of Positive Psychology, 3*(2), 137–152. https://doi.org/10.1080/17439760701756946

Peterson, B. E., & Duncan, L. E. (2007). Midlife women's generativity and authoritarianism: Marriage, motherhood, and 10 years of aging. *Psychology and Aging, 22,* 411–419.

Peterson, C. (2000). The future of optimism. *American Psychologists, 55,* 44–55.

Peterson, C., & Seligman, M. E. P. (2004). *Character strengths and virtues. A handbook and classification.* New York: Oxford University Press.

Piliavin, J. A. (2003). Going well by doing good: Benefit for the benefactor. In C. Keyes & J. Haidt (Eds.), *Flourishing: Positive psychology and the live well-lived* (pp. 227–248). Washington, DC: APA.

Reich, K. H. (2000). What characterizes spirituality? A comment on Pargament, Emmons and Crumpler, and Stifoss-Hansen. *The International Journal for the Psychology of Religion, 10*(2), 125–128.

Rittenour, C. E., & Colaner, C. W. (2012). Finding female fulfillment: Intersecting role-based and morality-based identities of motherhood, feminism, and generativity as predictors of women's self satisfaction and life satisfaction. *Sex Roles, 67,* 351–362.

Rothrauff, T., & Cooney, T. M. (2008). The role of generativity in psychological well-being: Does it differ for childless adults and parents? *Journal of Adult Development, 15,* 148–159.

Ryff, C., & Keyes, C. L. M. (1995). The structure of psychological well-being revisited. *Journal of Personality and Social Psychology, 69,* 719–727.

Ryff, C. D. (1989). Happiness is everything, or is it? Explorations of the meaning of psychological well-being. *Journal of Personality and Social Psychology, 57,* 1069–1081.

Sandage, S. J., Hill, P. C., & Vaubel, D. C. (2011). Generativity, relational spirituality, gratitude, and mental health: Relationships and pathways. *International Journal for the Psychology of Religion, 21*(1), 1–16.

Savikko, N., Routasalo, P., Tilvis, R., Strandberg, T., & Pitkälä, K. (2005). Predictors and subjective causes of loneliness in an aged population. *Archives of Gerontology and Geriatrics, 41,* 223–233. https://doi.org/10.1016/j.archger.2005.03.002

Sawatzky, R., Ratner, P. A., & Chiu, L. (2005). A meta-analysis of the relationship between spirituality and quality of life. *Social Indicators Research, 72,* 153–188. https://doi.org/10.1007/s11205-004-5577-x

Scheier, M. F., & Carver, C. S. (1985). Optimism, coping, and health: Assessment and implications of generalized outcome expectancies. *Health Psychology, 4*, 219–247.

Scheier, M. F., & Carver, C. S. (1992). Effects of optimism on psychological and physical well-being: Theoretical overview and empirical update. *Cognitive Therapy and Research, 16*, 201–228.

Scheier, M. F., Carver, C. S., & Bridges, M. W. (1994). Distinguishing optimism from neuroticism (and trait anxiety, self-mastery, and self-esteem): A reevaluation of the Life Orientation Test. *Journal of Personality and Social Psychology, 67*, 1063.

Scheier, M. F., Carver, C. S., & Bridges, M. W. (2001). Optimism, pessimism, and psychological well-being. In E. C. Chang (Ed.), *Optimism and pessimism: Implications for theory, research, and practice* (pp. 189–216). Washington, DC: American Psychological Association.

Schnell, T. (2009). The Sources of Meaning and Meaning in Life Questionnaire (SoMe): Relations to demographics and well-being. *Journal of Positive Psychology, 4*(6), 483–499. https://doi.org/10.1080/17439760903271074

Schnell, T., & Becker, P. (2007). *Der Fragebogen zu Lebensbedeutungen und Lebenssinn (LeBe)*. Göttingen, Germany: Hogrefe.

Schnell, T., & Hoof, M. (2012). Meaningful commitment: Finding meaning in volunteer work. *Journal of Beliefs and Values, 33*(1), 35–53. https://doi.org/10.1080/13617672.2012.650029

Schweizer, K., Beck-Seyffer, A., & Schneider, R. (1999). Cognitive bias of optimism and its influence on psychological well-being. *Psychological Report, 84*, 627–636.

Scioli, A., Ricci, M., Nyugen, T., & Scioli, E. (2011). Hope: Its nature and measure. *Psychology of Religion and Spirituality, 3*(2), 78–97. https://doi.org/10.1037/a0020903

Seligman, M. E. P. (2011). *Flourish: A visionary new understanding of happiness and well-being*. New York: Free Press.

Slezáčková, A. (2017). *Hope and well-being. Psychosocial correlates and benefits*. Malta, Europe: University of Malta: Centre for Resilience and Socio-Emotional Health.

Slezáčková, A., & Krafft, A. (2016). Hope: A driving force of optimal human development. In J. Mohan & M. Sehgal (Eds.), *Idea of excellence: Multiple perspectives* (pp. 1–12). Chandigarh, India: Panjab University. ISBN 81-85322-59-7.

Smith, K. P., & Christakis, N. A. (2008). Social networks and health. *Annual Review of Sociology, 34*, 405–429.

Snyder, C. R. (1994). *The psychology of hope: You can get there from here*. New York: Free Press.

Snyder, C. R. (2000). *Handbook of hope: Theory, measures and applications*. San Diego, CA: Academic Press.

Snyder, C. R., Rand, K. L., & Sigmon, D. R. (2002). Hope theory: A member of the positive psychology family. In C. R. Snyder & S. J. Lopez (Eds.), *Handbook of positive psychology* (pp. 257–276). New York: Oxford University Press.

Stek, M. L., Vinkers, D. J., Gussekloo, J., Beekman, A. T., van der Mast, R. C., & Westendorp, R. G. (2005). Is depression in old age fatal only when people feel lonely? *American Journal Psychiatry, 162*(1), 178–180.

Umberson, D., & Montez, J. K. (2010). Social relationships and health: A Flashpoint for health policy. *Journal of Health and Social Behavior, 51*(Suppl), 54–66. https://doi.org/10.1177/0022146510383501

Veenhoven, R. (2016a). *Happiness in Czech Republic (CZ)*, World Database of Happiness, Erasmus University Rotterdam, The Netherlands. Viewed on 2016-06-16 at http://worlddatabaseofhappiness.eur.nl

Veenhoven, R. (2016b). *Happiness in Malta (MT)*, World Database of Happiness, Erasmus University Rotterdam, The Netherlands. Viewed on 2016-06-16 at http://worlddatabaseofhappiness.eur.nl

Victor, C., Scambler, S., Bowling, A., & Bond, J. (2005). The prevalence of, and risk factors for, loneliness in later life: A survey of older people in Great Britain. *Ageing and Society, 25*, 357–375.

Visser, A., Garssen, B., & Vingerhoets, A. (2010). Spirituality and well-being in cancer patients: A review. *Psycho-Oncology, 19*, 565–572. https://doi.org/10.1002/pon.1626

Werner, S. (2012). Subjective well-being, hope, and needs of individuals with serious mental illness. *Psychiatry Research, 196*(2-3), 214–219. https://doi.org/10.1016/j.psychres.2011.10.012

Westburg, N. G. (2001). Hope in older women: The importance of past and current relationships. *Journal of Social and Clinical Psychology, 20*(3), 354–365. https://doi.org/10.1521/jscp.20.3.354.22307

Windsor, T. D. (2009). Persistence in goal striving and positive reappraisal as psychosocial resources for ageing well: A dyadic analysis. *Aging & Mental Health, 13*(6), 874–884. https://doi.org/10.1080/13607860902918199

Wojciechowska, L. (2011). Basic hope and generativity in middle adulthood. *Polish Psychological Bulletin, 42*(4), 188–197. https://doi.org/10.2478/v10059-011-0025-7

Yildirim, Y., & Kocabiyik, S. (2010). The relationship between social support and loneliness in Turkish patients with cancer. *Journal of Clinical Nursing, 19*(5-6), 832–839. https://doi.org/10.1111/j.1365-2702.2009.03066.x

Zullig, K. J., Ward, R. M., & Horn, T. (2006). The association between perceived spirituality, religiosity, and life satisfaction: The mediating role of self-rated health. *Social Indicators Research, 79*, 255.

Chapter 9
Hope and Education: Role of Psychological Capital and Cultural Differences

Valle Flores-Lucas, Raquel Martínez-Sinovas, and Rajneesh Choubisa

Introduction

Educational organizations have always emphasized academic and curricular achievements, but when it comes to character education, a majority of educational organizations avoid paying necessary attention to individual development of their members (Parks & Peterson, 2009). Fortunately, this scenario is changing and in recent years, a growing body of research has led to a spontaneous interest in developing the skills, abilities and well-being of educational stakeholders in different countries. For instance, Hoy and Tarter (2011) pointed out that the goal of educational administrators should be exploring the pedagogical actions and elements that lead to healthier, more engaged, significant and happier classrooms. In this sense, positive educational approach focuses on the development and management of our personal resources such as strengths of character, including the well-being of all education related agents (i.e. students, teachers, etc.). Incidentally, positive psychology education has also shown its usefulness to find out what personal resources have an impact on the student's academic achievement, engagement to the school, and mental health. Moreover, this is also assumed to be a case for hope which has shown to be a good predictor of relevant academic and other outcome variables.

The predictive power of hope on some relevant academic outcomes and its protective role in students' mental health and wellbeing are the main reasons that provoked us to explore the explicable. Needless to say, there is no unique and consensual

V. Flores-Lucas (✉) · R. Martínez-Sinovas
Department of Psychology, University of Valladolid, Valladolid, Spain
e-mail: mariavalle.flores@uva.es

R. Choubisa
Department of Humanities and Social Sciences, Birla Institute of Technology & Science (BITS), Pilani, Rajasthan, India

© Springer International Publishing AG, part of Springer Nature 2018
A. M. Krafft et al. (eds.), *Hope for a Good Life*, Social Indicators Research
Series 72, https://doi.org/10.1007/978-3-319-78470-0_9

theory and conceptualization of hope and most of the approaches differ with respect to its basic elements. There are even differences between approaches that conceptualize hope like an emotion or as a personality trait or cognitive process (see Delas, Martin-Krumm, & Fenouillet, 2015 for a revision). Despite such discontinuities, one of the most accepted theory of hope and probably the most relevant from the purview of education is Snyder's hope theory (1994). Snyder's hope theory (1994, 2002) conceptualizes hope as a cognitive-motivational process and the theory has generated a big amount of relevant research around its role in affecting students' well-being, mental health, social relationships and above all, their academic achievements and outcomes. Hope is seen like the perceived ability to create pathways to reach the desired goals and the ability to motivate oneself to use those pathways and reach those goals in spite of possible obstacles (Snyder, 2002). In Snyder's conceptualization of hope, both types of thinking (agency and pathways) are equally important and essential to get the goal, however, agency thinking is even more necessary when obstacles and difficulties arise or when our goal is actually long term and hard to reach (for example, get a university degree or develop a successful career development).

Irrespective of any intricacies or discontinuities, our main agenda behind this chapter is to capture and present the predictive character of the concept of hope in a holistic manner. The chapter in fact attempts to draw parallels to provide a food for thought in a bid to consider the overarching construct of Psychological Capital (PsyCap) that can potentially predict educational success. We contend that promoting academic *PsyCap* not only helps achieve academic success but appropriate integration of academic PsyCap above and beyond one' life could have far reaching consequences. We substantiate our assumptions in light of results of Hope-Barometer survey by considering a cultural continuum and highlight the significant relationships between hope, *PsyCap* and other relevant variables that impact educational and future life success.

Hope and Education

Hope, according to this conceptualization, has been shown to act as a good predictor for some relevant variables in the personal and academic development of students. Moreover, hope has shown to have a positive influence in several relevant dimensions of mental health and coping, so, next we reiterate the main findings about the influence of hope on academic outcomes and variables related to students' well-being and academic success. The following section summarizes the major findings of hope with respect to prominent variables related to students and education.

Hope, Subjective Well-Being and Life Satisfaction

Subjective well-being is the subjective perception of happiness or the capacity to reflect on the life satisfaction and the positive and negative affectivity which is experienced (Sánchez-Cánovas, 2007). Research proves that hope is a good predictor of subjective well-being (better than optimism), and agency thinking is better predictor of subjective well-being than the pathways component (Bailey & Snyder, 2007; Magaletta & Oliver, 1999). In a study conducted in university counselling centres, it was found that clients who reported higher levels of hope also reported higher subjective wellbeing and lower symptom distress (Magyar-Moe, 2004, cit. in Werner, 2012). In other study with adolescents, results confirmed that hope is a cushion against adverse and stressful experiences and promotes psychological and subjective well-being (Valle, Huebner & Suldo, 2006).

Satisfaction with life is defined as an overall assessment which the person makes about his life, comparing what one has achieved (achievements) and what one expects to obtain (expectations) (Diener, Emmons, Larsen, & Griffin, 1985). In this case, hope has shown to act as an important predictor of satisfaction with life (Bailey, Eng, Frisch, & Snyder, 2007; Bailey & Snyder, 2007; Rand, Martin, & Shea, 2011). Moreover, this predictive power of hope has been confirmed at different levels of education and with different student typologies such as law students (Rand et al., 2011), secondary school and high school students (Gilman, Dooley, & Florell, 2006; Gilman & Huebner, 2006; Valle et al., 2006) and students with learning difficulties (Heiman & Shesmesh, 2012).

A possible cause of the relationship between hope and satisfaction with life as well as subjective well-being could be that people with a hopeful vision tend to think more about life experiences which are in effect 'satisfactory' (Rose, Elkis-Abuhoff, Goldblatt, & Miller, 2012). Furthermore, the higher predictor power of hope (as compared to optimism) in these variables could be because hope is future-oriented and focuses on individual goals and a strong determinant of behaviour whereas optimism is not rooted in specific goals (Shorey, Little, Snyder, Kluck, & Robitschek, 2007).

Hope, Academic Engagement and Achievement

Hope has also been shown as a good predictor of two of the most important academic variables viz., academic engagement and achievement (e.g. Levi, Einav, Ziv, Raskind, & Margalit, 2014; Snyder, et al., 2002). One of the most accepted conceptualization of academic engagement is proposed by Christenson, Reschly, and Wylei

(2012), according to which, academic engagement is the students' active participation in academic and school-related activities and their commitment to their educational goals and learning. Quite a few studies relate engagement with the construct of hope, of which, one confirms the predictive character of hope on engagement as well as its indirect effect on positive emotions (Ouweneel, Le Blanc, Schaufely, & Van Wijhe, 2012).

Besides, there exist a number of studies conducted by corporate firms such as Gallup organization. These studies have focused on studying measures that predict success in students and that promote the best conditions to develop learning and personal growth. Gallup organization has developed the *Gallup Student Poll Scale* which examines three different constructs at the theoretical and psychometric levels viz., hope, engagement and well-being (Lopez, Agrawal, & Calderon, 2010). The data obtained after the application of the scale reveals that the students who are high on engagement, approximately 75% of them show high hope (Gallup, 2012). Also, these data seems to be congruent with the results obtained by Van Ryzin (2011). Other research has shown that the three dimensions of engagement (vigour, dedication and absorption) correlate positively with academic performance when measured with the number of passed exams relative to the total number of exams in the previous term (Schaufeli, Martínez, Marques, Salanova, & Bakker, 2002).

As far as academic achievement is concerned, there exists strong evidence in the scientific literature that hope predicts academic results (Gallagher & Lopez, 2017). Research carried out with grade school, high school, and college students suggests that hope is correlated reliably with higher academic performance (Snyder, Cheavens, & Michael, 1999). The reasoning behind this could be that people with higher hope levels strive hard to achieve their goals and when an obstacle appears they perceive it as a challenge. They look for alternatives to achieve their goals with success because they tend to have more positive thoughts (success thoughts) than negative thoughts (failure thoughts) (Snyder, et al., 2002). Gallagher, Marques, and Lopez (2017) published a meta-analysis that analyzed the strength of the association between hope and academic achievement. Their results prove that hope accounts for 12% of the variance in academic performance. The meta-analysis not only included work that relates hope with higher scores on subsequent achievement tests for grade school children (Snyder, et al., 1997), higher overall grade point averages (GPAs) for high school students (Snyder, et al., 1991) for frontline researchers, but, even included studies conducted by other researchers that relate hope to higher achievement test scores for grade school children (Marques, Lopez, Fontaine, Coimbra, & Mitchell, 2015) and higher semester grade point averages for college students (Buckelew, Crittendon, Butkovic, Price, & Hurst, 2008; Curry, Snyder, Cook, Ruby, & Rehm, 1997).

In addition to these correlational paradigms when Snyder's Hope Model (2002) was used as an intervention to increase hope, there were significant improvement in variables related to academic achievement and development of personal well-being. Marques, Lopez, and Pais-Ribeiro (2011) applied a hope intervention to Portuguese primary students (aged between 10 and 12 years) where the impact assessment results showed increased levels of hope, satisfaction with life and self-esteem while keeping these results 18 months as follow up. However, they did not find significant improvements in mental health or academic achievement. Other study by Feldman and Dreher (2012) applied a single session hope program to college students. Participants in hope intervention showed more improvements of their levels of hope, life purpose, and vocational calling, from pre- to post-test than control participants. This suggests that students' hope level can be increased with interventions programs since studies have shown positive effects on personal and academic variables (Bouwkamp & Lopez, 2001; Madden, Green, & Grant, 2011; Pedrotti, Edwards, & Lopez, 2008).

It is explicitly for this reason that we think it is worthy to carry out more intensive research investigations involving education related interventions that can potentially improve not only students' hope levels, but, other personal resources which would be useful to their successful academic adjustment and development. Thus, we believe that, the construct of Psychological Capital (*PsyCap*) which best encapsulates these principles and personal resources should be utilized in an educational scenario for effective career development of students. In the next section we introduce *PsyCap* construct and the necessary justification to apply it in the educational context and also discuss the controversial points of our proposition.

Psychological Capital in Educational Context: Beyond Hope

Psychological capital has been defined as a positive psychological state of individual development that requires: having confidence to assume and make efforts to be successful in difficult tasks; having positive expectations of success in the present and for the future; persevering in the pursuit of goals and standing up and recovering through problems and adversities in order to reach success (Luthans, Youssef, & Avolio, 2007). Luthans, Avey, Avolio, and Peterson (2010) defined *PsyCap* as a set of resources rather than distinct set of personality traits despite the fact that according to *Values in Action* (VIA) model, hope and resilience are considered strengths or positive personality traits (Carr, 2011). As per definition, *PsyCap* is composed of personal resources and skills such as self-efficacy, hope, resilience and dispositional optimism. In strong theoretical sense, personal resources are not considered static (like personality traits) and therefore can be developed and improved.

Of late, this construct has turned into one of the central themes of research in Positive Organizational Behaviour (POB) as it has been found to be a good predictor of desirable attitudes and behaviour (citizenship) in employees and other positive outcomes. *PsyCap* has also shown to be negatively related to undesirable attitudes and inappropriate behaviour in different types of personnel (e.g. Avey, Patera, & West, 2006; Avey, Reichard, Luthans, & Mhatre, 2011; Choubisa, 2009; Norman, Avolio, & Luthans, 2010). Furthermore, in order to provide good academic foundation that incorporates students' academic achievement, including their technical and conceptual knowledge, higher education institutions ought to indulge in the career development of their students with a much wider perspective.

Owing to such benefits, universities should endorse the development of some personal resources and skills (such as *PsyCap*) that are relevant to students' academic success and future job integration and job success i.e. their integral career development.

We cannot deny the fact that the world of work is constantly changing whereby rapid innovation and new challenges requires oneself to be competitive in the contemporary market. This mandates that employees must not only possess good technical knowledge but also other types of knowledge, experiences, skills and resources a.k.a. "human capital" (Luthans, Luthans, & Luthans, 2004). Although, human capital and social capital are vital to the success of organizations, *PsyCap* has been proposed as a new complementary concept that remains viable nowadays and even in future organizational success. Even though, a number of studies exist, there are some aspects of this construct that require some discussion and research.

As we pointed out in the introduction of this chapter, Snyder's hope model is no unique and consensual conceptualization of Hope. Also, Snyder's hope model and his trademark *Dispositional Hope Scale* have been validated in so many countries and languages. Still, there seems to be a scarcity of studies that have compared the possible cultural differences in hope. Hence, it could be interesting to explore and highlight possible cultural or ethnic differences in manifestation and expression of hope with special reference to the field of education. More importantly, the components of *PsyCap* have become a point of contention because of close similarities between hope and self-efficacy and between hope and optimism, yet, none of them have answered the question of up to what extent these resources were similar or different than personal resources. Therefore, in the next paragraphs, we present the main research findings by reviewing hope conceptualization in light of possible similarities and differences and then present the results of our exploratory cross-cultural study.

Hope: Cultural and Ethnic Differences

Some researchers have highlighted that Snyder's hope model does not cater to the cultural and ethnic differences in its conceptualization of hope. As such, his model mainly reflects the western cultural conceptualizations and does not necessarily reflect other cultural or ethnic conceptualizations. Fortunately, a couple of specifications to this model have been pointed out in the literature.

Of the many possible cultural differences, one is concerned with the sources of goals. Snyder's hope conceptualization on the other hand excludes the idea that goals and motivating thoughts could come from other people or hope sources different to one-self. Nevertheless, Bernardo (2010) has clarified through the usage of the *Dispositional Hope Scale* (Snyder, Harris, et al., 1991) that hope is generated from one's own believes, expectancies, abilities and commitment to get goals and own ability to keep motivated until the goal is achieved. Juxtaposing these contrasting thoughts results in a disjointed model wherein goals, positive actions or thinking are defined independently of others. As such, this disjointed model could not be a representative of other cultures that are less individualistic than dominant American culture. Therefore, Bernardo has formulated an extension to Snyder's hope model by appending locus of hope as a dimension. He proposes four loci of hope: internal; external-family; external-peers and external-spiritual and subsequently validated these four loci of hope dimensions. In other words, his proposition meant that agency could also refer to the commitment and support of other external agents and pathways could imply goals and actions of external agents.

In a bid to rationalize the abovementioned thought, empirical results are presented via data that was collected through an international cross-sectional Internet survey called Hope-Barometer. To substantiate our point, we present preliminary descriptive and mean differences from three participating countries which differ in terms of level of individualism v/s collectivism. In the literature, generally, Eastern cultures are considered more collective than Western cultures (Leung, Olomolaiye, & Chen, 2006). Although collectivism vs individualism is not a uni-dimensional construct (Triandis, 2004) and individualism and collectivism are not the opposite sides of one dimension, yet both sides can coexist in the same culture like in India (Sinha, 2014).

Of all the countries participated in the Hope-Barometer survey, we have deliberately chosen three counties. First of all, Germany was considered owing to its individualistic culture. Second choice was Spain which is considered to be a collectivistic culture in relation to other European countries, except Portugal, but an individualistic culture in comparison to other world countries. And lastly, Indian subcontinent which is considered both collectivistic and individualistic country with less scores than Spain and Germany, but very close to Spain in terms of Hofstede's ranking. We think comparing these countries was plausible as three of them were representing a continuous gradient (on a continuum) without being extreme in terms of collectivism v/s individualism. Besides, it would be interesting to see especially the comparative picture of Spain and India because they have more or less similar status on this continuum as compared to other countries. In addition, another reason for choosing these three countries was due to the fact that homogenous university student sample was captured majorly for these three countries. Since the chapter focuses on an educational context, we use a subset of student population of N = 290 university students from these three countries (106 from Germany, 143 from India and 41 from Sapain). The selection criterion for inclusion in the final sample was age between 18 and 30 years. The mean age was 21.72 years for German students, 20.86 years for Indian students and 20.90 years for Spanish students.

Our study analyses the possible differences in university students from the chosen countries on following dimensions: *Sources of Hope (Personalities)*; *Dispositional Hope*; *Perceived Hope*; *Physical and Psychological Health*; *Positive and Negative Affects* and *Depression*. We used the non-parametric test called *Kruskal-Wallis test* for independent samples to compare the means of the three countries with respect to different variables. The pairs were also compared through *Mann Whitney U-test* for two independent samples to find out statistically significant differences. In order to showcase the cultural and ethnic differences, we present

Table 9.1 Sources of hope (Providers): country-wise descriptive data (N = 290)

Item parameters	Germany (n = 106)		India (n = 143)		Spain (n = 41)	
	M	SD	M	SD	M	SD
Physicians, therapists, etc.	1.49	1.09	1.22	1.03	1.44	.98
Bankers, financial advisers, etc.	.77	.88	.78	.94	.49	.68
Experts, scientists, researchers, …	1.54	1.09	1.17	1.03	1.15	1.09
Politicians, the government	1.44	1.06	.98	1.05	.49	.81
Teachers, educators, professors, …	1.88	1.03	1.89	.92	1.88	.87
God	1.02	1.21	1.69	1.13	.34	.66
I give myself hope …	2.15	.88	2.47	.67	2.34	.79
The many ordinary people …	1.58	1.05	1.83	.96	1.27	.95
Entrepreneurs, businessmen, …	.66	.81	1.17	.98	.34	.53
Priests, spiritual leaders, gurus, …	.55	.89	1.08	1.04	.12	.33
Wife, husband, partner	2.21	1.01	1.77	1.16	1.90	1.14
Parents, grandparents	2.17	.98	2.34	.84	2.49	.81
Friends	2.30	.85	2.04	.93	2.34	.86
Children, grandchildren	1.37	1.21	1.31	1.12	1.44	1.36
Colleagues, business partners	1.40	.91	1.39	.99	1.71	1.10
The boss, employer, …	1.37	1.02	1.27	1.00	.66	.76

M-Mean; SD-Standard Deviation

country-wise descriptive data for the variable: sources of hope personalities i.e. the types of personalities upon which we entrust our hopes or sources that help draw us inspiration for our hopes. A four point Likert scale was used to assess the level of strength of these sources of hope (the rank on this scale was 3).

The results shown in Tables 9.1 and 9.2 reveal that the chosen countries differ in the relevance that the different sources of hope have for the participants. We specifically found significant differences between Germany and India about the relevance of these source of hope viz., Scientists/researches/engineers (U = 6140.000; p < .01), politicians/government (U = 5702.500; p < .01), wife/husband (U = 5993.500; p < .01) and friends (U = 6385.500; p < .05) are stronger hope sources for German students. On the other hand, God (U = 5154.500; p < .01), oneself (U = 6148.500; p < .01), businessmen (U = 5332.500; p < .01) and spiritual leaders (U = 5287.000; p < .01) are stronger hope sources for Indian students. Likewise, significant differences between German and Spanish students were found in the domains viz., politicians/government (U = 1060.000; p < .01), God (1537.500; p < .05), spiritual leaders (U = 1662.500; p < .01), businessmen (U = 1757.500; p < .05) and boss/supervisor (U = 1326.000; p < .01) wherein these domains were stronger sources of hope for German students. Finally, differences between Indian and Spanish students were found on the domains viz., Politicians/government (U = 2160.500; p < .01), businessmen (1494.000; p < .01), God (U = 1025.000; p < .01), common people (U = 2017.000; p < .01), spiritual leaders (U = 1347.000; p < .01) and boss/supervisor (U = 1940.000; p < .01) which were found to be stronger sources of hope for Indian students as compared to their Spanish counterparts.

Table 9.2 Country-wise paired comparisons for the sources of hope (N = 290)

	Germany v/s India		Germany v/s Spain		India v/s Spain	
	U	p	U	p	U	p
Physicians, therapists, etc.	6526.5	.52	2113.5	.790	2556.0	.194
Bankers, financial advisers, etc.	7481.5	.851	1818.0	.093	2517.0	.130
Experts, scientists, researchers, ...	6140.0	.008**	1743.5	.055	2886.0	.875
Politicians, the government	5702.5	.001**	1060.0	.000**	2160.5	.006**
Teachers, educators, professors, ...	7493.0	.872	2119.0	.807	2896.0	.901
God	5154.5	.000**	1537.5	.002**	1025.0	.000**
I give myself hope ...	6148.5	.005**	1925.5	.250	2730.5	.452
The many ordinary people...	6579.0	.064	1810.0	.104	2017.0	.001**
Entrepreneurs, businessmen, managers	5332.5	.000**	1757.5	.042*	1494.0	.000**
Priests, spiritual leaders, gurus, ...	5287.0	.000**	1662.5	.005**	1347.0	.000**
Wife, husband, partner	5993.5	.003**	1852.0	.135	2746.5	.521
Parents, grandparents	6953.0	.222	1780.5	.062	2624.0	.251
Friends	6385.5	.023*	2104.5	.745	2398.5	.059
Children, grandchildren	7375.5	.706	2093.0	.717	2764.5	.563
Colleagues, business partners	7515.5	.906	1806.0	.098	2442.0	.091
The boss, employer, direct supervisor	7170.0	.449	1326.0	.000**	1940.0	.001**

**p ≤ .01; *p ≤ .05

The analysis support Bernardo's (2010) statement that people have distinct sources of hope different to oneself and other people could also be relevant sources of hope. Our data specifically supports the idea that spiritual leaders and God could be important sources of hope for many people. However, our data does not support the hypothesis that individualistic societies, especially, non-extreme individualistic society like Germany or Spain, rely on oneself as the major source of hope. It also shows significant differences in the relevance of one-self as source of hope, but surprisingly it was stronger for Indian students than for German students and we did not found any difference in this item between Spanish students and other students. Thus, with the comparative analysis one cannot conclude with certainty that more individualistic societies rely on oneself (vis-a-vis other people) as a main source of hope. The results also showed that Spanish students gave less relevance as a hope source to politicians and government than Indian or German students. This could be due to the special political situation in Spain in the last years that might have generated a climate of disappointment and lack of trust among the general population. German students rely heavily on technical professionals, scientists and researchers as sources of hope in comparison to Indian and Spanish students. Also, Indian students draw hope from spiritual personalities (i.e. God, spiritual leaders, etc.) that reflect a major role of spirituality in Indian culture. On the contrary, Spanish students are not at all impacted by spiritual personalities in instilling hope. This could

Table 9.3 Descriptive data for selected hope scales-country wise (N = 290)

	Germany (n = 106)		India (n = 143)		Spain (n = 41)	
	M	SD	M	SD	M	SD
Perceived hope	3.248	0.889	3.384	0.942	2.919	1.079
Dispositional hope	3.432	0.772	3.486	0.732	3.466	0.661
Agency	3.375	0.835	3.301	0.895	3.463	0.770
Pathways	3.488	0.866	3.671	0.767	3.469	0.861

be due to the Spanish history that has nurtured Catholic ethics and Catholic institutions, especially during the dictatorship.

As far as other possible racial/ethnic or cultural differences in hope are concerned, a previous study has shown that different ethnic groups present significant differences in hope components (Chang & Banks, 2007). For instance, Latinos depict higher levels of agency thinking than European-Americans and Africans-Americans, and Latinos and African-Americans depict higher levels of pathways thinking than European-Americans and Asian-Americans. Their study pointed out that global function of hope variable tends to remain same across different cultural/ ethnic or racial groups but their components vary between different cultural/ethnic groups. Thus, in order to check out possible cultural and ethnic differences, we compared levels of hope across university students from the three selected countries. We used the *Adult Dispositional Trait Hope Scale* (*ADTHS*: Snyder, Harris, et al., 1991) and also the *Perceived Hope Scale* (*PHS*: Krafft, Martin-Krumm, and Fenouillet, 2017) to check for the differences among their central tendencies. The six item PHS scale was rated on a 6-point Likert-type scale (0 = strongly disagree to 5 = strongly agree) to measure perceived hope. We decided to use PHS in addition to ADTHS mainly for comparison and also because this scale is a direct measure of level of hope as perceived by respondents while having a much broader scope than dispositional hope. Also, it takes into account aspects not pointed out in other hope models (see Krafft et al., 2017). Table 9.3 shows the descriptive data in terms of variables assessed.

Besides, we ran appropriate tests to check for mean differences calculated through non-parametric tests. Tables 9.4 and 9.5 shows the *Kruskal-Wallis* analysis and the *Mann-Whitney U test* values through which datasets were compared. Our results did not confirm the Chang and Banks (2007) analysis since significant differences in Dispositional Hope or any of its components (agency and pathways thinking) were not evident. Nevertheless, these results were congruent with a previous study involving Portuguese, Spanish and Romanian University Students in which no significant differences on Dispositional Hope or among any of their components was found (cf., Flores-Lucas et al., 2013). The variations in results could be due to the fact that study participants were from different geographical locations in our study whereas considerable acculturation might have happened to ethnically diverse sample in Chang and Banks' (2007) study.

Table 9.4 Mean country-wise comparisons among hope variables (N = 290)

	χ^2	p (GI = 2)
Perceived hope	7.167	.028*
Dispositional hope	0.105	.949
Agency	2.328	.312
Pathways	3.058	.217

*p ≤ .05

Table 9.5 Country-wise paired comparisons for the hope variables (N = 290)

	Germany vs. India		Germany vs. Spain		India vs. Spain	
	U	p	U	p	U	p
Perceived hope	6739.5	0.134	1871.0	0.191	2144.0	**0.009****
Dispositional hope	7497.5	0.884	2093.5	0.731	2869.0	0.835
Agency	7017.5	0.316	1994.5	0.438	2526.5	0.176
Pathways	6664.0	0.102	2154.5	0.936	2605.5	0.276

**p ≤ .01

The life experiences and challenges of living in a multicultural and ethnically diverse country such as USA with the presence of a dominant ethnic group (such as Latino participants in the Chang and Banks study) could be as different or similar in case with the three comparison groups. Besides, we found only one significant difference between Indian and Spanish students in the *PHS*, in which Indian student's depicted higher levels of perceived hope than their Spanish counterparts. Leaving aside the possible cultural and ethnic differences in hope, the function of hope in terms of its relationships and its effects on people behavior is the same in all populations studied (cf. Chang & Banks, 2007). Thus, we strongly recommend that empirical studies that can potentially explore the radical cross-cultural differences in hope should be carried out in near future.

As with the discussion on the conceptual delimitation between the components of the PsyCap, many research findings have clarified the questions related to its similarities and differences. Therefore, we next elaborate the main empirical evidence around that clarification.

Hope, Optimism and Self-Efficacy

A plethora of studies have tried to analyse the relationships, including the similarities and differences between hope, optimism and self-efficacy, but none had justified their role in education. To substantiate, we present a brief summary of the major conclusions of the empirical evidence that reflect the significance, plausibility and scope of using PsyCap in an educational scenario.

Hope and Optimism

Optimism and hope are closely related because both include personal beliefs (like forward-thinking) and are generally stable personality traits that reflect the extent to which one believes that his or her own future will be prosperous and favourable (Alarcon, Bowling, & Kahazon, 2013; Bryant & Cvengros, 2004; Gallagher & Lopez, 2009; Scheier & Carver, 1985; Snyder, Harris, et al., 1991). But, there are differences between them that have been scientifically documented (Rosenstreich, Feldman, Davidson, Maza, & Margalit, 2015). One of the main differences is that the optimism theory emphasizes the motivational component (referred to as expectation of outcomes) whereas the theory of hope puts more emphasis on the interaction of pathways and agency components (Alarcon et al., 2013; Snyder et al., 1999). Although both theories are cognitive in nature and explain behaviour through different situations, both of them are oriented towards future in a unique and different way. Whilst hope focuses more directly on the personal attainment of specific goals, optimism focuses more on the expected quality of future outcomes in general (Bryant & Cvengros, 2004; Snyder, Ilardi et al., 2000).

Other studies have analysed the influence of hope and optimism on few more variables whereby findings suggest that both are good predictors of psychological well-being (Gallagher & Lopez, 2009; Magaletta & Oliver, 1999; Shorey et al., 2007) and satisfaction with life (Bailey et al., 2007; Rand et al., 2011). With respect to coping as a strategy, optimism is a better predictor than hope (Bryant & Cvengros, 2004) whereas hope is a better predictor for the variable of self-efficacy (Bryant & Cvengros, 2004) and academic achievement (Rand et al., 2011). As a matter of fact, hope has been shown to be a learnable skill that can be instilled and even enhanced through intervention (Feldman, Davidson, & Margalit, 2015; Feldman & Dreher, 2012) whereas optimism has been considered as a relatively stable trait (Ronsenstreich et al., 2015).

Self-Efficacy and Hope

Self-efficacy (Bandura, 1977) is one of the constructs that has more similarity with hope (Snyder et al., 2006). Bandura (1977) posits that self-efficacy comprises of the expectation of efficacy or feelings of confidence in one's own abilities and the expectation of a result. In spite of the presumed similarities between the two concepts, one of the main differences between self-efficacy and hope is that self-efficacy is the most important step in order to carry out the actions required to achieve a specific goal (Bandura, 1977) whereas hope theory emphasizes that both pathways and agency thoughts are equally important before and during the entire process (Snyder, 2002). Other difference is that hope conceptualization gives an explicit description of the etiology of emotions but this does not occur in the theory of self-efficacy (Snyder, 2002). Besides, one more prominent difference between both resources is that agency predicts well-being better than general self-efficacy (Snyder, Shorey, Cheavens, Pulvers, Adams, & Wiklund, 2002).

It has also been pointed out that a positive relationship exists between the agency pathway and self-efficacy which suggests that both constructs share a common emphasis on persistence (Magaletta & Oliver, 1999). A study by Robinson and Rose (2010) suggested that trait hope measure has correlated positively with self-efficacy to explain 30.9% of the variance whereas dispositional hope measure has correlated to explain 35.9% of the variance in predicting self-efficacy. In addition to the variances the results also suggested that specific measures of both constructs (hope and self-efficacy) are more predictive for the academic/educational domain. Moreover, research on students with learning difficulties has found that the predictive power is less for this group as compared to group without learning difficulties (Lackaye & Margalit, 2008; Lackaye, Margalit, Ziv, & Ziman, 2006). Overall, the studies suggest that hope, optimism and self-efficacy are different human resources with close relationships between them.

Despite the fact that PsyCap was defined in the field of Organizational Psychology and it has mainly been applied in the work context, recently, Luthans, Luthans, and Avey (2014) have formulated the concept of "Academic PsyCap" that has application in the field of education. *Academic PsyCap* provides students with relevant resources to their academic success and prepares them to be successful in their future working life. Although, the dimensions of *PsyCap* have turn out to be good predictors of academic success, academic engagement and achievement, prior research has shown *PsyCap* as a higher order construct and it has predicted performance and satisfaction better than its individual components. Once research confirms the validity of the components of academic PsyCap (like different personal resources), one can move forward in applying *PsyCap* to the field of education.

As far as inculcation of academic *PsyCap* is concerned, one study has reported the development and deployment of a short psycho-educational intervention program to develop *PsyCap* in business students' with promising results (Luthans et al., 2014). So we think that future research in the field of academic *PsyCap* is desirable and need of the hour in order to understand the development of these resources better and the effect of this construct on many academic variables. Therefore, we think that educational institutions have to promote the development and implementation of educational or psycho-educational interventions to develop *academic PsyCap* in students.

Conclusion

Snyder's Hope model has generated a huge amount of research that has demonstrated its validity as a construct. Also, there are enough empirical studies that have shown the relationships between hope and other relevant personal variables. The available review is limited and suggests that hope function and its relationships with other variables are undeniably same across different countries, cultures or ethnic groups. However, more research is necessary in order to establish if hope components vary between different ethnic or cultural groups.

Hope has also proved to be a very important personal resource or trait and found to be a good predictor of mental health, well-being and academic success. There is plethora of empirical evidence that have shown the relationships between hope and the most relevant academic variables and outcomes in almost all the stages of education in one's life. Besides, there also exist studies that showcase the effectiveness of intervention programs to improve hope in different phases of one's educational life. Therefore, we think and profess that positive education research needs to further investigate and develop the academic *PsyCap* construct. We believe that this will ensure future research could unequivocally focus on an in-depth exploration of its positive effects on constructs such as well-being, academic success and most importantly, future work success of our students.

References

Alarcon, G. M., Bowling, N. A., & Khazon, S. (2013). Great expectations: A meta-analytic examination of optimism and hope. *Personality and Individual Differences, 54*, 821–827.

Avey, J. B., Patera, J. L., & West, B. J. (2006). Positive psychological capital: A new lens to view absenteeism. *Journal of Leadership and Organizational Studies, 13*, 42–60.

Avey, J. B., Reichard, R. J., Luthans, F., & Mhatre, K. H. (2011). Meta-analysis of the impact of the positive psychological capital on employee attitudes, behaviors and performance. *Human Resource Development Quarterly, 22*(2), 127–152.

Bailey, T. C., Eng, W., Frisch, M. B., & Snyder, C. R. (2007). Hope and optimism as related to life satisfaction. *The Journal of Positive Psychology, 2*(3), 168–175.

Bailey, T. C., & Snyder, C. R. (2007). Satisfaction with life and hope: A look at age and marital status. *The Psychological Record, 57*(2), 233–240.

Bandura, A. (1977). Self-efficacy: Toward a unifying theory of behavioral change. *Psychological Review, 84*(2), 191–215.

Bernardo, A. (2010). Extending hope theory: Internal and external locus of trait hope. *Personality and Individual Differences, 49*, 944–949.

Bouwkamp, J., & Lopez, S. J. (2001). *Making hope happen: A program for inner-city adolescents* (Unpublished master's thesis). University of Kansas, Lawrence.

Bryant, F. B., & Cvengros, J. A. (2004). Distinguishing hope and optimism: Two sides of a coin, or two separate coins? *Journal of Social and Clinical Psychology, 23*(2), 273–302.

Buckelew, S. P., Crittendon, R. S., Butkovic, J. D., Price, K. B., & Hurst, M. (2008). Hope as a predictor of academic performance. *Psychological Reports, 103*, 411–414.

Carr, A. (2011). *Positive psychology: The science of happiness and human strengths*. New York: Routledge.

Chang, E. C., & Banks, K. H. (2007). The color and texture of hope: Some preliminary findings and implications for hope theory and counseling among diverse racial/ethnic groups. *Cultural Diversity and Ethnic Minority Psychology, 13*(2), 94–103.

Choubisa, R. (2009, August). POB: A comparative analysis of positive psychological capital amongst public & private sector employees. *AIMA Journal of Management & Research, 3*(3/4), 1–9.

Christenson, S. L., Reschly, A. L., & Wylie, C. (Eds.). (2012). *Handbook of research on student engagement*. New York: Springer.

Curry, L. A., Snyder, C. R., Cook, D. L., Ruby, B. C., & Rehm, M. (1997). Role of hope in academic and sport achievement. *Journal of Personality and Social Psychology, 73*(6), 1257–1267.

Delas, Y., Martin-Krumm, C., & Fenouillet, F. (2015). La théorie de l'espoir: une revue de questions. *Psychologie Française, 60*, 237–262.

Diener, E. D., Emmons, R. A., Larsen, R. J., & Griffin, S. (1985). The satisfaction with life scale. *Journal of Personality Assessment, 49*(1), 71–75.

Feldman, D. B., Davidson, O. B., & Margalit, M. (2015). Personal resources, hope, and achievement among college students: The conservation of resources perspective. *Journal of Happiness Studies, 16*(3), 543–560.

Feldman, D. B., & Dreher, D. E. (2012). Can hope be changed in 90 minutes? Testing the efficacy of a single-session goal-pursuit intervention for college students. *Journal of Happiness Studies, 13*(4), 745–759.

Flores-Lucas, V., Marujo, H. A., Neto, L. M., Tutu, A., & Martínez-Sinovas, R. (2013). *Hope, optimism and humor sense in university grades. A cross-cultural study between Spanish, Portuguese and Romanian students.* Symposium presented at 3rd World Congress on Positive Psychology. L.A. United States, 27–30 June.

Gallagher, M. W., & Lopez, S. J. (2009). Positive expectancies and mental health: Identifying the unique contributions of hope and optimism. *The Journal of Positive Psychology, 4*(6), 548–556.

Gallagher, M. W., & Lopez, S. J. (2017). *The Oxford handbook of hope. Oxford library of psychology.* New York: Oxford University Press.

Gallagher, M. W., Marques, S. C., & Lopez, S. J. (2017). Hope and the academic trajectory of college students. *Journal of Happiness Studies, 18*, 341–352.

Gallup. (2012). *Gallup student poll manual.* Gallup, Inc. Retrieved from http://www.gallupstudentpoll.com/home.aspx

Gilman, R., Dooley, J., & Florell, D. (2006). Relative levels of hope and their relationship with academic and psychological indicators among adolescents. *Journal of Social and Clinical Psychology, 25*(2), 166–178.

Gilman, R., & Huebner, E. S. (2006). Characteristics of adolescents who report very high life satisfaction. *Journal of Youth and Adolescence, 35*(3), 293–301.

Heiman, T., & Shemesh, D. O. (2012). Students with LD in higher education use and contribution of assistive technology and website courses and their correlation to students' hope and well-being. *Journal of Learning Disabilities, 45*(4), 308–318.

Hoy, W. K., & Tarter, C. J. (2011). Positive psychology and educational administration: An optimistic research agenda. *Educational Administration Quarterly, 47*(3), 427–445.

Krafft, A. M., Martin-Krumm, C., & Fenouillet, F. (2017). Adaptation, further elaboration, and validation of a scale to measure hope as perceived by people: Discriminant value and predictive utility vis-à-vis dispositional hope. *Assessment, 13*, 1–16.

Lackaye, T., & Margalit, M. (2008). Self-efficacy, loneliness, effort, and hope: Developmental differences in the experiences of students with learning disabilities and their non-learning disabled peers at two age groups. *Learning Disabilities: A Contemporary Journal, 6*(2), 1–20.

Lackaye, T., Margalit, M., Ziv, O., & Ziman, T. (2006). Comparisons of self-efficacy, mood, effort, and hope between students with learning disabilities and their non-LD-matched peers. *Learning Disabilities Research & Practice, 21*(2), 111–121.

Leung, M. Y., Olomolaiye, P., & Chen, D. Y. (2006). *Cross-cultural study for the stress of estimators in Hong Kong and the United Kingdom.* The Joint International Conference on Construction Culture, Innovation and Management. Sustainable Development through Culture and Innovation, Dubai.

Levi, U., Einav, M., Ziv, O., Raskind, I., & Margalit, M. (2014). Academic expectations and actual achievements: The roles of hope and effort. *European Journal of Psychology of Education, 29*(3), 367–386. https://doi.org/10.1007/s10212-013-0203-4

Lopez, S. J., Agrawal, S., & Calderon, V. J. (2010). *The Gallup Student Poll technical report.* Washington, D.C.: Gallup.

Luthans, B. C., Luthans, K. W., & Avey, J. B. (2014). Building the leaders of tomorrow: The development of academic psychological capital. *Journal of Leadership & Organizational Studies, 21*(2), 191–199.

Luthans, F., Avey, J. B., Avolio, B. J., & Peterson, S. J. (2010). The development and resulting performance impact of positive psychological capital. *Human Resource Development Quarterly, 21*(1), 41–67.

Luthans, F., Luthans, K. W., & Luthans, B. C. (2004). Positive psychological capital: Beyond human and social capital. *Business Horizons, 47*(1), 45–50.

Luthans, F., Youssef, C. M., & Avolio, B. J. (2007). *Psychological capital*. New York, NY: Oxford University Press.

Madden, W., Green, S., & Grant, A. M. (2011). A pilot study evaluating strengths-based coaching for primary school students: Enhancing engagement and hope. *International Coaching Psychology Review, 6*(1), 71–83.

Magaletta, P. R., & Oliver, J. M. (1999). The hope construct, will, and ways: Their relations with self-efficacy, optimism, and general well-being. *Journal of Clinical Psychology, 55*(5), 539–551.

Marques, S. C., Lopez, S. J., Fontaine, A. M., Coimbra, S., & Mitchell, J. (2015). How much hope is enough? Levels of hope and students' psychological and school functioning. *Psychology in the Schools, 52*(4), 325–334.

Marques, S. C., Lopez, S. J., & Pais-Ribeiro, J. L. (2011). "Building Hope for the Future": A program to foster strengths in middle-school students. *Journal of Happiness Studies, 12*(1), 139–152.

Norman, S. M., Avolio, B. J., & Luthans, F. (2010). The impact of transparency and positivity on trust in leaders and their perceived effectiveness. *The Leadership Quarterly, 21*(3), 350–364.

Ouweneel, E., Le Blanc, P. M., Schaufeli, W. B., & van Wijhe, C. I. (2012). Good morning, good day: A diary study on positive emotions, hope, and work engagement. *Human Relations, 65*(9), 1129–1154.

Park, N., & Peterson, C. (2009). Character strengths: Research and practice. *Journal of College and Character, 10*(4), 1–10.

Pedrotti, J. T., Edwards, L., & Lopez, S. J. (2008). Promoting hope: Suggestions for school counselors. *Professional School Counseling, 12*(2), 100–107.

Rand, K. L., Martin, A. D., & Shea, A. M. (2011). Hope, but not optimism, predicts academic performance of law students beyond previous academic achievement. *Journal of Research in Personality, 45*(6), 683–686.

Robinson, C., & Rose, S. (2010). Predictive, construct, and convergent validity of general and domain-specific measures of hope for college student academic achievement. *Research in the Schools, 17*(1), 38–52.

Rose, S., Elkis-Abuhoff, D., Goldblatt, R., & Miller, E. (2012). Hope against the rain: Investigating the psychometric overlap between an objective and projective measure of hope in a medical student sample. *The Arts in Psychotherapy, 39*(4), 272–278.

Rosenstreich, E., Feldman, D. B., Davidson, O. B., Maza, E., & Margalit, M. (2015). Hope, optimism and loneliness among first-year college students with learning disabilities: A brief longitudinal study. *European Journal of Special Needs Education, 30*(3), 338–350.

Sánchez-Cánovas, J. (2007). *Manual Escala de Bienestar Psicológico* (2nd ed.). Madrid, Spain: TEA Ediciones, S. A.

Schaufeli, W. B., Salanova, M., González-Romá, V., & Bakker, A. B. (2002). The measurement of engagement and burnout: A two sample confirmatory factor analytic approach. *Journal of Happiness Studies, 3*(1), 71–92.

Scheier, M. F., & Carver, C. S. (1985). Optimism, coping, and health: Assessment and implications of generalized outcome expectancies. *Health Psychology, 4*(3), 219–247.

Shorey, H. S., Little, T. D., Snyder, C. R., Kluck, B., & Robitschek, C. (2007). Hope and personal growth initiative: A comparison of positive, future-oriented constructs. *Personality and Individual Differences, 43*(7), 1917–1926.

Sinha, J. B. P. (2014). *Psycho-social analysis of the Indian mindset*. New Delhi, India: Springer.

Snyder, C. R. (1994). *The psychology of hope: You can get there from here*. New York: Free Press.

Snyder, C. R. (2002). Hope theory: Rainbows in the mind. *Psychological Inquiry, 13*(4), 249–275.

Snyder, C. R., Cheavens, J., & Michael, S. T. (1999). Hoping. In C. R. Snyder (Ed.), *Coping: The psychology of what works* (pp. 205–231). New York: Oxford University Press.

Snyder, C. R., Harris, C., Anderson, J. R., Holleran, S. A., Irving, L. M., Sigmon, S. T., et al. (1991). The will and the ways: Development and validation of an individual-differences measure of hope. *Journal of Personality and Social Psychology, 60*(4), 570–585.

Snyder, C. R., Hoza, B., Pelham, W. E., Rapoff, M., Ware, L., Danovsky, M., et al. (1997). The development and validation of children's hope scale. *Journal of Pediatric Psychology, 22,* 399–421.

Snyder, C. R., Ilardi, S. S., Cheavens, J., Michael, S. T., Yamhure, L., & Sympson, S. (2000). The role of hope in cognitive-behavior therapies. *Cognitive Therapy and Research, 24*(6), 747–762.

Snyder, C. R., Lehman, K. A., Kluck, B., & Monsson, Y. (2006). Howpe for rehabilitation and vice versa. *Rehabilitation Psychology, 51*(2), 89–112.

Snyder, C. R., Shorey, H. S., Cheavens, J., Pulvers, K. M., Adams, V. H., III, & Wiklund, C. (2002). Hope and academic success in college. *Journal of Educational Psychology, 94*(4), 820–826.

Triandis, H. C. (2004). The many dimensions of culture. *The Academy of Management Executive (1993–2005), 18*(1), 88–93.

Valle, M. F., Huebner, E. S., & Suldo, S. M. (2006). An analysis of hope as a psychological strength. *Journal of School Psychology, 44,* 393–406.

Van Ryzin, M. J. (2011). Protective factors at schools: Reciprocal effects among adolescents' perceptions of school enviroment, engagement in learning and hope. *Journal of Youth and Adolescence, 40*(12), 1568–1580.

Werner, S. (2012). Subjective well-being, hope, and needs of individuals with serious mental illness. *Psychiatry Research, 196*(2–3), 214–219.

Printed by Printforce, the Netherlands